MULTIMODAL RETINAL IMAGING

Amresh Chopdar, FRCSEd, FRCOphth
Formerly Consultant Ophthalmologist
Surrey and Sussex NHS Trust
Redhill, Surrey
UK

Tin Aung, MBBS, MMed(Ophth), FRCS(Ed), FRCOphth, FAMS, PhD(Lond)
Senior Consultant and Head
Glaucoma Service, Singapore National Eye Centre
Deputy Director, Singapore Eye Research Institute
Professor, Department of Ophthalmology
Yong Loo Lin School of Medicine
National University of Singapore
Singapore

JP medical publishers

London • Philadelphia • Panama City • New Delhi

Published by JP Medical Ltd, 83 Victoria Street, London, SW1H 0HW, UK
Tel: +44 (0)20 3170 8910 Fax: +44 (0)20 3008 6180
Email: info@jpmedpub.com Web: www.jpmedpub.com

ISBN: 978-1-907816-60-4

British Library Cataloguing in Publication Data
A catalogue record for this book is available from the British Library

Library of Congress Cataloging in Publication Data
A catalog record for this book is available from the Library of Congress

JP Medical Ltd is a subsidiary of Jaypee Brothers Medical Publishers (P) Ltd, New Delhi, India.

Publisher:	Richard Furn
Development Editor:	Gavin Smith
Editorial Assistant:	Sophie Woolven
Design:	Designers Collective Ltd

Typeset, indexed, printed and bound in India.

Foreword

It is with great honour and pride that I have the opportunity to write the foreword for this unique textbook, *Multimodal Retinal Imaging*. It contains fifteen chapters on all aspects of retinal imaging. Each chapter is ordered in a consistent format; for example, the technique-based chapters all include appropriate information on the anatomical and physiological background as well as aspects of the optical, physical and biochemical principles behind the imaging techniques.

Although this is a book with multiple authors, it is particularly gratifying that all the clinical chapters take a similarly uniform approach to the description of normal and abnormal patterns and characteristics of retinal images and their interpretation. I believe this approach facilitates better understanding of retinal conditions and imaging. It has been used in other texts and seminars by the lead editors, particularly Dr Chopdar, for many years and it has stood the test of time.

The field of retinal diagnostic imaging is a fast-changing one and the editors, Amresh Chopdar and Tin Aung, have chosen a fine team of experts who are also good communicators and teachers. They provide an up-to-date review of the common and less common retinal conditions, describing how these are diagnosed and recognised in their different stages of evolution using a whole range of modern imaging equipment. I commend the authors not only for their hard work in writing the excellent chapters but also for their efforts over many years in carefully selecting and collecting clinical cases which they use for teaching purposes. Many of them serve regularly as speakers for the fellowship level teaching seminars run by the Royal College of Ophthalmologists in the UK and share a common drive and interest in fostering the learning and teaching of skills in imaging, diagnosis and therapy of retinal diseases.

I therefore recommend this book to all those who want to improve their understanding of and skill in performing retinal imaging, especially those in training and also those from the allied health professions involved in community- or hospital-based retinal services who want to further their knowledge of this field.

Yit Yang
Consultant Ophthalmologist
Wolverhampton Eye Infirmary
Royal Wolverhampton Hospitals NHS Trust
Wolverhampton, UK
and
Visiting Professor
School of Life and Health Sciences
Aston University
Birmingham, UK

Preface

Retinal imaging techniques have expanded in leaps and bounds from the early days of colour fundus photography and fundus fluorescein angiography to a multitude of newer techniques. Ophthalmologists need to continually update their skills to adapt to these newer techniques. This book provides both trainee and practising ophthalmologists, as well as ophthalmic photographic technicians, with the skills needed to apply the varied techniques used in everyday clinical practice and accurately interpret the results obtained.

This book was conceived in line with the Skills Transfer Retinal Imaging course run by the Royal College of Ophthalmologists. Some of the contributors also lecture and participate in running the course. The book describes the techniques of fundus fluorescein angiography, indocyanine green angiography, echography, and also includes newer techniques such as optical coherence tomography, autofluorescence and Heidelberg retinal tomography.

The content is divided into two sections: techniques (chapters 1–7) and interpretation of retinal disorders (chapters 8–15). Each chapter is generously illustrated to help the reader become familiar with the technical aspects of both image acquisition and disease recognition.

Amresh Chopdar
Tin Aung
November 2013

Acknowledgements

The editors are grateful to the many authors who have donated their precious time to write chapters in their areas of expertise.

Our thanks are due to JP Medical Ltd, who have been patient and taken great care in producing this high quality book.

Contents

Contributors

Hatem Riad Atta, FRCSEd, FRCOphth, DO
Consultant Ophthalmologist
Vitreo-Retinal Surgeon
Aberdeen Royal Infirmary
Aberdeen
UK

Tin Aung, MBBS, MMed(Ophth), FRCS(Ed), FRCOphth, FAMS, PhD(Lond)
Senior Consultant and Head
Glaucoma Service, Singapore National Eye Centre
Deputy Director
Singapore Eye Research Institute
Professor, Department of Ophthalmology
Yong Loo Lin School of Medicine
National University of Singapore
Singapore

Carol Y Cheung, PhD
Research Scientist and Assistant Professor
Singapore Eye Research Institute
Singapore National Eye Centre
Singapore

Victor Chong, MD, FRCS, FRCOphth
Consultant Ophthalmic Surgeon
Oxford Eye Hospital
Oxford University Hospitals NHS Trust
Oxford
UK

Amresh Chopdar, FRCSEd, FRCOphth
Formerly Consultant Ophthalmologist
Surrey and Sussex NHS Trust
East Surrey Hospital
Redhill, Surrey
UK

John Mark S de Leon, MD
Glaucoma Clinical Research Fellow
Singapore Eye Research Institute
Singapore

Sushma Dhar-Munshi, MBBS, MS, DipNBE, FRCSEd
Consultant Ophthamologist and Medical Retina Specialist
Department of Ophthalmology
Sherwood Forest Hospitals NHS Foundation Trust
Sutton-in-Ashfield, Nottinghamshire
UK

Vishali Gupta, MD
Advanced Eye Centre
Postgraduate Institute of Medical Education and Research
Chandigarh
India

Heinrich Heimann, MD, FRCOpht
Consultant Ophthalmic Surgeon
Ocular Oncology Unit
Royal Liverpool University Hospital
Liverpool
UK

Raeba Mathew, MS, FRCS
Specialty Doctor, Medical Retina
Department of Ophthalmology
King's College Hospital NHS Trust
London
UK

Geeta Menon, FRCS(Ophth), FRCOphth
Consultant Ophthalmic Surgeon
Department of Ophthalmology
Frimley Park Hospital NHS Foundation Trust
Surrey
UK

Shamira Perera, BSc(Hons), MBBS (Hons), FRCOphth
Senior Consultant
Singapore National Eye Centre
Singapore

Ethan R Priel, FOPS
Ophthalmology Department
MOR
Bnei Brak
Isreal

Sobha Sivaprasad, FRCS, DM
Consultant Ophthalmologist
Moorfields NIHR Biomedical Research Centre
London
UK

Yih-Chung Tham, BSc(Hons)
Singapore Eye Research Institute
Singapore National Eye Centre
Singapore

Chapter 1 Fundus fluorescein angiography

Amresh Chopdar

INTRODUCTION

Currently, fundus fluorescein angiography is an indispensable and key diagnostic aid in the diagnosis and management of many retinal vascular, degenerative, and neoplastic disorders. In recent years, the analogue form has almost universally been replaced with digital angiography. This requires greater expertise in recording and interpretation skills.

The aim of fundus fluorescein angiography is to visualize and record fluorescence emanating from both the intra- and extravascular compartments following intravenous injection of fluorescein dye. The basic principle of fluorescence is that the dye becomes excited by absorbing light energy from one wavelength and emits light at a different wavelength. The emitted light, the fluorescence, is less intense; therefore, a highly sensitive optical system equipped with appropriate filter combination is necessary to record the fluorescence. Current digital fluorescein cameras do not need film but record straight onto the hard disk of a computer via a digitizing board. Fluorescein angiography displays the microvascular structural detail to illustrate the pathophysiological changes. A thorough knowledge of the pathophysiology of eye diseases is a prerequisite for correct interpretation of abnormalities on the angiograms.

EARLY DEVELOPMENT

In 1961 Novotny and Alvis were the first to introduce the modern-day fluorescein angiography. The introduction of fundus cameras by Zeiss made fundus fluorescein angiography a practical reality.

Camera

Currently, a number of manufacturers are marketing various fundus cameras capable of carrying out fundus fluorescein angiography. All have a compact and integrated electronic power pack, have versatile mobility, and are capable of capturing fundus views at several magnifications. The best result is obtained when photography is performed through dilated pupils. The digital imaging technique converts images into arrays of numerical figures that can be manipulated and stored on a computer's hard disk. Images are made up by dots called pixels. Each pixel represents information as a numerical value and collectively the pixels form a composite picture of the fundus. All the images are acquired and stored as Tagged Image File Format (TIFF). However, to optimize disk space and ease of transmission through the internet, it is necessary to convert and store these images on Joint Photographic Experts Group (JPEG) file interchange format, which compresses the data. This slightly reduces the quality of the image although it is not obvious when displayed on a modern high-resolution monitor.

Filters

The contemporary filter is a set of matched interference filters, which sharply cuts off wavelengths between the exciter and the barrier filters. The exciter filter must allow the optimum transmission of light of between 400 and 495 nm wavelengths, to allow maximal absorption in order to excite the circulating fluorescein in the blood. Similarly the barrier filter must block all light below 500 nm, but allows all emitting wavelengths up to 530 nm through. There should be no overlap between the wavelengths of exciter and emission filters. The modern range of filter combination of 490 nm for the exciter filter and 530 nm for the barrier filter was recommended by Delori et al. (1976) (**Figure 1.1**).

Dye

Fluorescein dye ($C_{20}H_{12}O_5$) is synthesized by a reaction between phthalic acid anhydride and resorcinol between 195°C and 200°C. A

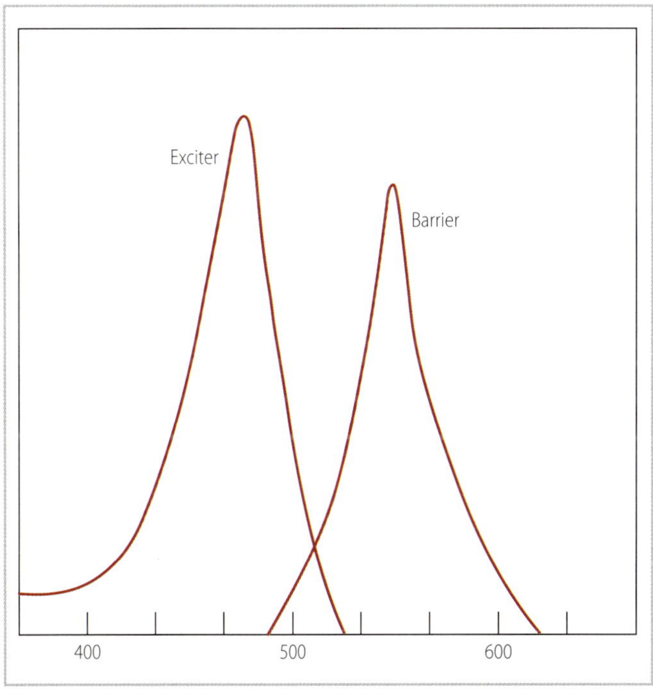

Figure 1.1 Fundus fluorescein angiography filter. The graph shows the exciter and barrier filter combination for fundus fluorescein angiography. The exciter filter cuts off at 490 nm wave band, whereas the barrier filter cuts off at 520 nm wave band. This combination allows maximum contrast for recording of the fluorescein angiogram. They are usually known as cross-matched filters and should be replaced as pair when required.

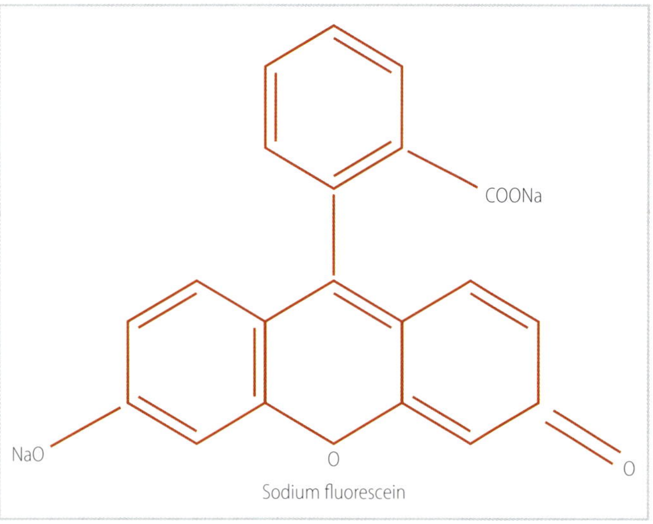

Figure 1.2 Chemical formula of fluorescein. The chemical formula of sodium fluorescein used in clinical practice is $C_{20}H_{10}O_5Na_2$.

sodium fluorescein solution is used in angiography ($C_{20}H_{10}O_5Na_2$) (**Figure 1.2**).

PROPERTIES OF FLUORESCEIN

Chemical properties

Sodium fluorescein is a water-soluble crystalline powder, with a molecular weight of 376.27 kD and a melting point of 315°C. The color of its aqueous solution varies from dark red to yellow-green according to its concentration. The color can be detected at a dilution as low as 1:1,000,000 by using ultraviolet light. Fluorescein may be detected by biomicroscopy at a concentration of $1{:}1 \times 10^9$. Fluorescence is shown only in the dissociated form. The intensity of fluorescence depends on the pH of the solution. The optimum fluorescence is seen at about pH 7.5. The optimum excitation takes place at 485 nm and emission at 530 nm. The intensity of the fluorescence is proportional to the concentration of dye up to about 10^{-3} g/100 mL–10^{-2} g/100 mL, after which the fluorescence decreases. When injected intravenously, the fluorescein is adsorbed on the albumin fraction of plasma protein. The maximum binding effect is achieved between pH 6 and pH 7. Fluorescein molecules deposit on the surface of the blood corpuscles, but show no evidence of diffusion into the cells.

Pharmacological properties

Fluorescein dye is well tolerated with very few side effects. The safety of the dye was first emphasized by Gifford in 1940. The lethal dose for rats is 600 mg per kg body weight when injected intraperitoneally. The dose used in man for fundus fluorescein angiography is usually 500–1000 mg in 20% concentration, corresponding roughly to 15 mg per kg body weight. As with any substance, caution is required in pregnancy and renal failure. The dye is excreted via urine. This may lead to a false-positive result when testing the urine in diabetic patients, and such patients should be warned not to readjust their insulin dosage for a day or two and to seek medical advice if necessary. The skin stains yellow for 4–6 hours.

Adverse effects

The complications and adverse effects of this dye have been extensively studied and can be classified as mild, moderate, or severe. The fluorescein is a mild photosensitizer; hence, patients should be warned not to expose themselves to strong sunlight while the skin remains yellow as this may result in sunburn. In a recent study, Kwan et al. (2006) reported 132 cases of adverse reactions out of 11,898 cases of angiography performed.

Mild

A mild reaction, seen in 5–10% of cases, is described as a transient effect that resolves fully without treatment. Nausea (4.6%), vomiting (1.3%) sneezing, and pruritus are very common. Extravasations of dye into the skin are painful but can be relieved by cold compression. Occasionally it may lead to sloughing of the skin. Inadvertent arterial injection is classified as a mild reaction, but if it is suspected the patient must be observed overnight in a cardiac unit.

Moderate

A moderate adverse reaction is also transient but needs medical treatment. The patient recovers fully without any sequelae. These reactions include urticaria, skin eruptions, thrombophlebitis, pyrexia, local tissue necrosis, transient nerve palsy, and syncopal attack.

Severe

A severe reaction is defined as prolonged effects requiring intensive medical treatment. It may threaten a patient's safety. Severe reactions include laryngeal edema, bronchospasm, anaphylaxis, shock, tonic seizure, myocardial infarction, and cardiac arrest. Studies by Butrus et al. (1999) and Fineschi et al. (1999) suggest that the most severe adverse reactions are mast cell dependent. Tryptase, a neutral protease of human mast cells, is a potentially important indicator of mast cell involvement in anaphylactic events. Additionally, b-tryptase levels can be assayed to detect anaphylactic reactions several hours after a precipitating event. A fatal reaction is rare but has been reported to occur. Yannuzzi et al. (1986) estimated the risk of death following fluorescein angiography to be 1:222,000.

PRINCIPLES OF FLUORESCEIN ANGIOGRAPHY

Anatomical principles

Choroid

The ophthalmic artery arises from the internal carotid artery and enters the orbit. It sends two, sometimes three, posterior ciliary arteries to form the choroid. The posterior ciliary arteries are named as the medial or lateral posterior ciliary artery according to their relationship to the optic nerve. When a third posterior ciliary artery is present, it runs above the optic nerve and is called the superior posterior ciliary artery. The lateral posterior ciliary artery supplies nearly two-thirds of the temporal choroid, while the medial posterior ciliary artery supplies the entire nasal half of the choroid. In some instances, the dividing lines between the medial and lateral posterior ciliary artery may be oblique. The watershed border between these two arteries usually passes across the optic disc. The medial and lateral posterior ciliary arteries divide into approximately 15–20 smaller branches before entering into the eye to supply the choroid. These are known as short posterior ciliary arteries. Most enter around the macula to form the choroid. The vortex veins lie 2.5–3.5 mm behind the equator and drain into the ampullae, which are dilated segments of the vortices lying within the sclera canals (Hayreh 1962) (**Figure 1.3**).

Choriocapillaris

This is a single layer of fine capillaries lying adjacent to Bruch's membrane. According to Hayreh (1975), terminal arterioles of the short posterior ciliary arterioles supply an independent lobule of the choriocapillaris comprising a central feeder arteriole and a series of peripheral draining venules. The lobular pattern is difficult to identify at the submacular and peripapillary region, but it is well developed at the posterior pole. The size of the lobule increases towards the periphery. The average lobule diameter is 515 × 450 µm at the equator and 645 × 550 and 955 × 670 µm at the periphery. The choriocapillaris has fenestrated endothelium (**Figure 1.4**).

Bruch's membrane

In 1884, Carl L W Bruch, an anatomist from Zurich, demonstrated a structureless membrane between the choroid and retinal pigment epithelium. Electron microscopy shows five different layers. The membrane plays a key role in various eye pathologies. The innermost and outermost layers are the basement membrane of the retinal pigment epithelium and the choriocapillaris, respectively. In between lies the elastic membrane sandwiched between the two collagen layers.

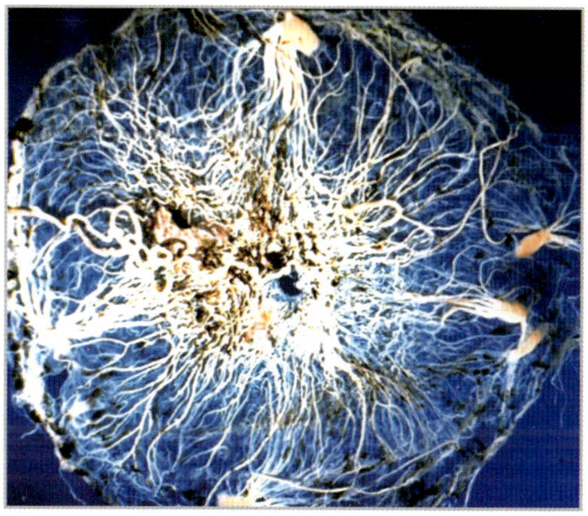

Figure 1.3 Blood supply of choroid. Dissection of the choroid seen from the scleral side shows many different sizes of choroidal vessels. At the center of the specimen, the void is the entrance of the optic nerve. The dense capillary with pigment seen to the left hand side of it is the macular area. The vortex veins are seen to drain blood from the choroid in an orderly segmental fashion. The long lateral posterior ciliary artery is seen to run from the left of the macular area in an anterior direction.

Retinal pigment epithelium

This is a monolayer of hexagonal cells in intimate contact with the Bruch's membrane outside and the outer segment of photoreceptors inside. It plays a critical role in the visual function of the photoreceptors. The retinal pigment epithelium maintains a fluid barrier between the retina and the choriocapillaris due to the tight junction between the cells called the zonula occludentes. The retinal pigment epithelium absorbs light energy via the melanin granules found within the cells. This helps to minimize light scatter and improves image resolution.

Central retinal artery

The central artery of the retina not only arises as the first branch of the ophthalmic artery in 77.45% of people but it also arises as a branch independent from the ophthalmic artery. It enters into the optic nerve and travels through it to emerge at the optic disc inside the eye. The central artery divides into the superior and inferior divisions, which in turn divide to form the nasal and temporal branches. Further branching takes place to supply the entire retina. Occasionally, a cilioretinal artery may emerge from the posterior ciliary system, supplying a variable portion of the retina between the optic disc and the macula. The retinal arteriole forms two sets of capillary networks: one superficial at the level of the nerve fiber layer and another at a deeper level that may extend as deep as the outer aspect of the inner nuclear layer. A further study by Hankind (1967) on flat ink injection of the human retina has shown that a separate, fine network of capillaries is seen on the retina close to the optic disc known as radial peripapillary capillaries. These are most prominent immediately around the disc and the superior and inferior temporal part of the retina adjoining the optic disc. These capillaries are not as noticeable on the nasal side of the fundus. They lie superficial to all retinal capillaries. They run a fairly long straight course radiating outward from the optic disc following the curve of the nerve fiber. These superficial radial capillaries are derived from the retinal arterioles lying deeper in the retina. From their origin they travel upwards to reach the superficial layer. They form parallel rows of elongated capillaries that occasionally bifurcate, but they rarely

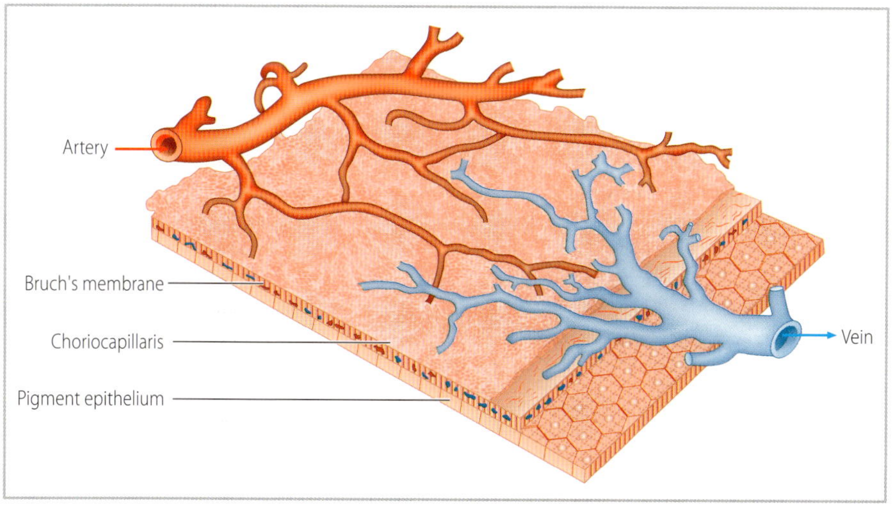

Figure 1.4 Choriocapillaris. The vascular arrangement of choriocapillaris as described by Dr. S S Hayreh.

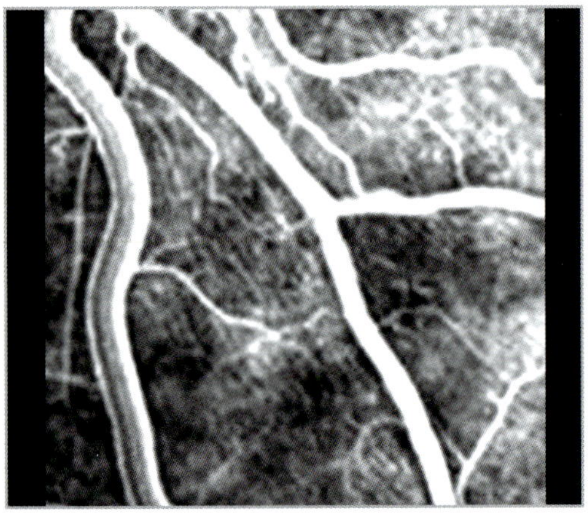

Figure 1.5 Radial peripapillary capillaries. The arteriovenous phase of the inferior temporal area of the left eye near the inferior pole of the optic disc and nearby retina shows radial peripapillary capillaries running parallel to the grooves of the optic nerve fibers.

anastomose with each other. After traveling superficially for a variable distance, the capillaries appear to enter into the deeper tissues where they are commonly joined by the venules (**Figure 1.5**).

Central retinal vein

The retinal circulation is drained by venules from all quadrants. The upper and lower halves of the retina drain their respective nasal and temporal quadrants. They follow a similar pattern to their counterpart, the central retinal artery. The upper temporal and nasal tributaries join to form the superior division and the inferior tributaries join to form the inferior division. These two major divisions join together in front of the lamina cribrosa to form the central retinal vein that pierces into the optic nerve and later joins the ophthalmic vein. A congenital abnormality of the venous arrangement at the optic disc, first described by Hayreh and Hayreh (1980) and later investigated by Chopdar (1984), confirms that two independently separate retinal veins may enter into the lamina cribrosa in 20.5% of people, preserving the characteristics of a central retinal vein, and thus deserve to be called a dual-trunked central retinal vein. Occasionally, they have been seen to emerge out of the optic nerve separately. Lieberman et al. (1976) have also seen similar anatomical variations in monkeys (**Figure 1.6a** and **b**).

Macula

According to Spitznas (1973), the macula is a 5.5 mm diameter area that begins at the temporal margin of the optic disc. The macula is divided into four zones: perifovea, parafovea, fovea, and foveola. The central 1.5 mm diameter area is the fovea, and the depression within it is the foveola. The foveola is only 0.35 mm in diameter. Here the retina is at its thinnest and contains only the photoreceptors and their nuclei. The axons of the outer plexiform layer form the Henle's layer that gives the typical appearance of cystoid macular edema on fluorescein angiography. Within the fovea, there is a capillary-free zone of 0.4 mm in diameter, as seen on fluorescein angiography. This is often referred to as the foveal avascular zone (FAZ). A 1.5 mm zone surrounding the fovea is the parafovea. The area outside this is the perifovea, measuring 2.5 mm in diameter (**Figure 1.7**).

Optic nerve head

Hayreh (1969) has given a full description of the blood supply of the optic nerve head and its role in various ocular pathologies. It recieves its blood supply both from the retinal and posterior ciliary circulation. For descriptive purposes, the optic nerve head can be divided into four different zones.

1. The lamina cribrosa region: the centripetal branches from the circle of Zinn and Haller or more directly from the posterior ciliary artery supply this region.
2. The prelaminar region: the blood supply to this part comes from the centripetal branches of the peripapillary choroidal plexus. The temporal side is more vascular than the nasal side.
3. The retrolamina: this area is supplied directly by the posterior ciliary arteries from the peripapillary choroid. This area may also receive its blood supply from the pial branches of the circle of Zinn and Haller.

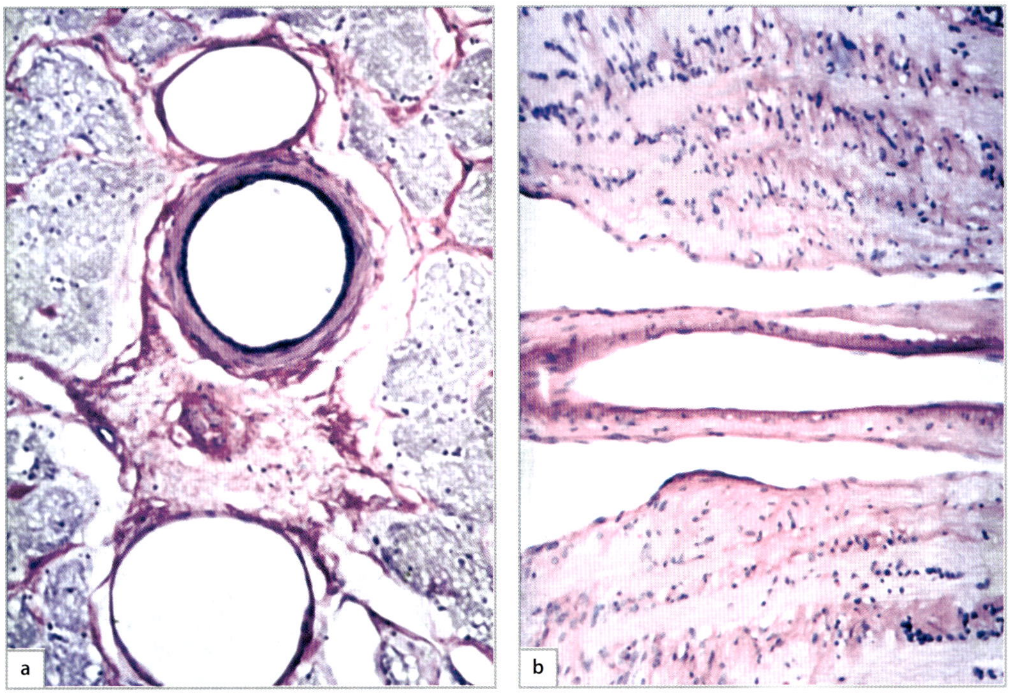

Figure 1.6 (a) Transverse section through the optic nerve. This section from a monkey's eye shows two central retinal veins remaining independent well within the optic nerve. The central retinal artery maintains its central position in between the two veins. (b) Sagittal section through the optic nerve. The sagittal section from a monkey's optic nerve shows the typical central position of the central retinal artery between the two separate retinal veins. Photos supplied by RW Green, Baltimore, USA.

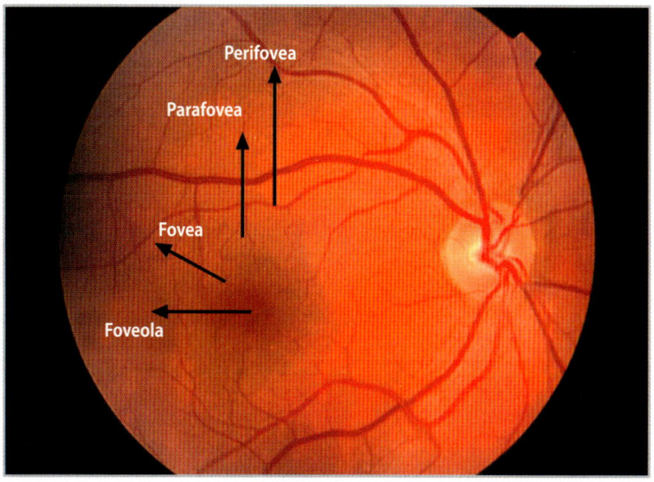

Figure 1.7 Macula of the right eye, showing the different macular zones.

4. Surface layer: the surface layer of the optic nerve head is supplied by the retinal arterioles—the branches of the retinal artery.

The prelaminar region draines into the choroidal veins. There is no corresponding venous channel for the circle of Zinn and Haller. The central retinal vein communicates with choroidal circulation in the prelamina (**Figure 1.8**).

Physiological principles

Blood–retina barrier

The central retinal artery is an end artery without anastomosis. The endothelial cells of retinal vessels possess a unique property that prevents the passage of solids including fluorescein molecules from plasma across the vascular wall in normal physiological circumstances, whereas the choroidal vessels are freely permeable to small molecules. The resulting extravascular fluorescein stains the choroidal connective tissues, Bruch's membrane, and any colloid bodies on it.

Retinal pigment epithelium

The tight junctions of retinal pigment epithelium, provided by the zonulae occludentes in healthy retinal pigment epithelium, prevent fluorescein passing beyond Bruch's membrane. The amount of melanin pigment present within the pigment epithelium is critical to the degree of background choroidal fluorescence reflected during fluorescein angiography. Excess pigment will mask, whereas a lesser amount of pigment will unmask, the background fluorescence during angiography utilizing the visible band of light. Indocyanine green angiography using the infrared band of light wave penetrates freely through the retinal pigment epithelium, thus allowing reasonable visibility of choroidal vasculature.

TECHNIQUES

Fluorescence angiography is an invasive procedure. The dye is prone to cause several adverse effects, some of which may be serious. It is essential that a selection of emergency drugs are kept readily accessible for use. Such a list can be drawn up in consultation with the accident and emergency and pharmacy departments. It is essential for the user to be familiar with emergency resuscitation methods. Make sure you are aware of the location of the cardiopulmonary resuscitation trolley and how to summon help in an emergency.

Patient selection

A full medical history including an inquiry for any allergy should be taken before considering fluorescein or indocyanine green angiography. A history of recent myocardial infarction and congestive cardiac failure is not an absolute contraindication, but caution must be exercised. Patients with respiratory illnesses such as chronic bronchitis, asthma, hay fever, and atopy may require a test dose prior to full injection. Individuals with hepatic and renal failure should be excluded from such a study unless it is vital for management. Fluorescein angiography should not be performed during the first trimester of pregnancy, and thereafter only with the utmost caution. Nursing mothers must be warned that fluorescein may be secreted into the milk. If fluorescein angiography is performed in a nursing mother, it is best to store the breast milk for one or two feedings before injecting fluorescein to replace the newly secreted milk (which can be discarded).

Patient preparation

The procedure must be explained to the patient in detail so that a trouble-free session can be achieved and good quality photographs can be obtained. It is important the patient is aware that the test will be carried out in dark. He/she will hear a series of clicking noises

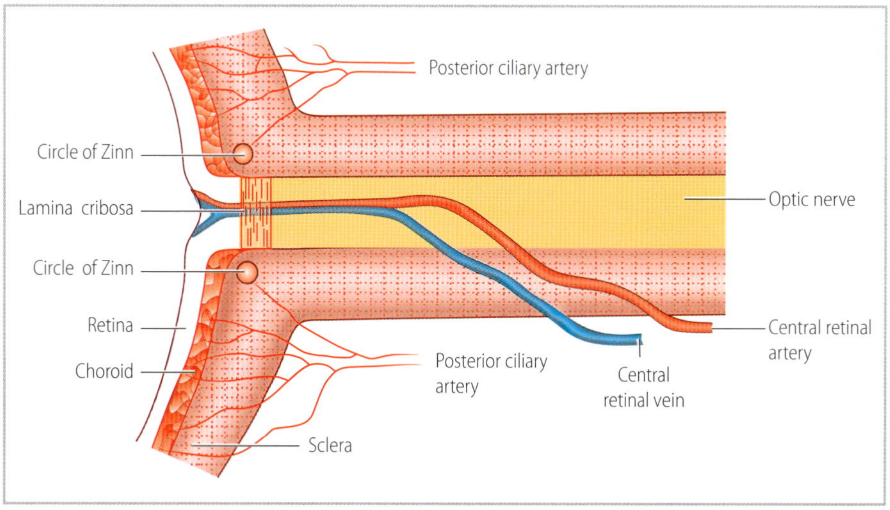

Figure 1.8 Blood supply of the optic disc. Modified from an original idea of Dr. S S Hayreh.

caused by the flashlights, but should be told not to sit back until finally asked to do so. Many patients sit back after the first flash, thinking the test is finished. It is a good practice to inform patients of the possible adverse reactions beforehand. This is an invasive procedure and many hospitals require signed consent. The pupils must be fully dilated with cycloplegics to avoid contraction due to bright flashlights.

The patient is comfortably seated in front of the camera so that the chin rests comfortably on the chinrest and the forehead presses firmly against the forehead bar.

Dye injection

A 5 mL amount of 20% fluorescein is drawn into a 5 mL syringe. Most practitioners use the whole 5 mL, but 2.5 mL can give good result. Usually, an antecubital vein is selected from either arm. A number 23-gauge butterfly cannula is inserted into the antecubital vein and held securely by adhesive tape. Once the cannula is secured within the vein, the preloaded syringe containing the dye is connected to the cannula. Once ready, a reasonably fast and continuous injection at a uniform speed without interruption is necessary for a compact bolus of dye to enter into the circulation.

Test dose

If the patient is suspected to have allergy, a test dose is vital. Normally 0.1 mL of the dye diluted with 1 mL of normal saline is injected into the inserted cannula. The patient is monitored for next 5 minutes for any untoward reaction. If there are any signs of adverse reaction, the angiography must be abandoned.

Oral fluorescein

Several authors have recommended fluorescein angiography following oral ingestion of fluorescein. The patient is asked to drink a mixture of fluorescein dye with orange juice. This technique is helpful where the early transit photographs are of little importance such as in detecting cystoid macular edema. A set of angiographic recordings is made approximately one and a half hours after the ingestion of the mixed drink.

Photography

Eyepiece adjustment

It is important that the operator fully relaxes his accommodation in order to focus the image sharply on the film. If you wear spectacles, or are prone to accommodate, then you should adjust the eyepiece as follows. You will see the eyepiece has several dioptric marks both in plus and minus signs. Also you will see a crosshair when looking down the tube. First rotate the eyepiece clockwise to the maximum plus sign, then looking through the eye piece bring the crosshair into focus by rotating the eyepiece in a counterclockwise direction. Repeat this procedure two or three times and adjust to the best focus. Remember that as you get fatigued during the course of the day, your accommodation may get worse. It is advisable to check accommodation again during an afternoon session.

Performing angiography

Now place the patient's chin as described above. Use the external or internal fixation as required. Move the whole camera toward the eye while looking from the side to observe the viewing lamp's filament, clearly focusing on the cornea. Make sure that lights from both filaments enter through the dilated pupil. Now, looking through the eyepiece, tune the fine-focusing knob to sharpen the retinal image. Ensure that there is no peripheral fringing. Finally trigger the flash switch to take the picture. First take a set of color photographs and then switch to load the filters for angiography. Ask the assistant to inject the dye both quickly and continuously in order to get a single bolus. Run the clock timer from the end of injection. Initially you will not see anything, but very soon a bright glow will appear in the choroidal circulation. Now you should start taking photographs, initially at 0.5-second intervals for the first 6 seconds, then increasing the time to one every 4–10 seconds for next few minutes. This marks the end of the transit period or the run. Once the patient has safely gone through this phase, the butterfly cannula may be removed. The patient is then asked to wait for 15–20 minutes while the late phase photographs should be taken. Do not forget to warn the patient about skin and urine discoloration and avoidance of direct exposure to sunlight for the next 24 hours. During the transit, you need to monitor the strength of exposure due to image blooming, which might require you to alter the gains of the exposure (Oosterhuis & Lammens 1965).

Pitfalls of photography

Wide-field and stereo photography need full dilatation of the pupil. The pupil must remain fully dilated throughout the period of angiography in spite of bright illumination from the flashlight. An undilated pupil makes the fundus picture appear dark. A peripheral orange halo indicates the camera being farther away from the eye, whereas a blue halo indicates it being closer. Longer eyelashes and blinking during photography usually show as ghosting of the upper half of the fundus picture. Clear ocular media is essential to obtain a good quality picture. Early lens opacity, thickening of the posterior capsule in pseudophakic eyes, vitreous opacities, and corneal opacities make images hazy. Sometimes it is possible to avoid peripheral lens opacity by suitably aligning the camera.

Nowadays the intraocular lens implant poses several technical difficulties. The reflection produced by the intraocular lens results in a white ring in the center of the field.

Grease marks on camera lens show gray splodges on the film. They may glisten at times. Clean the camera lens regularly with lens cleaning tissue. Never use cloth or ordinary tissue, as the fibers will stick to the lens due to static electricity.

The patient's blood pressure and circulation time are important factors to obtain good contrasting images. If the circulation time is slow due to reduced cardiac output or slower peripheral circulation, the dye does not concentrate well and the pictures become dull and lack contrast.

Normal fluorescein angiogram

The sequence of dye circulation through the vascular tree divides the angiogram into four different phases such as choroidal or prearterial, arterial, arteriovenous, and venous phase.

Choroidal phase

Because of the expeditious and numerous branching of the posterior ciliary artery, this phase is brief and the filling is often segmental and patchy. A distinct lobular pattern may be observed if the recording is obtained during the very early phase of circulation. Frequently, a watershed zone is seen passing across the optic disc revealing the demarcation line between the lateral and medial posterior ciliary artery supply (**Figure 1.9**).

Arterial phase

The dye first appears in the retina through the central retinal artery and quickly displays the architecture of the entire retinal vascular tree. It takes approximately 6–8 seconds for the dye to reach the retinal circulation (**Figure 1.10a** and **b**).

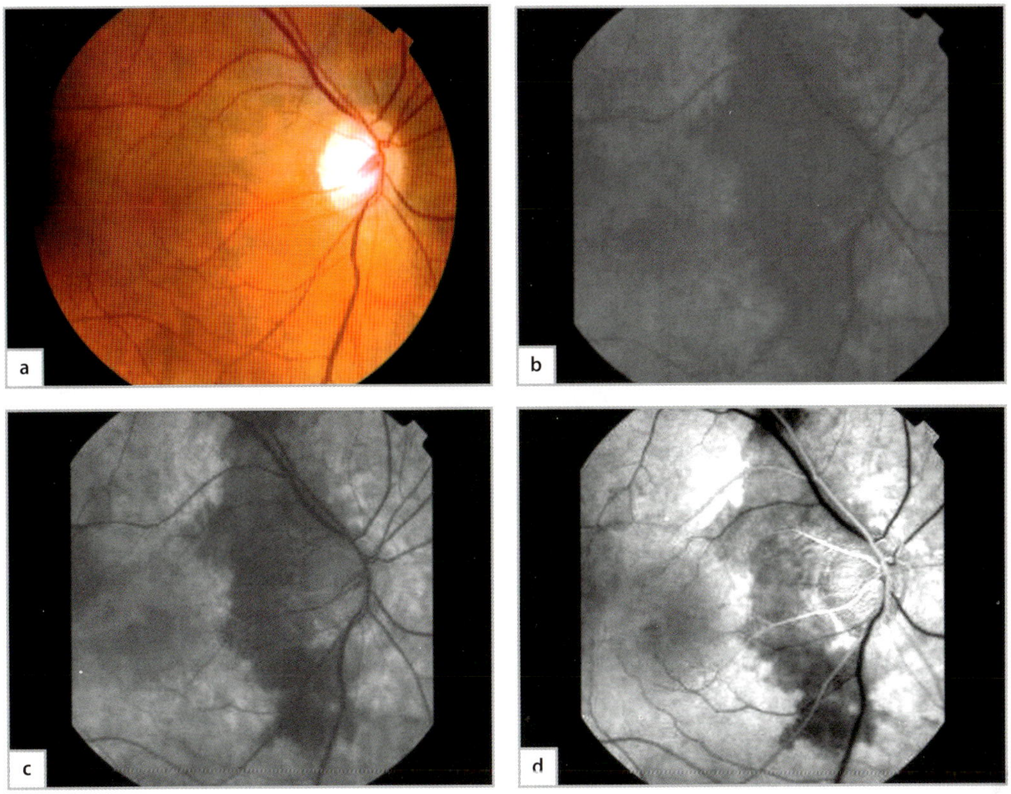

Figure 1.9 (a) The right eye shows a normal fundus. (b) Choroidal phase. The very early choroidal phase of the fluorescein angiogram shows the watershed zone passing across the optic disc. The lateral and medial posterior ciliary arteries seem to supply their specific zone. (c) The later frame still shows the dye limited to the choroidal circulation. The watershed zone is now clearly passing just lateral to the temporal border of the optic disc. (d) During the fully filled choroidal phase of the angiogram, the demarcation line remains visible.

Arteriovenous phase

During the arteriovenous phase, the dye is seen in both the retinal artery and vein. Although theoretically the dye must pass through the capillaries before reaching the veins, visualization of capillaries is not at its best until the venous phase. The earliest sign of the venous phase is marked by a lamellar flow of dye where the dye is seen sliding along the lateral wall of the veins (**Figure 1.10c**).

Venous phase

Soon the lamellar flow is lost and the entire blood column in the vein is mixed with the dye. The retinal arteries still retain a significant amount of dye during this stage. The intensity of fluorescence continues to increase within the veins and finally matches that of the arteries. During the late venous phase, the intensity of fluorescence begins to fade from the arteries but the concentration of dye builds up within the veins (**Figure 1.10d** and **e**).

Late phase

The late phase is normally recorded 15–20 minutes after the injection of the dye. This shows the ultimate fate of the dye. This phase is important for demonstrating the competency of the various barriers and interfaces (**Figure 1.10f**).

Areas of special interest

Macular area

The macular area exhibits several special features, for example masking of the choroidal background due to presence of xanthophyll pigment in the fovea. This generally corresponds to the so-called FAZ. The perifoveal arcade is best demonstrated during the venous phase. There is free anastomosis of retinal capillaries around the perifoveal arcade. This anastomosis leads to the formation of macular edema in diseases affecting the peripheral part of the retina even if disease is limited to one sector only (**Figure 1.11**).

Optic disc area

The optic disc and peripapillary area have two different capillary networks: the epipapillary and the radial peripapillary plexuses. As the name suggests, the first of these is seen on the surface of the disc and the second runs parallel to the major retinal vessels on the surface of the retina (**Figure 1.12 a–d**).

Abnormal fluorescence

Hypofluorescence

1. Masking a. Pigment	Melanin Choroidal nevus Choroidal malignant melanoma Retinal pigment epithelium hypertrophy Retinal pigment epithelium hyperplasia Dark fundus in some macular dystrophies Racial characters
b. Blood	Choroidal hemorrhage Retinal hemorrhage Subhyaloid hemorrhage
c. Xanthophyll	Macular pigment
d. Serous fluid in between interface	Central serous retinopathy Retinal detachment
2. Filling defects	Retinal vascular occlusion Choroidal infarct
3. Loss of tissues	Colobomas

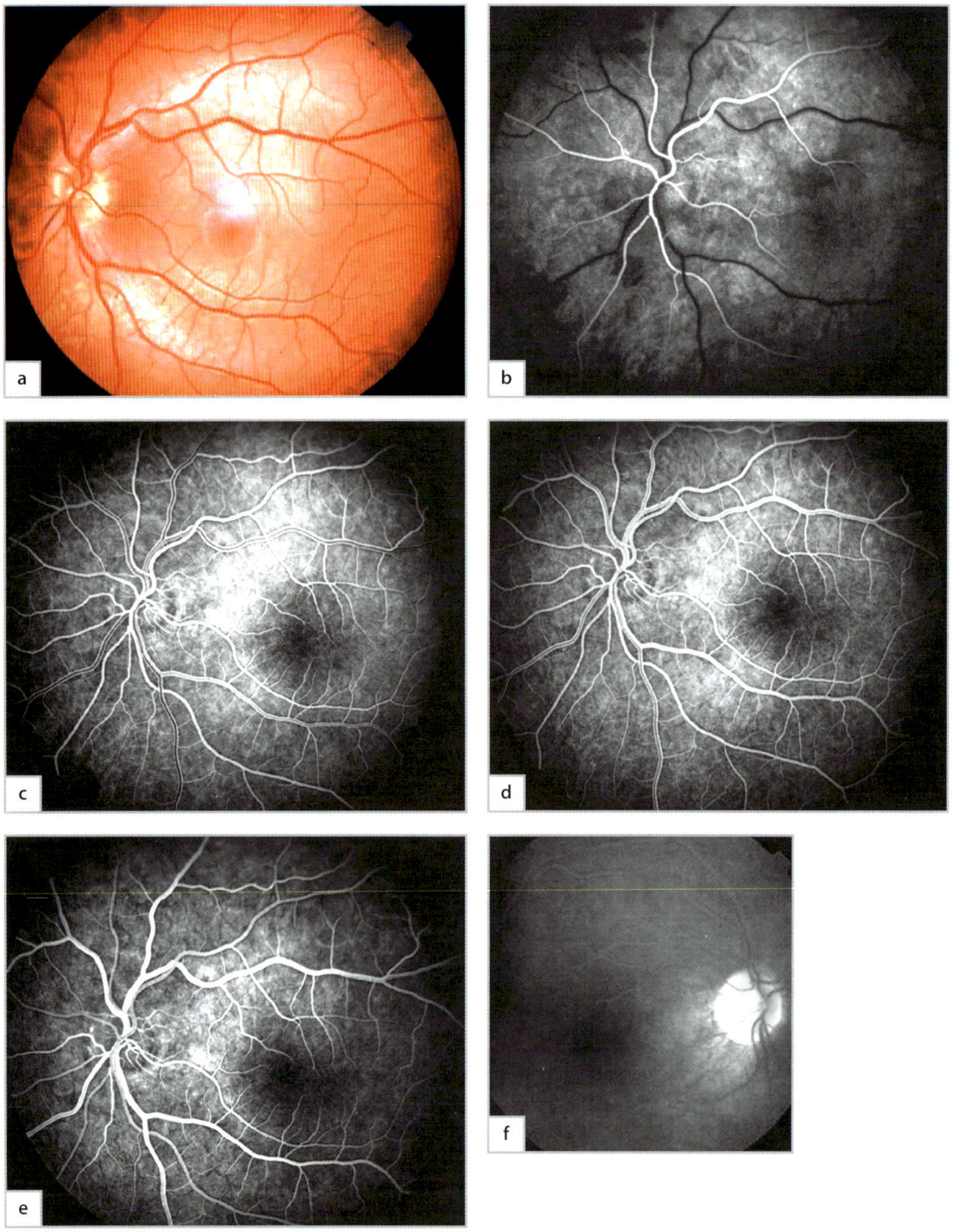

Figure 1.10 (a) Arterial phase. The left eye shows a normal fundus with normal branching of retinal blood vessels. (b) The arterial phase of the fluorescein angiogram shows filling of the main branches of the central retinal artery. (c) Arteriovenous phase. During the early arteriovenous phase, the choroidal background is well filled and so are the branches of the retinal artery. The veins are now beginning to return the dye. Note the hyperfluorescence on the lateral wall of the veins and relative hypofluorescence in the middle of the bloodstream. This is known as laminar flow. The plasma stained with the dye concentrates on the walls, whereas the cellular components in the central column have yet to take up the dye. (d) Mid venous phase. Both the arteries and the veins are now full. The intensity of fluorescence in each of the channels appears almost of similar strength. (e) Late venous phase. The late venous phase shows increased fluorescence from the veins. (f) Late phase. Approximately 30 minutes after the injection of the dye, there is disappearance of the dye from the choroid and retinal circulation. The optic disc may retain a slight amount of staining.

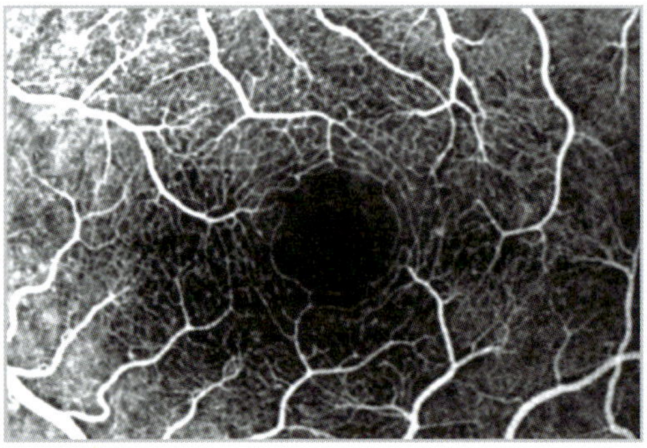

Figure 1.11 Macular area. The enhanced view during the arteriovenous phase of fluorescein angiography of the foveal area shows the perifoveal arcade. The center of the fovea remains hypofluorescence and devoid of any vascularity.

Hyperfluorescence

1. Window defect	Albinism Retinal pigment epithelium atrophy, angioid streaks
2. Morphologic change	Arteriosclerosis aneurysms Blood vessels: dilation tortuosity New vessels Tumor vessels: choroidal hemangioma Malignant melanoma Angiomatous retina, hamartoma
3. Leakage Pooling of dye in serous fluid	Disciform macular degeneration, retinal detachment Central serous retinopathy
4. Staining Seen during late phase of angiography	Retinal vasculitis, colloid bodies Disc drusen Soft exudate Chorioretinal scars

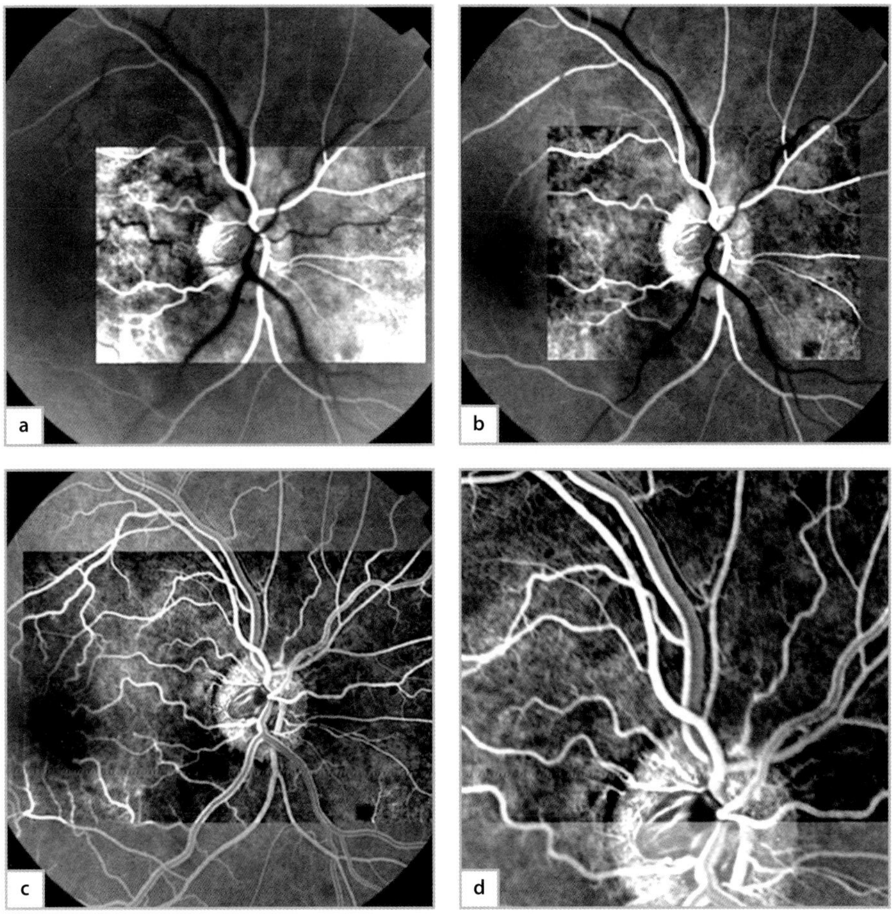

Figure 1.12 Optic disc area, enhanced view. (a) The early arterial phase of the fluorescein angiogram shows patchy filling of the choroid around the optic disc. There appears to be a cilioretinal artery emerging from the 8 o'clock position of the optic disc. (b) The late arterial phase shows the normally filled choroidal background. All the branches of the retinal arteries are full. The deeper surface of the optic disc shows filling of deeper vessels on the optic disc. (c) The early arteriovenous phase shows laminar flow in the veins and epipapillary vessels on the surface of the disc. (d) The enlarged view of frame C shows the epipapillary vessels on the surface of the optic disc and radial peripapillary vessels along the grooves of superior temporal quadrant. These are derived from the retinal arteriolar circulation.

REFERENCES

Bruch CLW. Untersuchungen zur Kenntniss des Kornigen Pigments der Wirbelthiere. In. Physiologischer und pathologischer Hinsicht, Zurich, Meyer u Zeller, 1884:1–62.

Butrus SI, Negvesky GJ, Rivera-Velazques PM, Schwartz LB. Serum tryptase: an indicator of anaphylaxis following fluorescein angiography. *Graefe's arch Clinic Exp Ophthalmol* 1999; **237**:433–434.

Chopdar A. Dual trunk central retinal vein: incidence in clinical practice. *Arch Ophthalmol* 1984; **102**:85–87.

Delori F, Ben-Sira I, Trempe C. Fluorescein angiography with an optimized filter combination. *Am J Ophthalmol* 1976; **82**:559–566.

Fineschi V, Monasterolo G, Rosi R, Turillazzi E. Fatal anaphylactic shock during a fluorescein angiography. *Forensic Sci Int* 1999; **100**:137–142.

Gifford H. Use of fluorescein intravenously as an aid to ophthalmic diagnosis and treatment. *Arch Ophthalmol* 1940; **24**:122–131.

Hayreh SS. Ophthalmic artery. III. Branches. *Br J Ophthalmol* 1962; **46**:212–247.

Hayreh SS. Blood supply of optic nerve head and its role in optic atrophy, glaucoma, and oedema of optic disc. *Br J Ophthalmol* 1969; **53**:721–748.

Hayreh SS. Segmental nature of the choroidal vasculature. *Br J Ophthalmol* 1975; **59**:631–648.

Hayreh SS, Hayreh MS. Hemi-central retinal vein occlusion pathogenesis, clinical features, and natural history. *Arch Ophthalmol* 1980; **98**:1600–1609.

Hankind P. Radial peripapillary capillaries of the retina. I. Artery. Human and comparative. *Br J Ophthalmol* 1967; **51**:115–123.

Kwan ASL, Barry C, McAllister IL, Constable I. Fluorescein angiography and adverse drug reactions revisited: the Lions Eye experience. *Clin Experiment Ophthalmol* 2006; **34**:33–38.

Lieberman MF, Maumenee AE, Green WR. Histologic studies of the vasculature of the anterior optic nerve. *Am J Ophthalmol* 1976; **82**:405–423.

Novotny HR, Alvis DL. A method of photographing fluorescence circulating blood in the human retina. *Circulation* 1961; **24**:82–86.

Oosterhuis JA, Lammens AJJ. Fluorescein angiography of ocular fundus. *Ophthalmologica* 1965; **149**:210–220.

Spitznas M. Der normale ophthalmoskopische und histologische Befund der Maculazone und seine varianten, Deutsche Ophthalmologischen Gesellschaft 1973; 73:26.

Yannuzzi LA, Roher KT, Tindel LJ, et al. Fluorescein angiography complication survey. *Ophthalmology* 1986; **93**:611–617.

Chapter 2 Indocyanine angiography

Heinrich Heimann

INTRODUCTION

Indocyanine green (ICG, $C_{43}H_{47}N_2NaO_6S_2$) is an artificial tricarbocyanine dye that is a component of color film. It was introduced into medicine in the 1950s when biocompatible dyes that could be injected into the bloodstream were first investigated. The primary medicodiagnostic applications of ICG were the quantification of cardiac output and liver function. The use of ICG for fundus angiography is based on unique optical and chemical properties that, compared with standard fluorescein angiography, allow a more detailed examination of the choroidal circulation and of retinal and choroidal lesions that are obscured by blood or fluid (Leys & Horsman 2009, Yannuzzi 2011).

The first fundus angiography using ICG in humans was performed by Flower and Hochheimer in the early 1970s. ICG was approved for the use in angiography by the US Food and Drug Administration (FDA) in 1975. The first clinical applications of infrared absorption choroidal angiography in humans were then reported in 1976 (Flower & Hochheimer 1976, Chopdar et al. 1978). The production of the first commercially available camera system in 1980 and the introduction of video angiography in the 1990s were further developments to improve this examination technique. However, it was not until the 2000s that ICG angiography found a more widespread use. The advents of digital photography and scanning laser ophthalmoscopes (SLOs) significantly improved the image capture, resolution, and contrast compared with earlier video angiography or film-based techniques. In addition, review and interpretation of the images are now greatly facilitated by the use of computer-based rather than conventional film-based or video imaging systems. ICG angiograms can be reviewed immediately following the procedure on networked, high-definition monitors with the option of further magnification or contrast enhancement of selected images. With multimodal imaging, previous examination results and images acquired by other methods is now standard and more productive than the time-consuming review of printed images or video sequences on different reviewing stations, as was done just 10 years ago.

Over the past decade, several clinical applications have emerged in which ICG angiography not only provides useful additional information regarding the pathophysiology of chorioretinal diseases but also has a direct impact on treatment pathways and outcomes. ICG angiography is considered by leading medical retina specialists to be an essential examination technique in defined clinical situations (Yannuzzi 2011). However, its use varies significantly between centers. On the one hand, some retinal specialists perform an ICG angiography on a routine basis in a large proportion of patients, and on the other hand a significant number of specialists rarely or never perform an ICG angiography. The critics of the more widespread use of ICG angiography argue that at present there is not enough evidence-based clinical research to justify the significant additional costs of this relatively time consuming and invasive diagnostic test. They are of the opinion that, compared to the recent developments and popularization of several noninvasive imaging techniques [spectral domain optical coherence tomography (OCT), enhanced depth imaging OCT, autofluorescence], the use of ICG angiography will decrease or even become obsolete in the near future. Proponents of ICG angiography proclaim that the unique abilities of ICG angiography to detect changes in the choroidal circulation cannot be met by any other current or emerging imaging technique. With the expanding knowledge about ICG angiography and the escalating number of treatment options, they foresee a future for ICG angiography as an established part of a state-of-the-art multimodal imaging service.

A synopsis of the most commonly used indications of ICG angiography and typical findings is listed in **Table 2.1**.

ANATOMICAL AND PHYSIOLOGIC PRINCIPLES

Fluorescence describes the ability of substances to emit light following excitation by light of a different wavelength. Fluorescence angiography of the eye is currently performed with two different dyes: fluorescein and ICG. Following intravenous injection, they fill the blood vessels of the eye via the ophthalmic artery. The dye molecules are excited with light sources of a defined wavelength. Their capability to fluoresce is then used as a light source that can be traced and located by photographic documentation. The resulting image detects the dye molecules within the vascular structures, thus providing an outline of the blood vessels of the eye and potential pathological structures with a much higher contrast compared to standard photographic techniques. In addition, changes of the dye's location can be monitored over time. This provides additional information about pathological changes when compared to normal eyes. The ophthalmologist reviewing the angiogram compares potential changes in the location of dye and the amount of detectable dye (hyper- or hypofluorescence) to normal angiograms. Together with the findings of the clinical examination, other imaging techniques, and previous angiograms, the angiography is then interpreted as part of the diagnostic process.

The chemical and optical properties of ICG differ significantly from those of fluorescein (Leys & Horsman 2009). ICG is excited by light in the near-infrared range of 790–805 nm wavelength, resulting in an emission of light between 770 and 880 nm. Modern SLO-based angiography systems use an infrared diode laser with a wavelength of 795 nm for excitation and barrier filters at 810 nm. Compared with fluorescein, the optical characteristics of ICG allow a better transmission of emitted light through the retinal pigment epithelium, fluid, and blood. In addition, ICG has a significantly higher molecular weight (775 kD vs. 375 kD of fluorescein), and almost all ICG molecules are rapidly bound to plasma proteins following injection. As a consequence, ICG extravasates more slowly and in significantly lower proportions through the choroidal vasculature or leaking blood vessels. With ICG, the choroidal vasculature and perfusion status are imaged in greater detail than with fluorescein angiography. Clinical examples, with significant alterations of the choroidal circulation, include diseases with significant alterations of the choroidal perfusion (e.g. polypoidal choroidal vasculopathy, choroiditis, choroidal tumors, or central serous retinopathy). Further, choroidal or retinal neovascularizations are easier to identify because they are not obscured by the leaking fluoresceine that acts like a smokescreen in the early phases of the

Table 2.1 Current indications for ICG angiography

Condition	Typical ICG findings	Advantage over FFA
Polypoidal choroidal vasculopathy (**Figures 2.20–2.22**)	Polypoidal dilatation of choroidal vessels Pulsating polyps on movie Branching vascular networks with points of focal dilatation	ICG necessary to diagnose polypoidal lesions
RAP (**Figures 2.23–2.25**)	Identification of retino-retinal or retinochoroidal anastomosis Significant leakage of ICG over RAP Movie demonstrates blood flow in RAP lesion Late hyperfluorescent spot over RAP lesion	Facilitates identification of RAP lesion
Occult AMD (**Figures 2.18–2.19**)	Identification of CNV Feeder vessel	May identify CNV not visible on FFA
Retinal pigment epithelial detachment	Identification of choroidal neovascularization	May identify CNV not visible on FFA
Non-AMD choroidal neovascularization	Identification of CNV	May identify CNV in ambiguous cases Definition of the extent of the CNV in areas covered by blood or exudates
Central serous retinopathy (**Figures 2.26–2.28**)	Focal leakage Staining of areas of previous hyperpermeability	Identifies areas of choroidal hyperpermeability not seen clinically or silent on FFA
Posterior uveitis (**Figures 2.13–2.17**)	Focal hypo- or hyperpermeability	Identifies disturbances of the choroidal circulation not visible clinically or on FFA
Choroidal hemangioma (**Figures 2.29–2.30**)	Early significant leakage Dye washout during the late phases	Higher sensitivity in identifying choroidal hemangioma

AMD, age-related macular degeneration; ICG, indocyanine green; FFA, fluorescein angiography; RAP, retinal angiomatous proliferation; CNV, choroidal neovascularization.

angiography. This is used for the identification of retinal angiomatous proliferations or choroidal neovascularizations in pigment epithelial detachments. And finally, vascular changes obscured by blood, lipids, or exudations in fluorescein angiograms can be identified with ICG angiography. This is of clinical importance in the identification of choroidal necovasularizations, polypoidal choroidal changes, or retinal macroaneurysms underlying a retinal hemorrhage that cannot be visualized with fluorescein angiography.

Following injection, ICG is not metabolized. It is exclusively excreted through the liver with a biphasic elimination curve. The initial half-life is 3–4 minutes, followed by a dose-related half-life of 60–80 minutes.

Although ICG provides an excellent outline of the retinal vasculature, it is mainly used for the detection of changes of choroidal blood flow. The choroid is situated between the retina and the sclera, thus forming the middle layer of the posterior segment. Anteriorly, it merges into the ciliary body and the iris. The thickness of the choroid varies between 0.25 mm in the macula and 0.1–0.15 mm at the equator (Richard 1992). It consists of several layers. Immediately attached to the basement membrane of the retinal pigment epithelium is Bruch's membrane. Bruch's membrane is only 2 µm thick and is composed of collagen and elastic fibers. Its composition and permeability seem to be important factors involved in the development of exudative and nonexudative age-related macular degeneration. Bruch´s membrane is bordered by the basement membrane of the choriocapillaris, which forms the next layer of the choroid. It consists of fenestrated capillaries that are organized in a unique segmental, lobular pattern. The size of the lobes varies with location and between patients. As a clinical guideline, the lobes average approximately 1/4 disc diameter in size. The lobes are fed by a central arteriole that then branches out into a meshwork of capillaries that run radially into the periphery of the lobe. The capillary diameter varies and is 9–20 µm at the posterior pole and 10–50 µm at the equator. Capillary size and number decrease with age. The endothelial cells of the capillaries are fenestrated with pores of 55–60 nm. The choriocapillaris blends into Sattler's layer (arterioles and venules of medium to small size) and then Haller's layer (larger arteries and veins). The arteries have a diameter of 40–90 µm, and the veins are around 20–100 µm in size. The vasculature is embedded in loose connective tissue that also incorporates melanocytes, lymphocytes, and nerve fibers. The outermost layer of the choroid is the lamina suprachoroidea that borders the sclera.

The blood supply of the choroid derives from the ophthalmic artery. Two to three branches of posterior ciliary arteries separate from the ophthalmic artery in the orbit (Richard 1992). They run near the optic nerve head and are divided, according to their anatomical location in relation to the optic nerve, into medial and lateral posterior ciliary arteries. In the majority of patients, the medial posterior ciliary artery arises together with the central retina artery as the first branch of the ophthalmic artery. The lateral posterior ciliary artery usually resembles the second branch. The lateral and the medial branches supply arterial vascular networks that are not connected. Thus, there is a 'watershed' of choroidal blood supply between the lateral and medial aspects of the choroid (Mori et al. 2008). The macula lies on the watershed between the lateral and medial blood supply. Before entering the globe, the medial and the lateral posterior ciliary arteries each divide into one long posterior ciliary artery and 10–20 short posterior ciliary arteries. The lateral short posterior ciliary arteries pierce through the sclera at the location of the macula and then run anteriorly in a radial fashion to supply the various segments of the choroid. The long posterior ciliary arteries run anteriorly to split at the level of the ora serrata and supply the major arterial circle of the iris.

The choroidal blood is drained via vortex veins. Venules arise at the edge of the lobes of the choriocapillaris, then unite into larger veins and finally form large vortex veins. In the majority of patients, four vortex veins (one in each quadrant) are present. They pierce the sclera posterior to the equator. In contrast to the arterial system, there are abundant anastomosis between different quadrants in the venous drainage system.

The choroid is also involved in supplying the blood supply to the optic nerve head. The prelaminar zone is supplied by branches of the peripapillary choroidal arteries. The lamina cribrosa is fed by short posterior ciliary arteries that form the vascular network of the circle of Zinn–Haller. Recurrent branches from the peripapillary choroid support the retrolaminar section of the optic nerve head. In contrast, the superficial nerve fiber layer on the optic nerve head is supplied by the branches of the central retinal artery.

TECHNIQUE

ICG angiography is an invasive and time-consuming diagnostic procedure that requires expensive equipment, specialized medical photographers, skilled ophthalmologists for interpretation of the angiogram, and the availability of emergency medical support in case of severe adverse reactions. Its use is, therefore, limited to tertiary centers specialized in the diagnosis and treatment of chorioretinal diseases. It should only be performed in selected cases to answer a particular clinical question based on the assessment of an ophthalmologist with significant experience in retinal disease.

There are no age restrictions, but patients must be fit and able to undergo the diagnostic procedure. This requires cannulation, pupillary dilatation, correct head positioning, and appropriate gaze at a slit lamp for several minutes. With the use of modern SLO imaging devices, there is relatively little light exposure. The examination causes only minor discomfort to the patient. However, patients may be apprehensive about the intravenous injection. A detailed explanation of the procedure, the nature, and low incidence of side effects and the required cooperation regarding head and eye positions are important prerequisites for obtaining high-quality angiograms. In most institutions, written consent is required. A comfortable positioning of the patient and the photographer should be assured before start of the angiography. Adequate pupillary dilatation and clear optical media are prerequisites for sufficiently good images, and reliable intravenous access is mandatory. If possible, the test should be performed before measurement of the intraocular pressure because this may negatively influence the clarity of the cornea and tear film. ICG angiography can be performed before or after fluorescein angiography. With multimodal imaging, the minutes between documentation of the various phases of the angiography are often used to capture additional images (e.g. OCT or color images). It must be kept in mind that autofluorescence images must be taken before fluorescein or ICG angiographies are performed (fundus autofluorescence before fluorescein angiography and near-infrared angiography before ICG angiography, respectively).

A point of ongoing discussion is whether ICG angiography is contraindicated in patients with known allergies to iodine-containing products (e.g. contrast media or disinfection products). Iodine is not part of the ICG molecule itself (Leys & Horsman 2009). However, the pharmacological product contains up to 5% sodium iodide required for the preparation of the product. These sodium iodide molecules are too small to cause an antibody response could trigger an allergic reaction. While most textbooks and manufacturer recommendations state that one should not perform an ICG angiography in patients who have a history of allergic reactions to iodine-containing products, this seems to be unjustified. Another myth is that patients with a known allergy to shellfish or seafood have a higher rate of allergic reaction to iodine-containing products than individuals with other known allergies.

In patients with hyperthyroidism, ICG angiographies should be performed with caution. The iodide uptake into the thyroid gland can be blocked by the application of sodium perchlorate 30 minutes before injection of the ICG. Radioactive iodine uptake studies should not be performed within 1 week after administration, as test results may be altered. Although ICG has been used in pregnant women without detectable side effects, ICG is classified as a 'pregnancy category C' drug with insufficient data to appraise the safety of ICG during pregnancy.

ICG is supplied as a sterile, lyophilized green powder in a vial. It is dissolved in sterile water and must be used within 5–8 hours. The manufacturer's guidelines recommend 0.1–0.3 mg ICG per kg body weight for diagnostic purposes (PULSION Medical Systems AG, Munich, Germany). However, it is common practice to use 25 mg ICG dissolved in 5 mL sterile water as a standard dose irrespective of body weight. In patients with increased pigmentation of the ocular fundus or for wide-angle angiographies, the dose can be increased to 50 or 75 mg. The drug is injected rapidly by the ophthalmologist or specialist nurse via a peripheral intravenous access, followed by a 5 mL saline flush.

Extravasated ICG is not associated with significant inflammatory reaction. Overall, ICG for angiography is associated with a low rate of minor side effects (< 1%) and is significantly better tolerated than fluorescein for angiography (Hope-Ross et al. 1994). Anaphylactic reactions are extremely rare, but fatal outcomes have been reported. The procedure must therefore be performed with appropriate safety measures under medical supervision.

PHOTOGRAPHY

ICG is less fluorescent than fluorescein. The resulting image is darker with less contrast than fluorescein angiographies. In addition, the time interval between choroidal arterial filling and arteriovenous transition via the choriocapillaris is much shorter than the retinal arteriovenous transition time and is almost impossible to capture with conventional angiography systems. Early applications of ICG angiography were flawed by dark, low-contrast angiograms that could not match the quality of fluorescein angiography and often missed useful images of the early phases of the angiography. This has changed dramatically since the introduction of SLO. Compared to the previously used film-based or video angiographies, amplification and modifications of the detectable fluorescence result in increasing brightness and contrast. In addition, high-speed photography (16 frames per second) allows the creation of digital angiography movie sequences. These can be used to analyze dye movement over time as well as review of every single image of the movie for a detailed analysis. Together with a higher image resolution and the reduction in reflections during image acquisition, the quality of ICG angiography has improved dramatically over the past decade.

ICG angiograms are nowadays almost exclusively captured on computer systems and stored in databases that enable review on multiple computer workstations within IT networks. With current multimodal imaging, considerable amounts of data are generated per patient session. When purchasing new imaging equipment, one has to realize that the IT network and backup structure are as important as the imaging system itself, to enable smooth and reliable review of high-quality images now and in the future.

The sequence and variables of image acquisition for ICG angiography depend on the underlying condition, the clinical question, the technical facilities, and the preferences of the reviewer. There is no standardized protocol. In order to obtain appropriate angiogram, the area of interest, the suspected diagnosis, and individual preferences regarding image acquisition should be communicated between the ophthalmologist and the medical photographer. Ideally, this is accompanied by a fundus drawing. Baseline demographic and clinical data are entered into the database to allow appropriate identification of the imaging session and comparison with previous and future examinations. The image is focused using the infrared setting of the imaging device (**Figure 2.1**). If needed, fundus autofluorescence and near-infrared autofluorescence images should be obtained before the angiography (**Figure 2.2**). Following dye injection, the timer is started and the initial arteriovenous dye transit is documented with high-speed photography during the first 10–30 seconds (**Figures 2.3–2.7**). Additional images are taken during the first minute (**Figure 2.8**). Most institutions routinely generate a movie sequence of the early transition phase. The venous and recirculation phases are documented with additional images at 5 and 10 minutes (**Figures 2.9–2.10**). Some specialists also perform late images, taken at 20 and 30 minutes, on a routine basis (**Figures 2.11–2.12**). In contrast to fluorescein angiography, the brightness of fluorescence shows greater variations during ICG angiography. The photographer commonly adjusts the camera settings during the angiography to obtain optimal results. This can cause variations in the intensity of the recorded fluorescence phenomena and has to be acknowledged when interpreting the results.

The size of the documented fundus area is determined by the choice of lens and varies with the clinical question. Most commonly, the three standard magnifications that are used for conventional fundus photography and fluorescein angiography are available. Setups vary with the cameras used, but usually consist of a 18–20° image (high magnification, detailed examination of the macula or optic nerve head), 30–35° (the posterior pole in between the vascular arcades) and 50–55° settings (the posterior pole with the macula, optic nerve head, and major vascular arcades). As a general rule, ICG

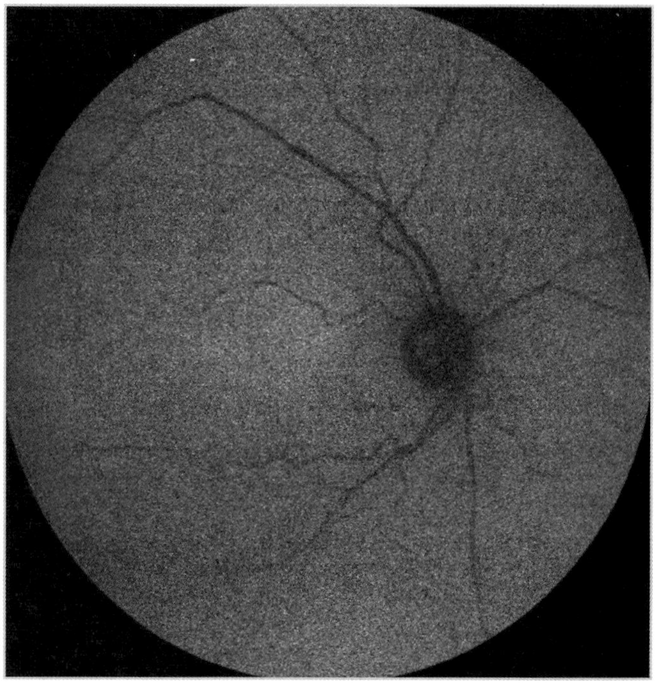

Figure 2.2 Normal near-infrared autofluorescence. In contrast to the autofluorescence images that are taken with the filters used for fluorescein angiography, the near-infrared autofluorescence is performed using the filter setting for indocyanine green (ICG) angiography. The main pigment depicted is melanin. The highest concentration is seen in the fovea, with decreasing intensity toward the periphery. The optic disc and retinal vessels show no autofluorescence. Near-infrared autofluorescence is performed before ICG angiography to identify areas of autofluorescence and pseudo-autofluorescence.

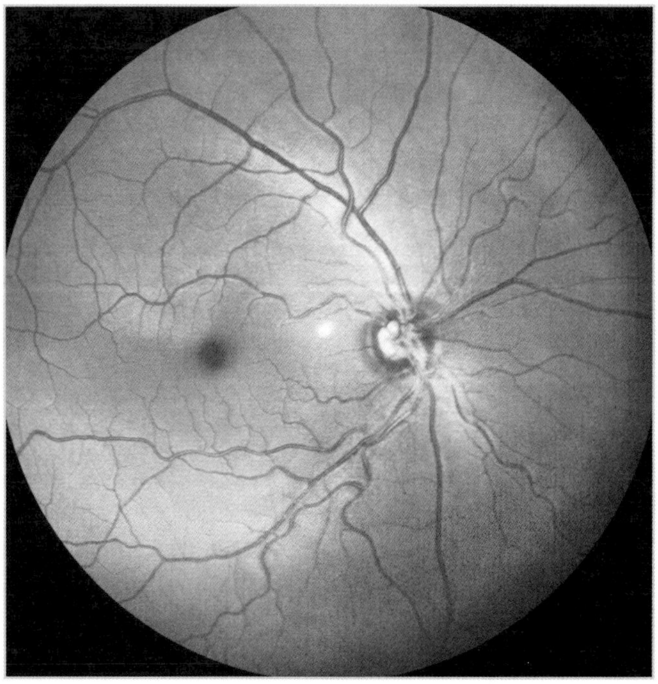

Figure 2.1 Near-infrared photography. This is a normal posterior pole image taken with the near-infrared photography setting of the scanning laser ophthalmoscope. This setting is used to focus the image and document a red-free fundus image for comparison with the images of the indocyanine green angiography.

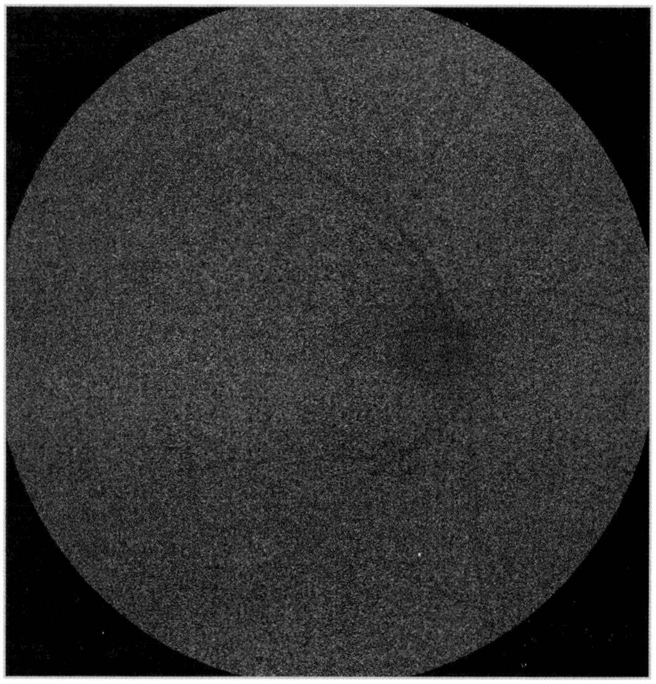

Figure 2.3 Normal indocyanine green (ICG) angiography (13 seconds; arterial phase). On a single image, the filling of the posterior ciliary arteries can only be guessed as a fuzzy fluorescence at the posterior pole around the macula. It is better appreciated on a movie sequence. The retinal arteries have not filled with ICG.

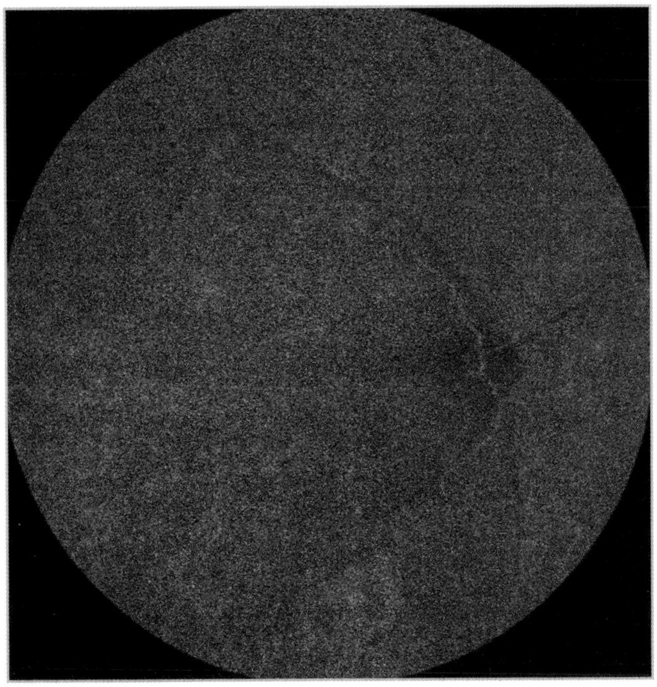

Figure 2.4 Normal indocyanine green angiography (20 seconds; early arteriovenous phase). The fluorescence is spreading radially in a lacelike pattern, filling the choroidal arterioles. The dye appears in the retinal arteries

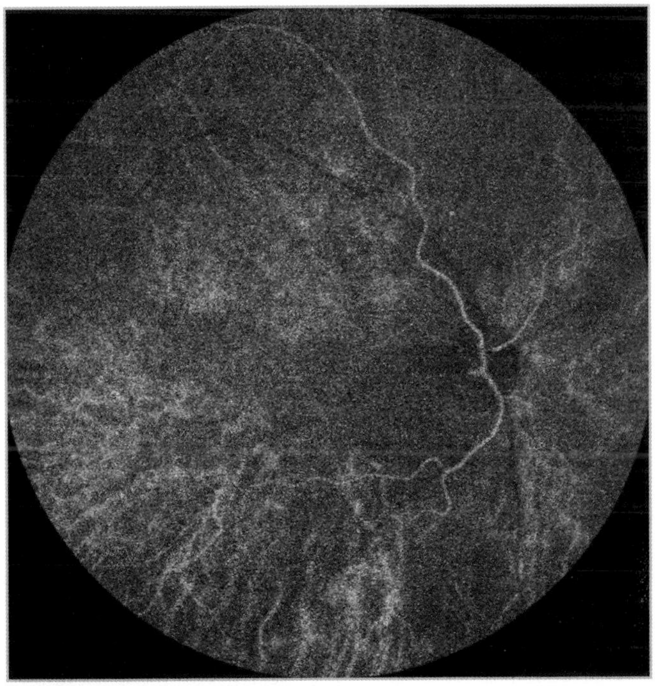

Figure 2.5 Normal indocyanine green angiography (21 seconds; arteriovenous phase). The dye has filled the choroidal arterioles and is entering the choroidal venules. Filling of the choriocapillaris is difficult to document on single frames but can seen on movie captures of the early phase.

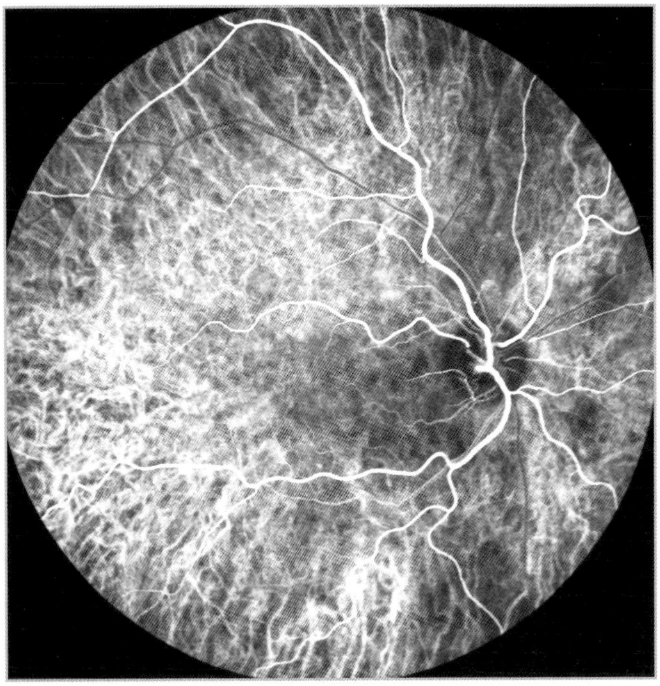

Figure 2.6 Normal indocyanine green (ICG) angiography (25 seconds; late arteriovenous phase). The choroidal venules are filling. There can be a blooming effect—the strong hyperfluorescence may obscure fundus details. A laminar flow of ICG can be detected in the retinal veins.

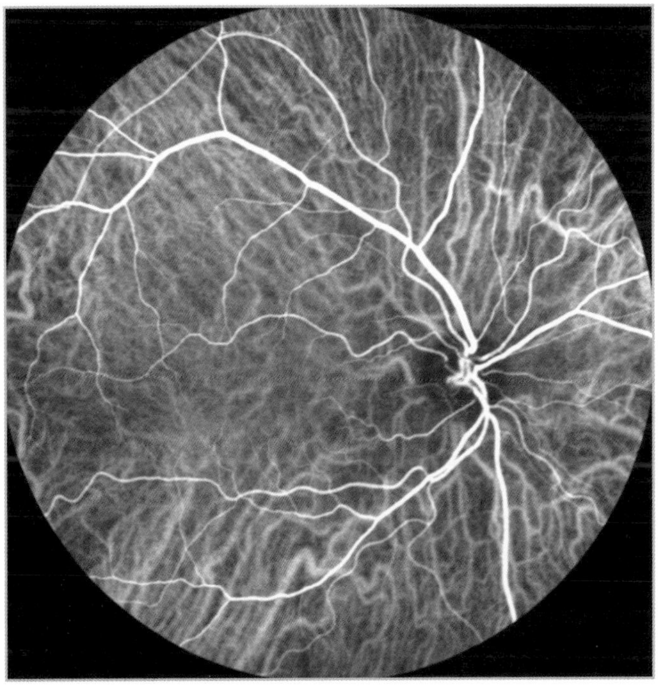

Figure 2.7 Normal indocyanine green (ICG) angiography (40 seconds; venous phase). The large choroidal venules are now filled with dye, draining toward the vortex veins. There is isofluorescence of ICG in retinal arteries and veins.

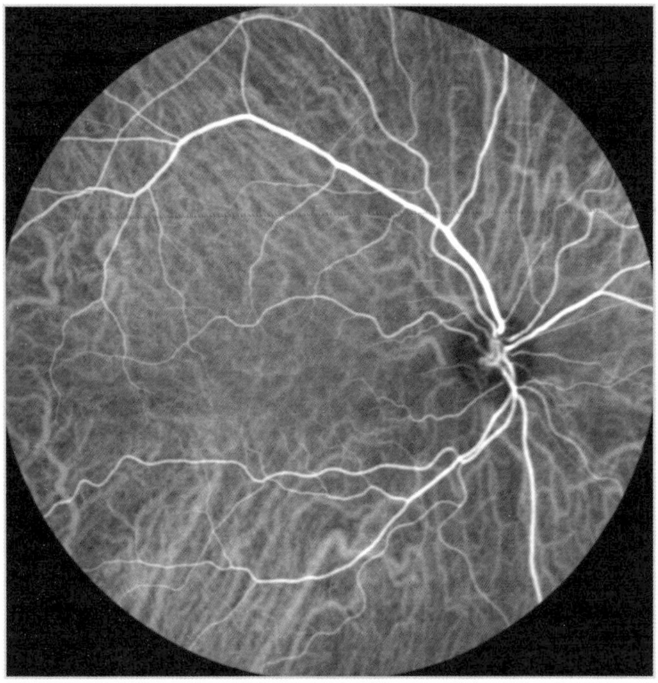

Figure 2.8 Normal indocyanine green angiography (1 minute; venous phase). There is a slight decrease in the fluorescence of the choroidal veins and less fluorescence in retinal arteries compared to retinal veins.

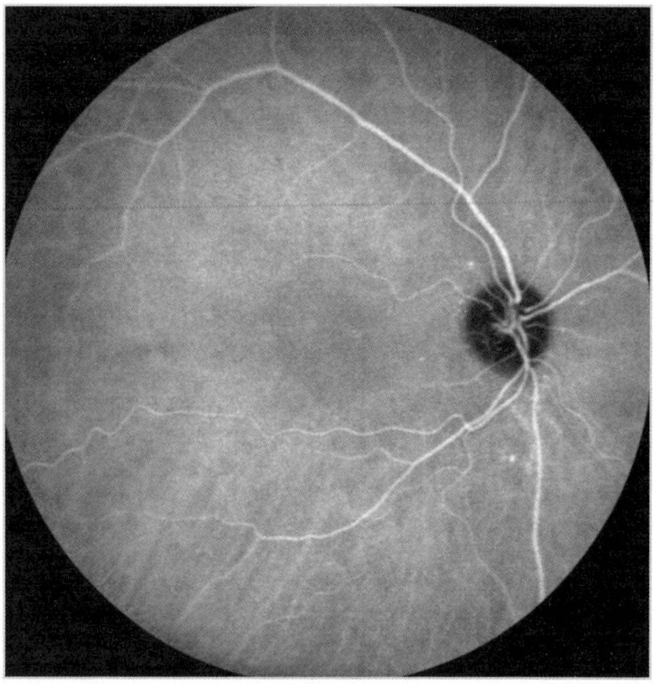

Figure 2.10 Normal indocyanine green (ICG) angiography (10 minutes). There is increasing background fluorescence, caused by extravasated ICG within the choroid. Intravascular ICG is still visible in the choroidal and retinal vasculature.

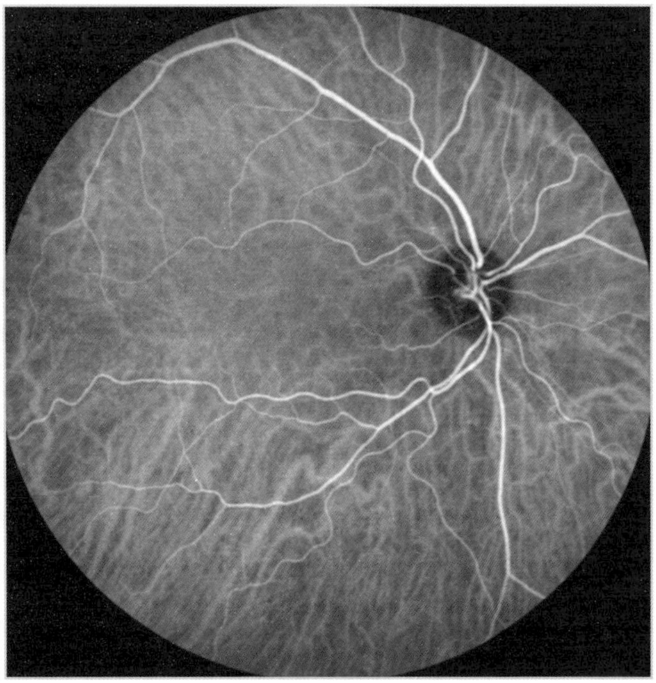

Figure 2.9 Normal indocyanine green angiography (5 minutes; venous phase). The choroidal veins, retinal arteries, and veins are still filled with dye. There is an overall decrease in the amount of fluorescence.

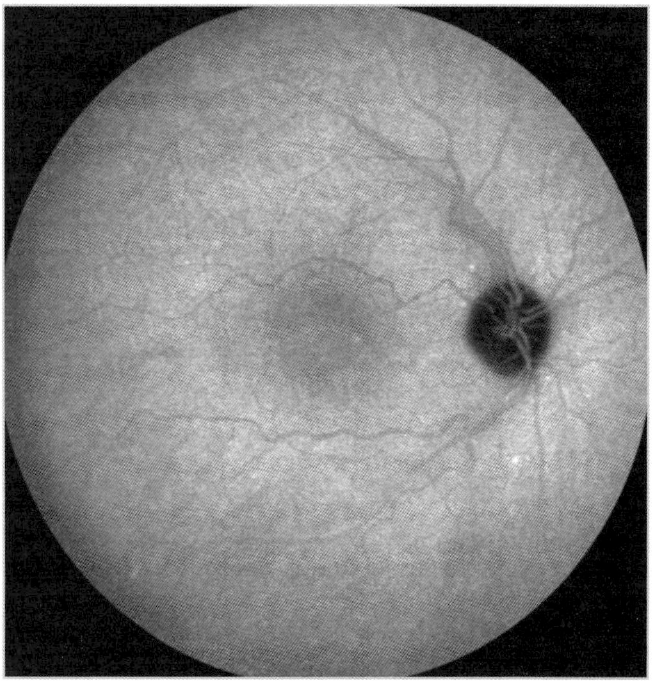

Figure 2.11 Normal indocyanine green (ICG) angiography (20 minutes). There is a decrease in background fluorescence. The choroidal vessels are outlined as shadows against the background fluorescence. A decrease in fluorescence of the retinal vessels is seen.

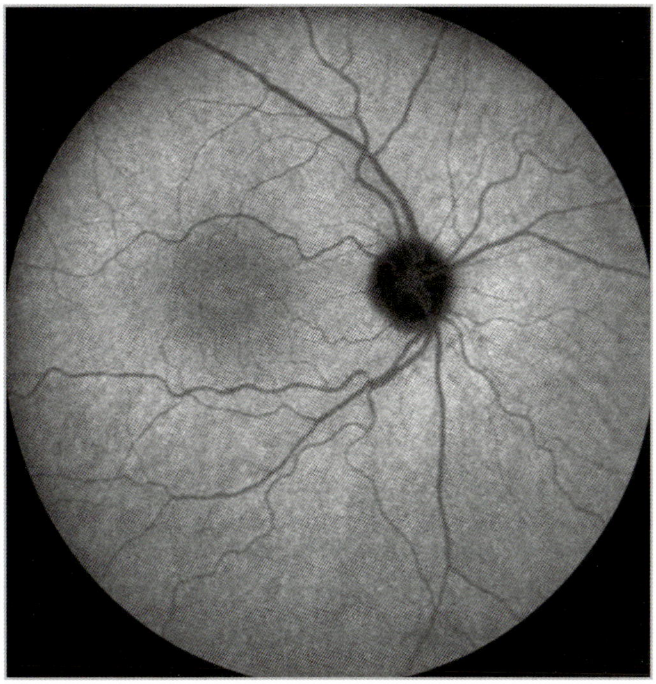

Figure 2.12 Normal indocyanine green angiography (30 minutes). There is a decrease in background fluorescence. The shadows of the choroidal vessels are still visible.

Figure 2.13 Indocyanine green angiography (early arterial phase). Radial filling of choroidal arteries is seen, beginning from the posterior pole and demarcating the watershed distribution between the medial and lateral choroidal vessels.

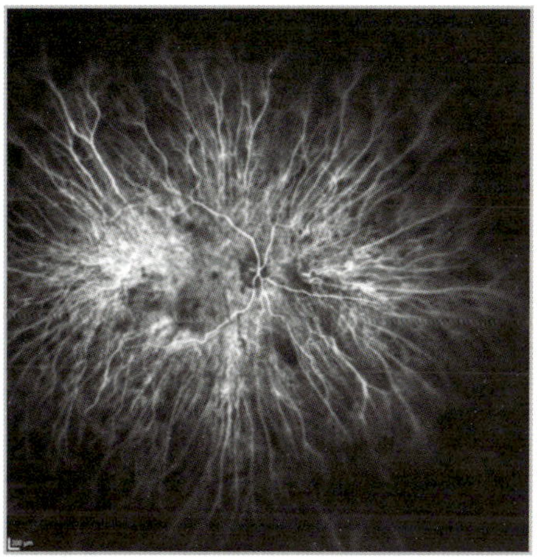

Figure 2.14 Indocyanine green angiography (arteriovenous phase). There is filling of choroidal arteries and veins. Areas of hypofluorescent spots are seen as an early indication of choroidal lesions.

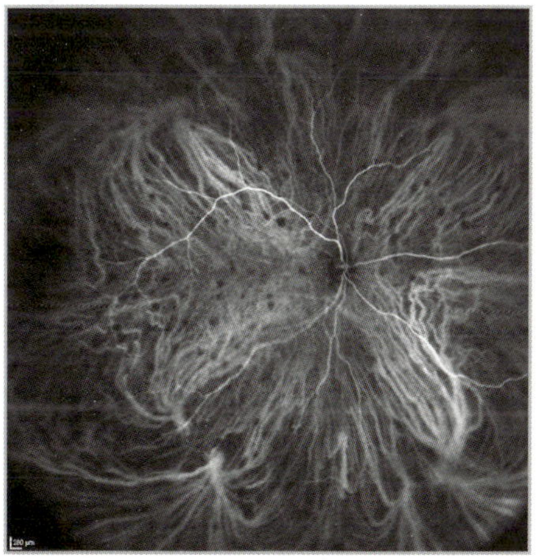

Figure 2.15 Indocyanine green angiography (venous phase). The choroidal veins are filled. The drainage to vortex veins in the mid-periphery of the fundus quadrants is clearly visible. Multiple hypofluorescent spots over the entire posterior pole are indicators of the choroidal pathology.

angiography is used more commonly to examine larger areas of the fundus than with fluorescein angiography. For example, polypoidal changes or choroidal filling defects are often located eccentrically or nasal to the optic disc. Our standard setting for ICG angiography is 55° compared with the most commonly used 30° for fluorescein angiography (**Figures 2.2–2.12**). Pseudo-stereo images are taken by varying the angle of the fundus camera in sequential images. Most imaging devices have a software and hardware option to generate, archive and review stereo images. The stereo effect is usually better with higher magnifications (30–35° images). An interesting option is to create a pseudo-stereo movie. By moving the angle of the camera during a movie capture of the venous phase of the ICG angiography, a pseudo-stereo effect is generated that can be appreciated during the review of the movie sequence.

An exciting new possibility is wide-angle ICG angiography. There are currently three ways to obtain such images. An increasing number of SLO-based imaging systems provide a montage software option that will stitch several images together to generate a wide-angle image. A 'true' wide-angle ICG angiogram over 150° can be performed using a contact lens (**Figures 2.13–2.17**). Finally, new lens optics are now available to provide ultra-wide ICG angiography with noncontact systems (**Figure 2.19**).

RECOGNIZING NORMAL RESULTS

ICG angiography is most commonly interpreted by dividing it into various phases (**Figures 2.2–2.12**). Following the conventional approach to interpretation of fluorescein angiographies, ICG angiography is separated into an early phase ('arterial phase,' from the first appearance of the dye in the ophthalmic circulation to arteriovenous transit, usually within 20 seconds), a mid phase ('venous phase,' between 20 seconds and 3 minutes), and a late phase ('recirculation phase,' 5–30 minutes). With the improvements in high-speed image capturing, the early phase can be subdivided into an arterial phase and an arteriovenous transit phase (Mori et al. 2008). This happens within few seconds following the initial appearance of the dye. Assessment of the early arteriovenous transit phase requires high-speed photography capabilities of modern imaging systems. Dynamic movies can be created and replayed at slower tempi. This enables the reviewer to assess the

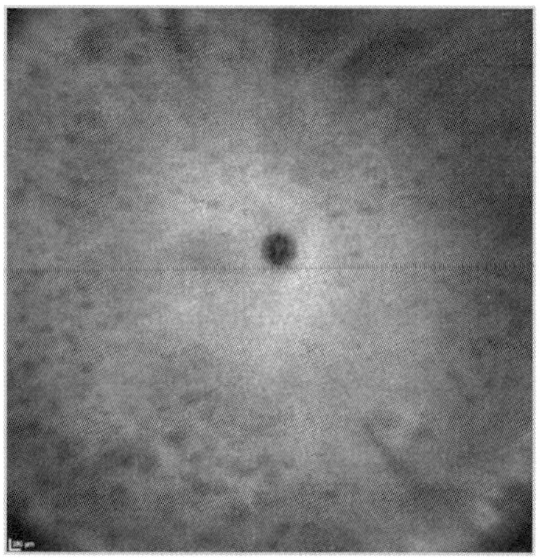

Figure 2.16 Indocyanine green (ICG) angiography (late phase). Numerous hypofluorescent spots are visible against the background fluorescence. There are significantly more spots identifiable than in the previous arteriovenous and venous phase. The ICG angiogram identifies the widespread choroidal pathology associated with the disease.

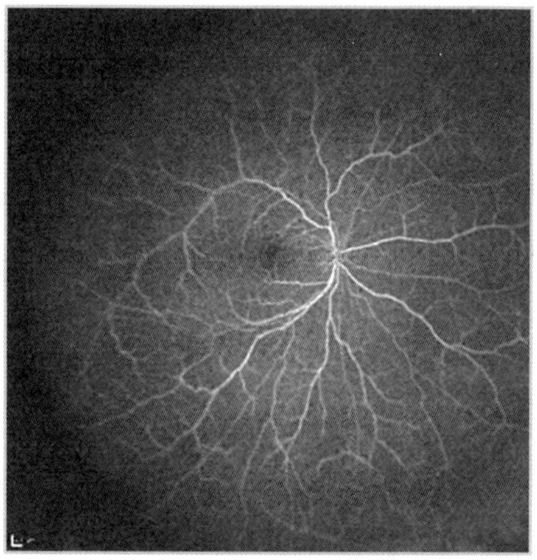

Figure 2.17 Fluorescein angiography (arteriovenous phase). In contrast to indocyanine green angiography, the choroidal lesions do not show up in fluorescein angiography. (Figures 2.13–2.17 patient with birdshot chorioretinopathy).

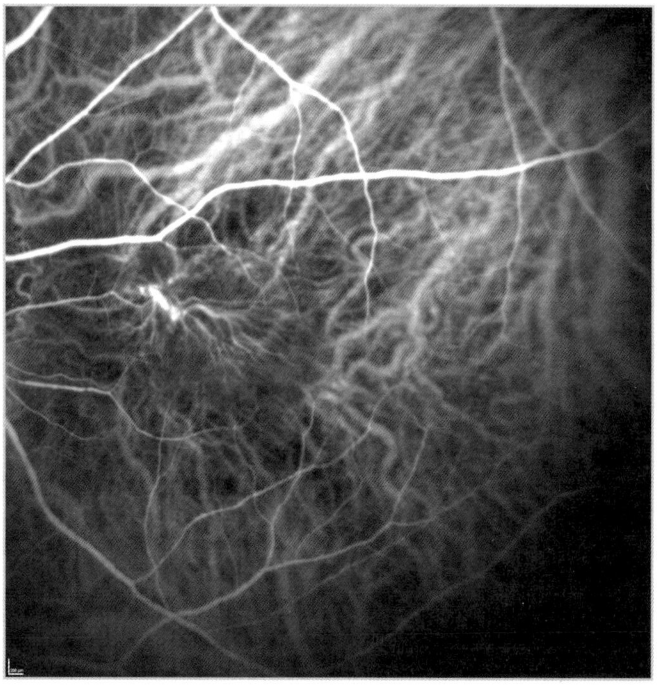

Figure 2.18 Indocyanine green (ICG) angiography (venous phase). This high-magnification view demonstrates the clear outline of the choroidal neovascularization and the feeder vessel at the posterior pole in a patient with age-related macular degeneration and occult choroidal neovascularisation.

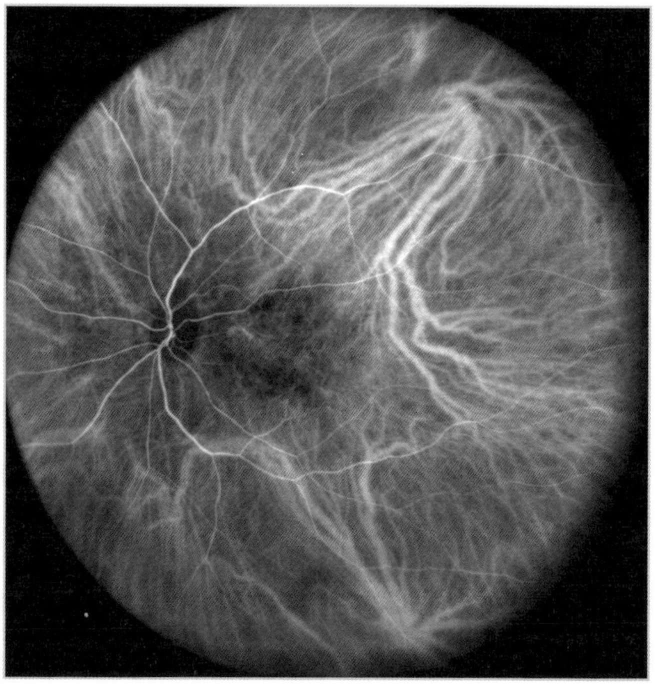

Figure 2.19 Indocyanine green (ICG) angiography (venous phase) using a new ultra-wide angiography with a noncontact lens. The neovascularization at the posterior pole as well as the vortex veins are visible (same patient as Figure 2.18).

early phase in greater detail, down to a frame-by-frame analysis. One of the difficulties of ICG angiography interpretation is that the three different vascular layers of the choroid (choriocapillaris, Sattler's and Haller´s layer) are superimposed on a two-dimensional image. Even with stereo angiography, the layers cannot be reliably separated in the majority of patients.

Before interpretation of the angiogram, preinjection images should be reviewed for signs of autofluorescence and pseudofluorescence. These can be caused by old hemorrhages, lipofuscin-like deposits, pigmented membranes, and long-lasting serous detachments (Piccolino et al. 1996). Artifacts can be caused by the blooming effect (increased fluorescence that obscures parts of the image during the initial filling of the choroidal vasculature). Increased fluorescence in the area of the crossing of blood vessels may be mistaken for hyperfluorescence and leakage.

After 12–15 seconds, ICG dye enters the choroidal circulation via the short posterior ciliary arteries. It can first be detected in the perimacular area, where it fills the posterior arterioles in a radial fashion toward the periphery. Corresponding to the variation in the diversion of the posterior ciliary arteries, watershed zones may be recognizable at this stage (Mori et al. 2008) (**Figure 2.13**). Filling of the choriocapillaris is difficult to detect. It most commonly appears as a 'haze' covering the previously filled arterioles. Shortly after the dye appears in the posterior ciliary arteries, ICG can be detected in the retinal circulation. The radial extension of retinal filling, arteriovenous transition, and laminar filling of retinal venules and veins corresponds to fluorescein angiography. After 15-20 seconds, the draining choroidal venules begin to fill with ICG. They appear larger than the arterioles. Typically, the venules and veins drain into four to six vortex veins. The intravascular amount of ICG fluorescence then decreases steadily during the mid phase due to extravasation, dilution, and clearance of the dye, resulting in lower contrast images between 5 and 10 minutes. During the late phase, the silhouettes of the hypofluorescent choroidal vessels can be observed against the hyperfluorescent extravascular space. At 20–30 minutes, an isofluroescent state (homogenous fluorescence) is reached. The optic disc remains hypofluorescent throughout the angiography.

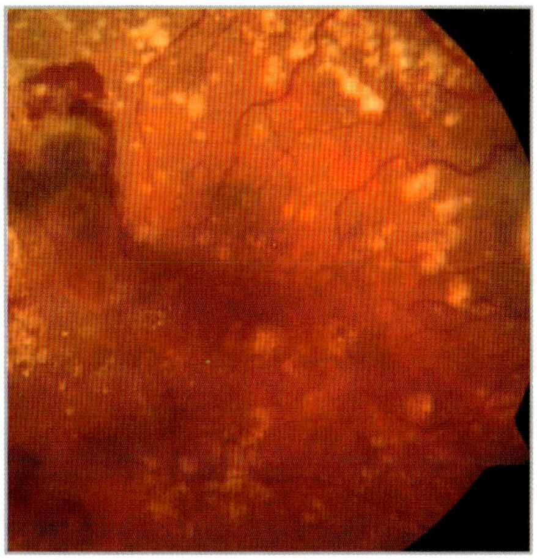

Figure 2.20 The right eye shows eccentric hemorrhages, pigment epithelial detachment and drusen at the posterior pole. (Figures 2.20–2.22 are from a patient with polypoidal choroidal vasculopathy).

INTERPRETING ABNORMAL SIGNS

The interpretation of ICG angiography is challenging even for experts in the field. Knowledge about pathological findings in various conditions is, compared with fluorescein angiography, still relatively limited, and there are much greater variations in the interpretation of results. However, due to improving imaging technology and more widespread use, knowledge of and clinical meaning of the test results are rapidly expanding.

When interpreting results of ICG angiography, it is advisable to interpret them in the context of the ophthalmologic history, the clinical picture, the OCT scan, and the fluorescein angiography to obtain as much information as possible about potential pathological changes. The interpretation of ICG angiograms begins with the identification of areas with an abnormally high (hyperfluorescence) or low (hypofluorescence) concentration of dye (**Figures 2.13–2.16**). In a second step, the anatomical location of these findings has to be identified. Finally, changes over the phases of the angiogram have to be assessed. Hyper- and hypofluorescence may increase or decrease in intensity or may change from hyper- to hypofluorescence and vice versa. An additional important step in ICG interpretation is review of early movie sequences to assess the dynamics of the occurring changes. Overall, the most important phase for interpretation of the angiogram is the mid or venous phase between 30 seconds and 3 minutes.

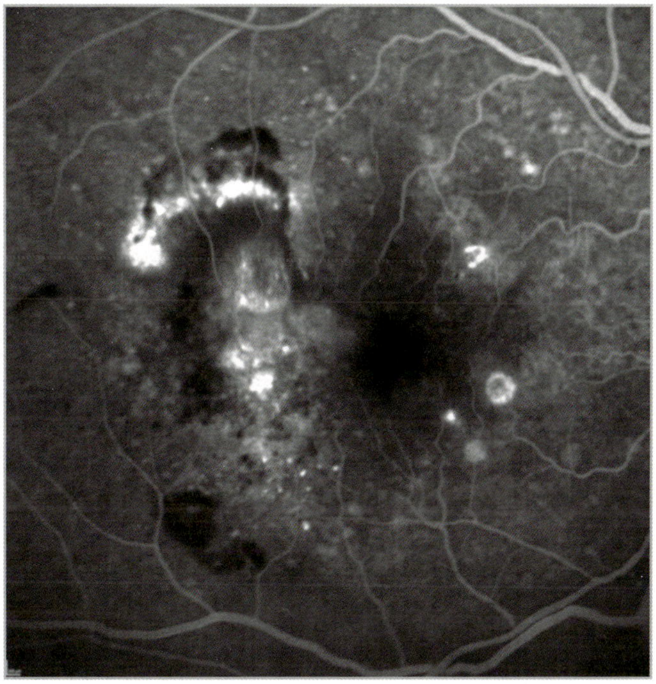

Figure 2.21 Fluorescein angiography. There is late leakage in the area of the fibrovascular pigment epithelial detachment, diffusely distributed over the posterior pole.

Compared with fluorescein angiography, hypofluorescent phenomena are less commonly observed and less pronounced. They are caused by blocked fluorescence (pigment, blood, exudations) or vascular filling defects. Because there is less blockage by blood or exudations in ICG angiography, hyperfluorescent spots underlying the blockage from neovascularizations or other pathology can often be visualized (**Figure 2.20–2.22**). Another unique feature of ICG angiography is the identification of hypofluorescent areas in the choroid that frequently cannot be detected on fluorescein angiography. This is used to identify areas of choroidal inflammation in the field of uveitis (**Figures 2.13–2.17**). Hyperfluorescence can be caused by abnormal retinal or choroidal vessels, leakage of dye, or an increased visibility through window defects. Compared to fluorescein, there is less leakage of ICG at sites of neovascularization. This facilitates the detection of vascular changes that may be missed on fluorescein angiography due to a 'smoke screen' effect from the leaking fluorescein.

At present, ICG angiography is most commonly used in the differential diagnosis of exudative age-related macular degeneration. It is particularly useful in identifying polypoidal choroidal vasculopathy, retinal angiomatous proliferations, and choroidal neovascularizations underneath pigment epithelial detachments. Additional indications include identification of choroidal neovascularization in ambiguous cases (high myopia, angioid streaks), central serous retinopathy, posterior uveitis, and choroidal tumors.

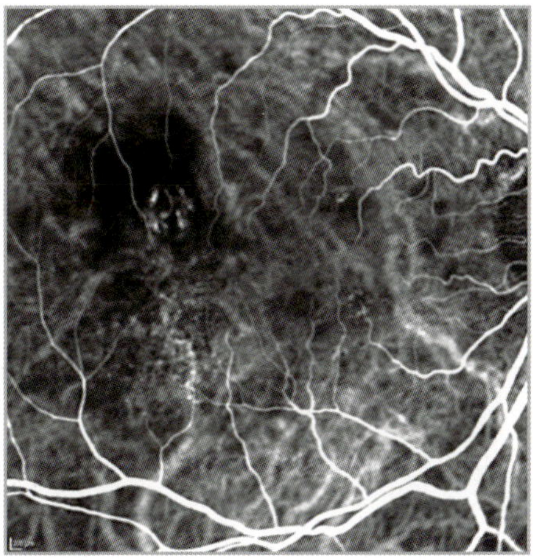

Figure 2.22 Indocyanine green (ICG) angiography reveals the underlying pathology of polypoidal choroidal vasculopathy.

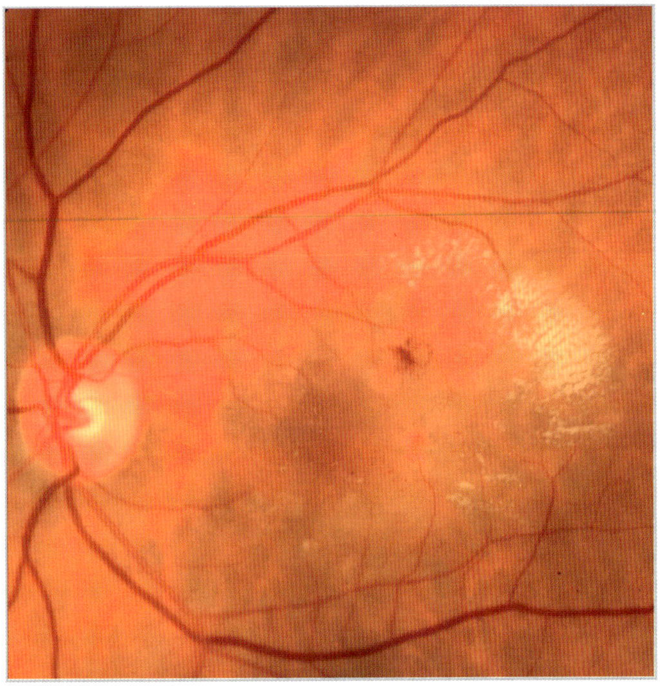

Figure 2.23 Retinal angiomatous proliferations (RAP lesions). The left eye shows eccentric hemorrhages and exudates suggestive of a possible retinal angiomatous proliferation lesion.

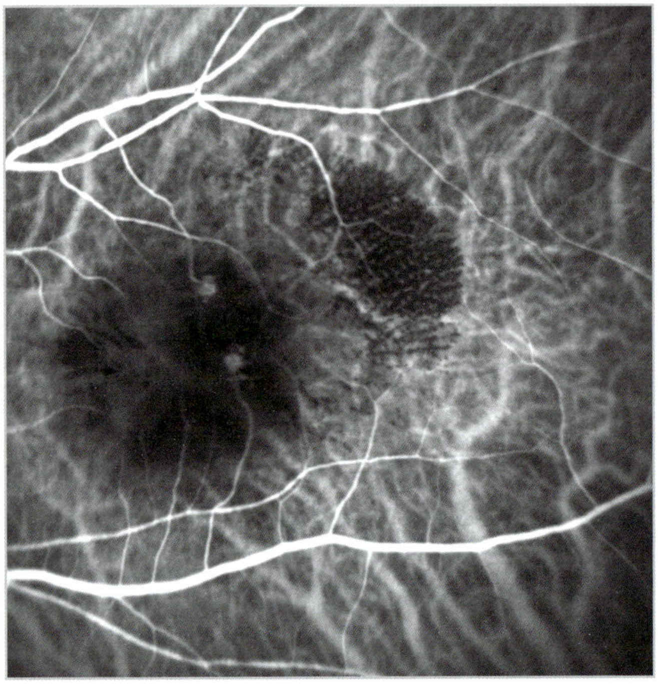

Figure 2.25 Retinal angiomatous proliferations (RAP lesions): indocyanine green (ICG) angiography. The multifocal retino-choroidal anastomosis can clearly be identified on ICG angiography.

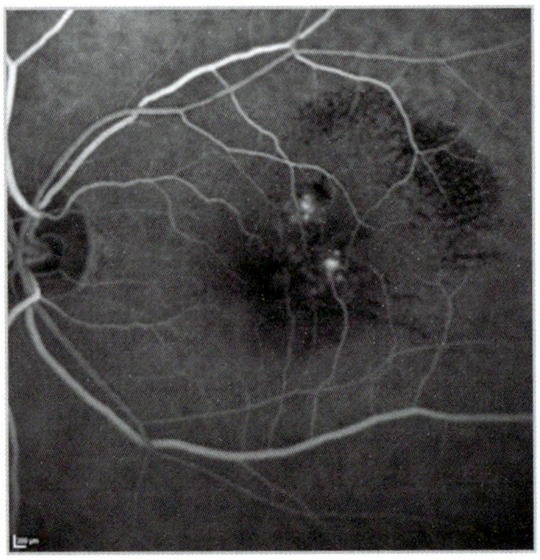

Figure 2.24 Retinal angiomatous proliferations (RAP lesions): fluorescein angiography. The late phase shows multifocal hyperfluorescent spots and late leakage.

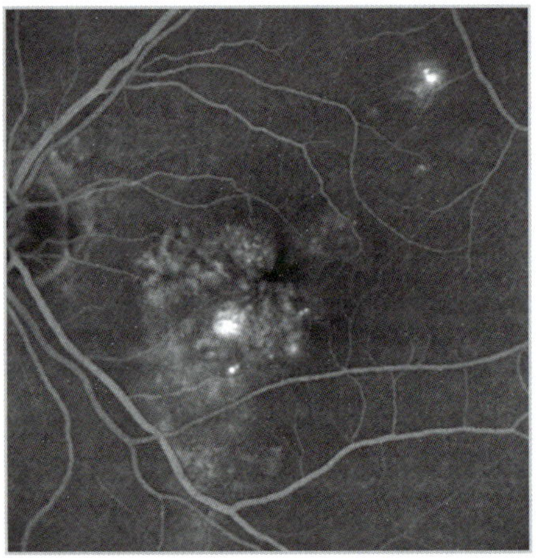

Figure 2.26 Central serous retinopathy: fluorescein angiography. There is an increase in multifocal hyperfluorescence in the actively leaking spots. Diffuse hyperfluorescence is seen in chronically damaged retinal pigment epithelium.

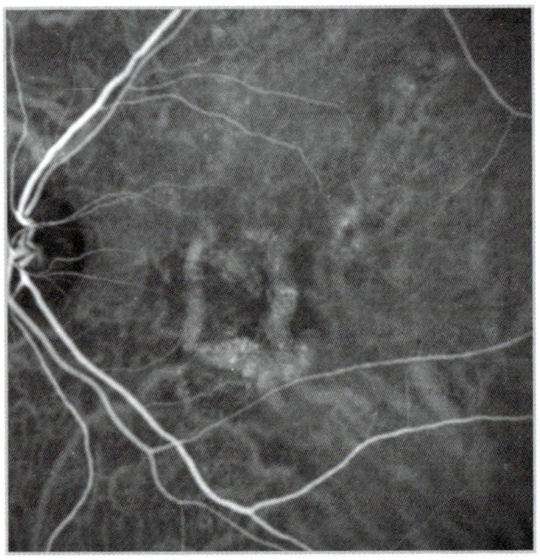

Figure 2.27 Central serous retinopathy: indocyanine green (ICG) angiography, venous phase. The actively leaking spots are surrounded by hypofluorescent choroid. There are ICG hyperfluorescent spots in the area of the active leakage as a sign of choroidal hyperpermeability underlying the defects in the retinal pigment epithelium.

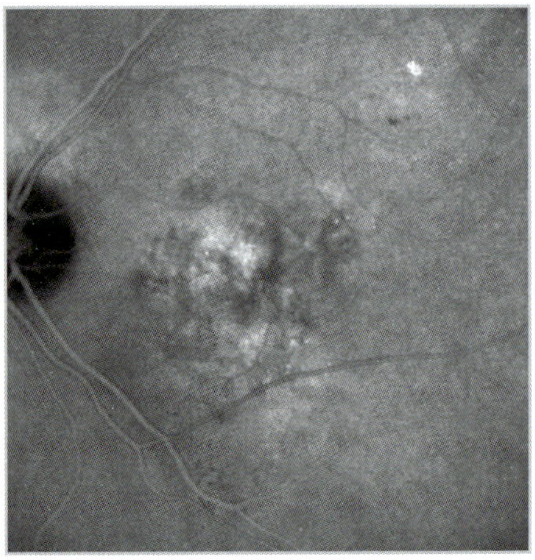

Figure 2.28 Central serous retinopathy: indocyanine green angiography (late venous phase). Diffuse hyperfluorescence surrounds the areas of active leakage and demonstrates the large areas of choroidal hyperperfusion and vascular pathology.

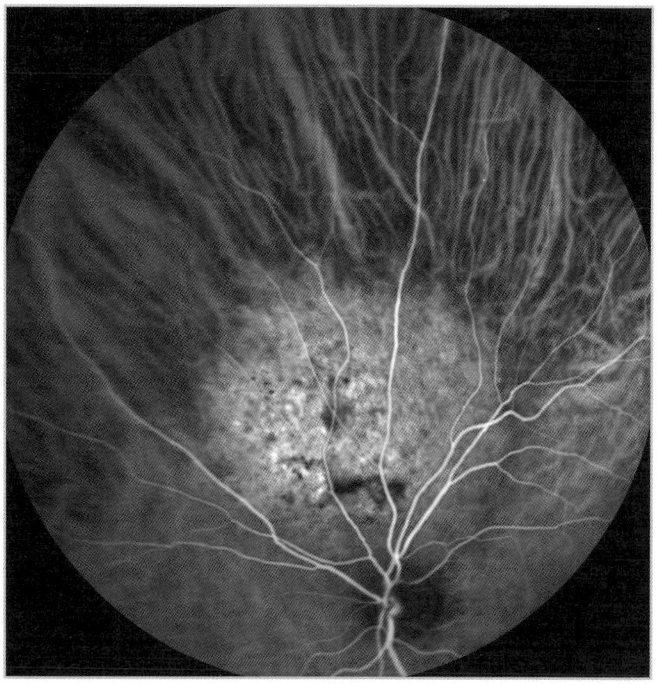

Figure 2.29 Circumscribed choroidal hemangioma, indocyanine green angiography (venous phase). Typical leakage is seen in the choroidal hemangioma during the early venous phase.

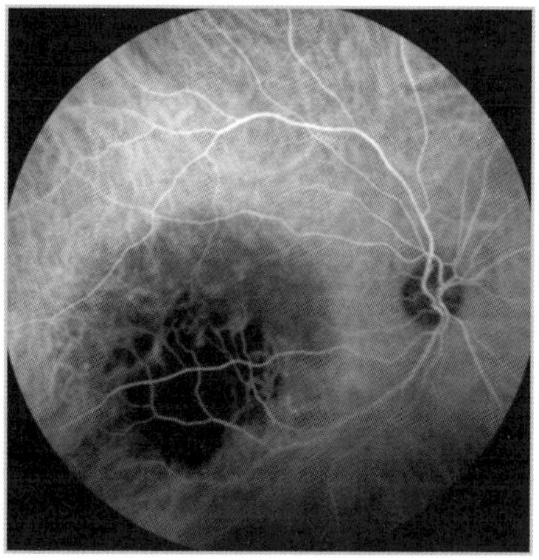

Figure 2.30 Circumscribed choroidal hemangioma after photodynamic therapy (PDT), indocyanine green (ICG) angiography (venous phase). This patient noticed a sudden visual loss 3 days following PDT for choroidal hemangioma. The ICG angiogram demonstrates a large area of hypofluorescence as an indicator of choroidal hypoperfusion corresponding to the area of PDT treatment.

REFERENCES

Chopdar A, Turk AM, Hill DW. Fluorescent infra-red angiography of the fundus oculi using indocyanine green dye. *Trans Ophthalmol Soc UK* 1978; **98**:142–146.

Flower RW, Hochheimer BF. Indocyanine green dye fluorescence and infrared absorption choroidal angiography performed simultaneously with fluorescein angiography. *Johns Hopkins Med J* 1976; **138**:33–42.

Hope-Ross M, Yannuzzi LA, Gragoudas ES, et al. Adverse reactions due to indocyanine green. *Ophthalmology* 1994; **101**:529–533.

Leys A, Horsman B (eds). Ophthalmic indocyanine green diagnostics study abstract book. Munich: PULSION Medical Systems, 2009.

Mori K, Yoneya S, Gehlbach PL. Indocyanine green angiography. In: Agrawal A (ed.), Fundus fluorescein and indocyanine green angiography. Thorofare, NJ: SLACK Incorporated, 2008:29.

Piccolino FC, Porgia L, Zinicola E, et al. Pre-injection fluorescence in indocyanine green angiography. *Ophthalmology* 1996; **103**:1837–1845.

Richard G. Choroidal circulation. New York: Thieme Medical Publishers, Inc., 1992:3–21.

Yannuzzi LA. Indocyanine green angiography: a perspective on use in the clinical setting. *Am J Ophthalmol* 2011; **151**:745–751.

Chapter 3 Optical coherence tomography for retinal diseases

Geeta Menon, Vishali Gupta

INTRODUCTION

Optical coherence tomography (OCT) was first suggested in the 1980s by James G. Fujimoto as a technology to measure zones of several structures within the body. Later David Huang processed the images created by axial scans to create a two-dimensional image in both axial and transverse directions. Further refinement in the technology led to the commercialization that has now developed into the two most common forms of scanning: the time domain and the spectral and Fourier domain OCT. The first generation of OCT technology was based on time domain OCT, while Fourier domain OCT is a more recent development.

The working principle of OCT is similar to that of ultrasound but there are two major differences. First, OCT uses light waves instead of sound waves. The speed of light being almost a million times faster than sound, OCT allows measurement of structures as small as 10 microns compared to 100 microns for ultrasound. Second, unlike ultrasound, OCT is contactless.

BASIC SCIENCE

Time domain OCT

OCT is a noncontact and noninvasive device where a broad bandwidth, near-infrared light beam composed of 820 nm is projected onto the retina. The incident light is reflected from the various boundaries between the retinal microstructures and tissues with distinct optical properties. The time delay of the light reflected from the various layers of the retina is compared with the time delay of the light reflected from a reference mirror at a known distance. The interferometer then combines the reflected pulses from the retina and the reflecting mirrors, resulting in a phenomenon known as interference. This interference is then measured by a photodetector, which determines the distance traveled by various light pulses by varying the distance to the reference mirror. This finally produces a range of time delays for comparison.

The interferometer integrates several data points over 2 mm of depth to construct a tomogram of retinal structures. It is a real-time tomogram using a false color scale. Different colors represent the grade of light backscattering from different depths of retina. The images thus produced have axial resolution of 10 microns and transverse resolution of 20 microns in time domain OCT.

Spectral domain OCT

Spectral/Fourier domain detection techniques measure the echo time delay of light by measuring the spectrum of the interference between light from the tissue and light from a stationary unscanned reference arm. Light returning from the sample and reference paths is combined at the detector, which in spectral domain OCT is a spectrometer. The spectrometer resolves the interference signals throughout the depth of each A-scan immediately by means of a Fourier transformation. It is possible because the spectrometer resolves the relative amplitudes and phases of the spectral components scattered back from all depths of each A-scan tissue sample, without varying the length of the reference path. Thus, eliminating the necessity of moving a mechanical reference arm makes it possible to acquire OCT images data about 70 times faster than conventional time domain OCT. The vast increase in scan speed makes it possible for the Cirrus HD OCT to acquire three-dimensional data sets, or entire cubes of data in about the same time (depending on the selected scan type) as conventional OCT (Gupta et al. 2012).

Technique in performing OCT

The OCT scans can be performed through an undilated pupil, though it is advisable to dilate the pupils for better quality scans. The Cirrus HD OCT by Carl Zeiss is one of the commercially available spectral domain OCTs, which provides internal fixation that is easy for the patient to use. A patient with poor visual acuity may use the external fixation device. For a new patient, the data entry is made before starting; for repeat patients, past records may be retrieved by searching the database. The patient is seated comfortably with his chin on the chinrest and is asked to look into the imaging aperture where he sees a green star-shaped target against a black background. When scanning begins, the background changes to bright flickering red. The patient must be instructed to look at the center of the green target throughout the scan acquisition period. The acquisition protocols are fairly standardized to obtain high-resolution line scans as well as acquire data in the macular cube so as to allow quantification. The scanning protocols may vary from machine to machine.

ANALYSIS AND INTERPRETATION

The screen enables anatomical structures to be viewed and depicted in the scan images. There are two types of analyses: objective analysis and image analysis.

Objective analysis

We are familiar with the interpretation of fluorescein angiograms where fluorescence is defined as hypo- or hyperfluorescent, and in ultrasound B scans the images are referred to as hypo- or hyperechoic. Likewise in OCT scans, we describe the reflectivity pattern of the scanned images. The best way to do this is to select the scan group, select the appropriate analysis protocol, and go to 'scan selection.' This gives a magnified view of the selected image for objective assessment. One can modify the image before studying it. In the image, one can make anatomic correlation, e.g. identify pigment epithelial detachment, and study the reflectivity patterns.

The following lesions show hyperreflective characteristics:

- Hard exudates – The hard exudates are seen as hyperreflective shadows in the neurosensory retina that completely block the reflections from the underlying retina.
- Blood – Blood causes increased scattering. In cases of small and thin hemorrhages, hyperreflectivity is seen whereas a thicker hemorrhage might block the reflections from the underlying structures.
- Scars – All the fibrotic lesions including disciform scars, choroidal rupture scars, and healed choroiditis are hyper-reflective.

The following lesions are hyporeflective:

- Serous fluid – Retinal edema is the commonest cause of reduced backscattering and one can actually pinpoint the site of fluid accumulation. The serous fluid devoid of any particulate matter produces an optically empty space with no backscattering.
- Hypopigmented lesions of retinal pigment epithelium (RPE)–Poor quality scans due to opaque media and refractive errors might be falsely interpreted as hyporeflective. However, hyporeflectivity in these situations is diffused resulting in an overall attenuation of the scan

Image analysis

The software offers the option of both qualitative and quantitative estimation protocols. To analyze the scan, one has to (a) select a patient, (b) select a scan group, (c) select an analysis protocol, and (d) then click analyze or scan selection. On selecting a protocol, the analysis can be performed immediately by clicking the analyze button or double clicking the protocol button. There are several quantitative analytic protocols for the retina, as follows.

Retinal thickness analysis, single eye

This scan group and the output graph depict retinal thickness with a black line. When the scroll bar is traced on the fundus image, the corresponding thickness at that A-scan location appears on the graph. The use of callipers gives the reading in microns. This protocol, when applied to the 'fast macular thickness scan,' shows the normative data color coded in each A-scan location. The normative database is applicable to the fast macular thickness map scan protocol. Normative data are age matched to the patient. Normative data appear only for patients over 18 years of age and whose records include their date of birth. The data use a different color range including light red-light yellow-green-yellow-red, indicating the normal distribution percentiles.

Retinal map, single eye

This protocol obtains two maps of retinal thicknesses: one showing the color code and the other giving numerical values in nine map sectors. The diameter of the map by default is adjusted to 1, 3, or 6 mm centered on the macula. Clicking on the 3.5 mm radial button changes the circle diameters of 1, 2.2, and 3.5 mm. This protocol, when applied to a fast macular thickness scan, shows the normative data color code in each A-scan location.

Retinal thickness and volume

This displays both the thickness and the volume for each eye, showing both eyes scan groups with radial lines or macular thickness map protocols. The upper maps show color-coded retinal thickness and lower maps show either average retinal thickness in microns or the volume in mm^3. On the lower right, the average foveal thickness (in microns +/– standard deviation for the center point) and the total macular volume in mm^3 are displayed.

Retinal thickness/tabular volume

This protocol, in addition to retinal thickness/volume analysis, also gives a data table that displays thickness and volume quadrant average, ratios, and differences among various quadrants and between the eyes. When applied to the fast macular thickness scan also shows the normative data color code in each A-scan location.

Change in thickness

This allows a comparison of thickness in all the nine subfields between different visits. In spectral domain OCT, the high-definition image analyses for 5-line raster scan analysis allow morphological study of the retinal layers (**Figure 3.1**).

Advanced interactive analysis presents an interactive multiplanar reformat (MPR) that enables a three-dimensional cross-sectional view. MPR allows the visualization of retinal layers at different depths by taking a transverse C-scan. Because of the curvature of the eye, various retinal layers would be arranged inside out, with the inner and outer retinal layers visible like onion rings (**Figure 3.2**). At the level of the ganglion and inner plexiform layers, the retinal vessels are easily recognized. They initially appear white in the more superficial layer and darker when OCT C-scans are taken at deeper layers of the retina (**Figure 3.3**). Three-dimensional maps allow better visualization of the vitreoretinal interface (**Figure 3.4**).

Quantitative data

Quantitative data are acquired by the inbuilt software that gives the central retinal thickness in nine subfields (**Figures 3.5** and **3.6**). In clinical practice, it is a combination of qualitative and quantitative analysis protocols that provide the useful information.

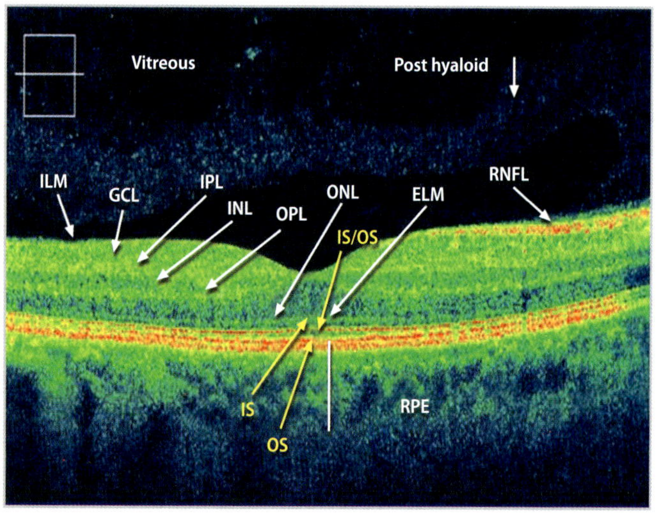

Figure 3.1 Normal raster line scan showing the different retinal layers. RPE, retinal pigment epithelium; IS, inner segment of photoreceptors; OS, outer segment of photoreceptors; ELM, external limiting membrane; IS/OS, inner and outer photoreceptor junction; ONL, outer nuclear layer; OPL, outer plexiform layer; INL, inner nuclear layer; IPL, inner plexiform layer; GCL, ganglion cell layer; ILM, inner limiting membrane; RNFL, retinal nerve fiber layer; post hyaloid, posterior hyaloid. Reproduced with permission from Uveitis Text and Imaging. Gupta A, Gupta V, Herbort CP, Khairallah M. Jaypee Brothers Medical Publishers (P) Ltd, New Delhi, 2009 chap 10; p. 216.

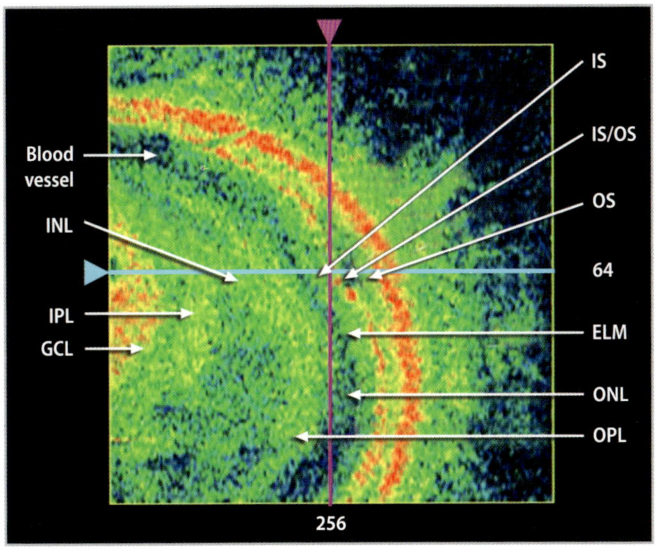

Figure 3.2 Transverse C-scan showing the different retinal layers. RPE, retinal pigment epithelium; IS, inner segment of photoreceptors; OS, outer segment of photoreceptors; ELM, external limiting membrane; IS/OS, inner and outer photoreceptor junction; ONL, outer nuclear layer; OPL, outer plexiform layer; INL, inner nuclear layer; IPL, inner plexiform layer; GCL, ganglion cell layer; ILM, inner limiting membrane; RNFL, retinal nerve fiber layer; post hyaloid, posterior hyaloids. Reproduced with permission from Uveitis Text and Imaging. Gupta A, Gupta V, Herbort CP, Khairallah M. Jaypee Brothers Medical Publishers (P) Ltd, New Delhi, 2009 chap 10; p. 216.

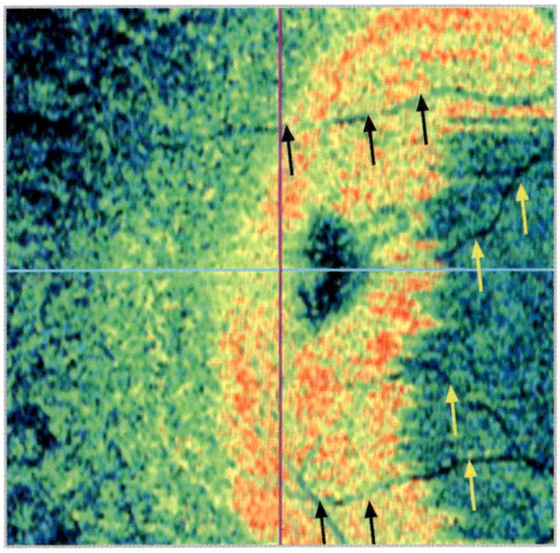

Figure 3.3 Transverse C-scan showing retinal blood vessels that appear as dark lines in the deeper layers of the retina (arrows). Reproduced with permission from Uveitis Text and Imaging. Gupta A, Gupta V, Herbort CP, Khairallah M. Jaypee Brothers Medical Publishers (P) Ltd, New Delhi, 2009 chap 10; p. 217.

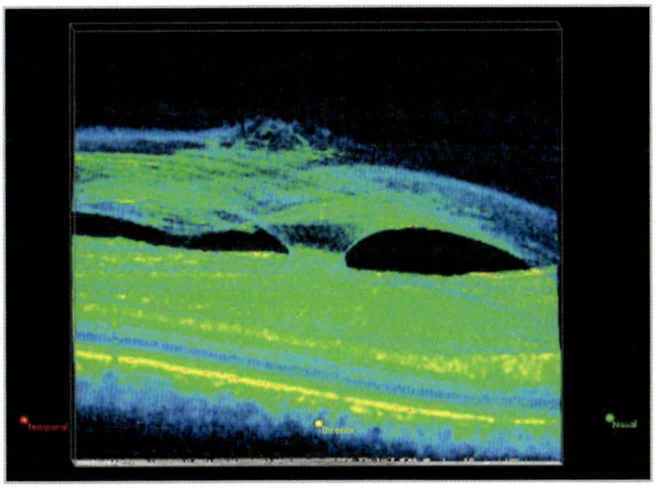

Figure 3.4 Three-dimensional optical coherence tomography of a patient with diabetic macular edema showing tractional forces on the vitreoretinal interface.

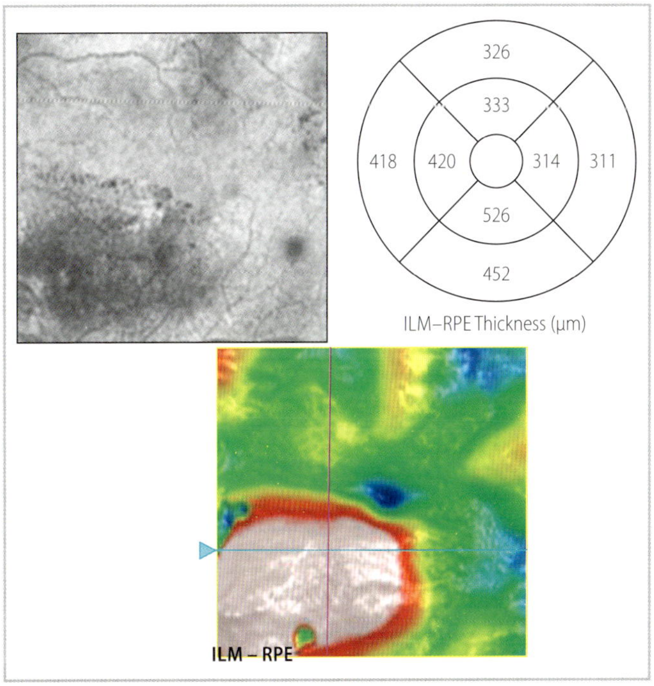

Figure 3.5 Color optical coherence tomography shows thickness of central 6 mm retina in microns in nine subfields.

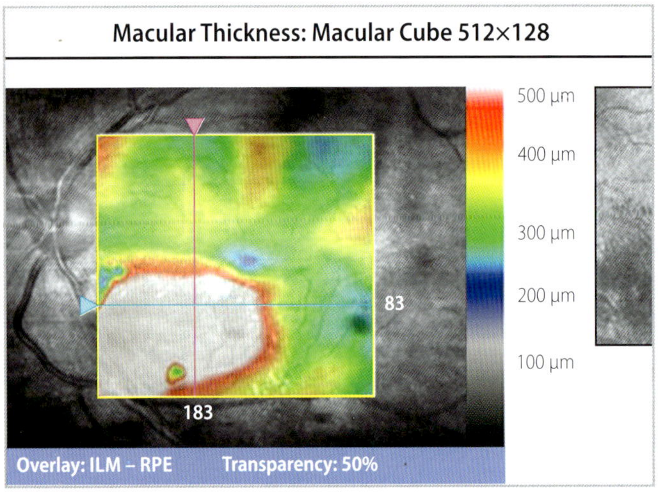

Figure 3.6 Superimposition of inner limiting membrane retinal pigment epithelium thickness map onto an optical coherence tomogram.

REFERENCE

Gupta V, Gupta A, Dogra MR. Atlas: Optical Coherence Tomography of Macular Diseases and Glaucoma. 4th Edn. Chapter 3, pp 7-9. Jaypee Brothers Medical Publishers (P) Ltd. New Delhi, India, 2012.

Chapter 4 Ocular echography

Hatem Riad Atta

TECHNIQUES

History and development

Two common methods are used to display ultrasound images. The first is A-scan (A for amplitude), and the second is B-scan (B for brightness). The introduction of ultrasound in medical diagnosis was a new field that had been greatly advantaged by the innovation of SONAR technology in the Second World War. In 1956, Mundt and Hughes were the first ophthalmologists to describe the use of A-scan in the detection of intraocular tumors. Further work on the technique of A-scan was carried out by Oksala and Lehtinen (1957). In 1965, Gernet pioneered the use of A-scan in axial eye length measurement. This investigation became the most common ultrasound application in ophthalmology, even to date, and paved the way for a more rewarding and successful experience in cataract surgery and artificial lens implantation.

Baum and Greenwood, in 1958, developed the first B-scan for ocular use, employing an immersion technique. A major advance came in 1972, when Bronson and Turner produced the first contact B-scan, rendering this examination modality easier and quicker for the operator, less invasive and more acceptable to patients (**Figure 4.1**). In the late 1960s and 1970s, Purnell (1969) and particularly Coleman with his coworkers in Cornell University (Coleman et al. 1977) produced numerous publications and undertook many refinements of B-scan instruments. Their contributions were significant in cementing the foundation of the modern ophthalmic B-scan.

In the meantime, and in parallel to the above, extensive and dedicated work on A-scan technology was undertaken by Ossoinig throughout the 1960s and 1970s (Ossoinig 1974, 1979). This resulted in the development of the standardized A-scan for ophthalmic tissue diagnosis. The combination of standardized A-scan, B-scan, and Doppler ultrasound employing well-prescribed examination methods is collectively known as standardized echography. This modality is considered, by many workers in this field, to be the most accurate and comprehensive method of ultrasound scanning for the eye and the orbit (Atta 1996, Byrne 2002).

In 1991, Pavlin et al. pioneered the application of high-frequency ultrasound (50 MHz) in anterior segment imaging. The result: astonishingly clear, near microscopic and in vivo images that hitherto it was impossible to create with the conventional 10 or 20 MHz scanners. The authors coined the term ultrasound biomicroscopy (UBM) to emphasize the highly magnified images that are similar to optical biomicroscopy. This technique increased the scope of indications of ultrasound to encompass those for anterior segment disorders including the diagnosis of (anatomical) types of glaucoma, iris and ciliary body masses, corneal and limbal abnormalities, and pars plana lesions.

Recent advances in transducer technology, image capture, and processing have resulted in a vast improvement in the quality of echograms. Other welcome facilities include image freeze frame, electronic measuring gates, video display, and digital storage. All these modern features have helped speed up the ultrasound examination and brought practical, safe, and cost-effective investigation into the day-to-day running of ophthalmic practices.

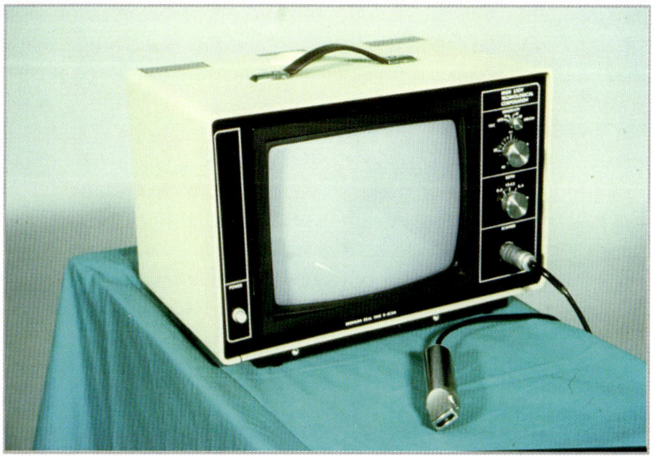

Figure 4.1 First contact B-scan, developed by Bronson and Turner in 1972.

Physics and principles of ultrasound

In this section, the physics and basic principles of diagnostic ultrasound will be discussed, not comprehensively, but in reference to the needs of the ophthalmic echographer. The workings of the instruments, conduction of examinations, and production of the most accurate results are discussed. Further details of the physics and instrumentation of diagnostic medical ultrasound can be found elsewhere (Lerski 1988, Fish 1990).

Ultrasound is acoustic wave energy with a frequency beyond the audible limit for a human (i.e. 20 KHz). In medical diagnosis, ultrasound frequencies range from 2 to 5 MHz for large and deep structures, e.g. abdominal organs, 10-20 MHz for conventional ultrasound of the eye and orbit and 50 MHz for high-frequency ultrasound (UBM) of the anterior eye segment. Similar to other wave forms, ultrasound waves follow the principle of the higher the frequency the less the penetration. Also, similar to light waves, ultrasound waves behave in a predictable pattern of reflection, refraction, and scatter when passing through the acoustic interface between tissues of different acoustic impedances. A portion of the ultrasound waves are not used for imaging as they are absorbed and converted into heat. The portion of the ultrasound waves that return from tissues back to the transducer are called echoes that are captured and displayed as an image. **Figure 4.2** is a flow chart showing the fate of ultrasound as it propagates through tissues.

The basic components of any diagnostic ultrasound instrument are diagrammatically displayed in **Figure 4.3**. These include the pulser that emits repeated pulses of electric energy that, in turn, generate pulses of returning echoes (pulse echo system). Essential components in all of the ultrasound instruments are the piezoelectric crystals at the tip of the transducer (probe). These naturally occurring materials, such as quartz, exhibit the unique property of transforming electrical energy into sound energy and vice versa, the piezoelectric effect. As the

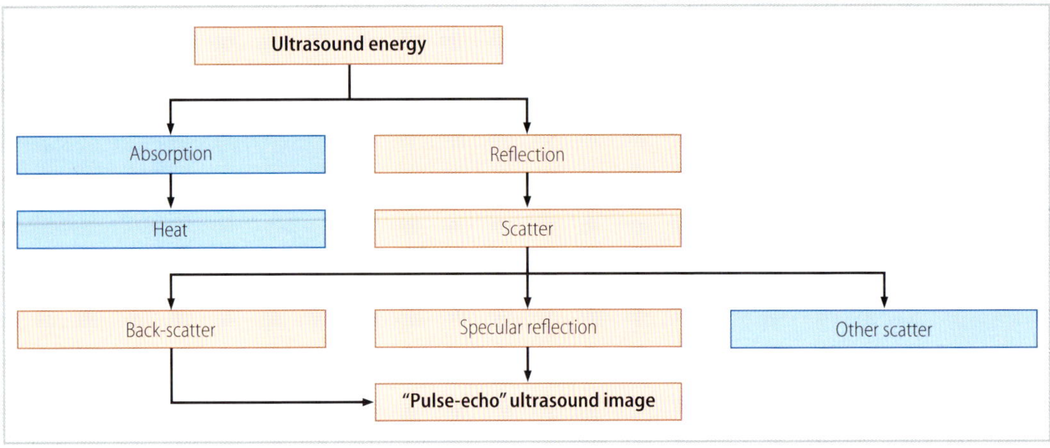

Figure 4.2 Fates of ultrasound energy.

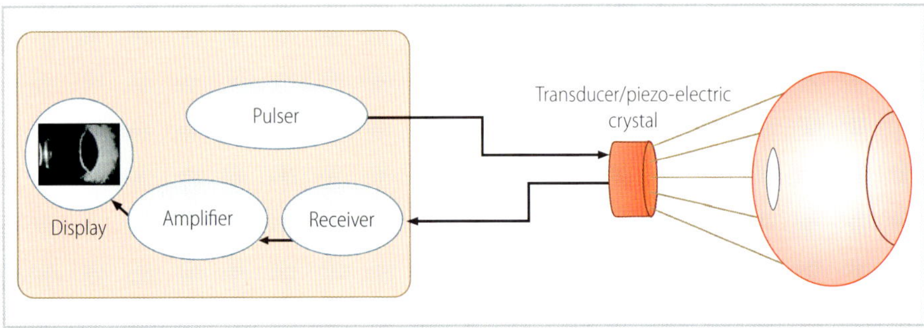

Figure 4.3 The principles of operation of an ultrasound instrument.

echoes return, they are processed by the receiver. Another important element of ultrasound instrument is the amplifier, since the returning echoes are normally very weak and they cannot be displayed without amplification. The type of amplification determines to a large extent the appearance of the displayed images. This is particularly important in A-scan and will be discussed in the section on standardized A-scan.

While A-scan is used less frequently in other disciplines, it remains a useful modality in ophthalmology as it is employed for biometry and tissue diagnosis. In A-scan, the returning echoes are displayed in one-dimensional series of waves (spikes) arising from a base line (**Figure 4.4**). The height of the spike represents the strength of the returning echo (the basis of tissue diagnosis). When the speed of sound in a medium is known, A-scan is used to calculate the distance between echo sources (the basis of biometry). **Table 4.1** shows the speed of sound in ocular structures.

B-scan is a two-dimensional image of a slice of ocular tissue. It is created from (numerous) A-scan spikes where each spike is converted to a dot on the display screen; the stronger the echo source the brighter the dot. Thus, the coalescence of numerous dots of various brightness creates the two-dimensional image of the familiar structure of the eye. **Figure 4.5** depicts the principle of B-scan.

The examiner needs also to be familiar with some terms and common functions that are available in scanners. These include time gain compensation, axial resolution, lateral resolution, gain, and gray scale. Manipulating these functions during examination will help produce the best images.

Time gain compensation (TGC) is an amplification function. As the sound waves penetrate deeper into the tissue, and due to attenuation, the returning echo signals from deeper interfaces are weakened and appear less reflective than similar interfaces placed more superficially. This is an undesirable effect in that identical tissues at different depths will not appear similar on the final image. TGC amplifies deeper signals disproportionally more than superficial signals in order to correct this anomaly. TGC is available on some scanners as a manual function at the disposal of the examiner. In other scanners, TGC function is automatically applied to the amplification process (**Figure 4.6**). Axial resolution is the ability of scanners to distinguish two separate echo sources along the beam path, while lateral resolution is the ability to distinguish two separate echo sources across the beam path (**Figure 4.7**). Normally axial resolution is increased when the gain is reduced and lateral resolution is increased when the frequency is increased.

Gain is an important function that is available to the examiner and changing it will significantly alter the appearance of echograms. Gain is a function of the receiver amplifier that directly affects the amplitude of displayed echoes. Its unit of measurement is the decibel (dB), which expresses the ratios of intensities in a logarithmic scale. The higher the dB gains, the higher spikes on A-scan and the brighter dots on B-scan. Very high gain will display weak signals better but will also produce unwanted noise artifacts and reduce resolution. Very low gain will suppress weak signals and prevent display of weak echo sources but has the advantage of enhancing resolution. Experienced echographers tend to adjust the gain control continuously during ultrasound examination to optimize the images. As a general guide, it is better to begin the examination with high gain in order to detect weak signals, e.g. mild vitreous hemorrhage (VH), and then reduce the gain to improve resolution, for example to detect and measure small elevation of the globe wall (**Figure 4.8**).

Gray scale is a function of B-scan. It is the ability to display dots in various degrees of brightness depending on the amplitude of echoes.

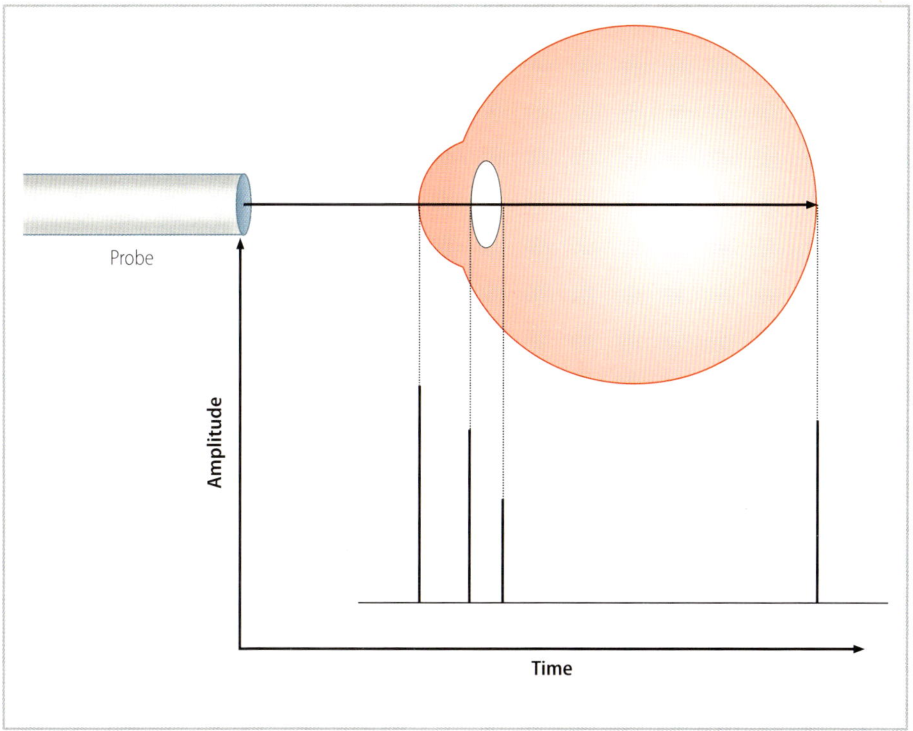

Figure 4.4 A-Scan principles (A for amplitude).

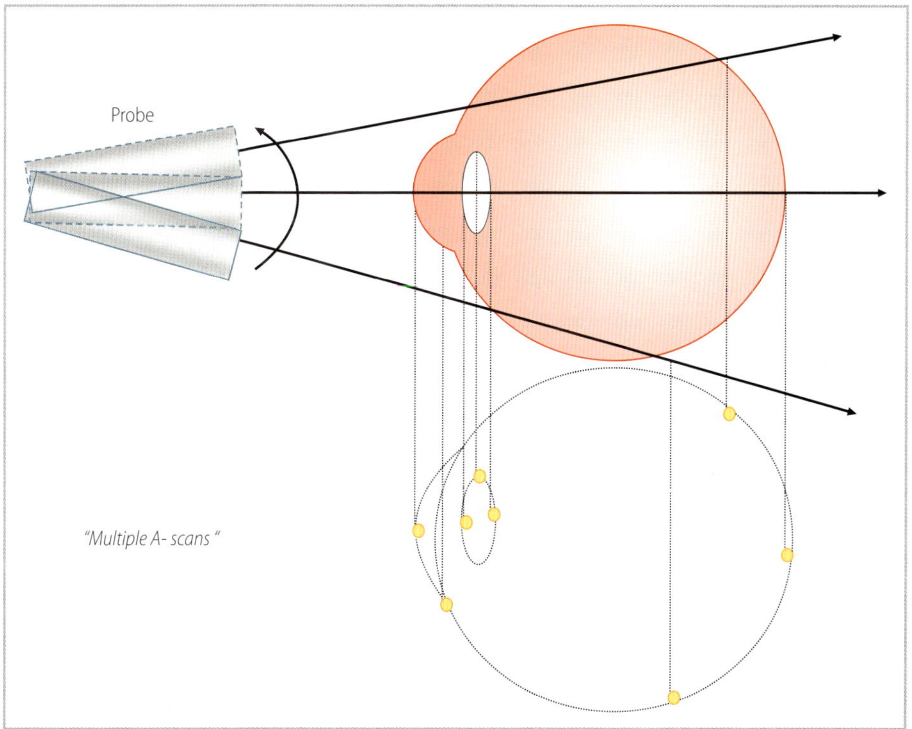

Figure 4.5 B-Scan principles (B for brightness).

Table 4.1 Speed of sound in ocular structures

Average (phakic) eye	1550 m/s
Aqueous and vitreous (aphakic eye)	1532 m/s
Lens	1641 m/s
Silicone oil-filled eye	990 m/s*

*Average figure.

High gray scale displays many shades of gray, from white (highest amplitude) to black (lowest amplitude). Low gray scale displays limited shades of gray. The examiner will alter the scale to produce the best pictorial image for a given echogram for diagnosis. As a general guide, it is better to start the examination with high gray scale. Once a diagnosis has been made, the gray scale is reduced to enhance the appeal of the image for recording and storage (**Figure 4.9**).

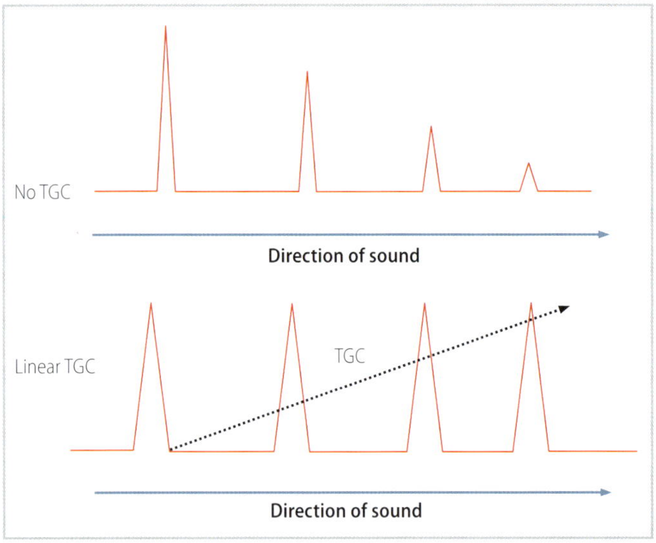

Figure 4.6 Time gain compensation.

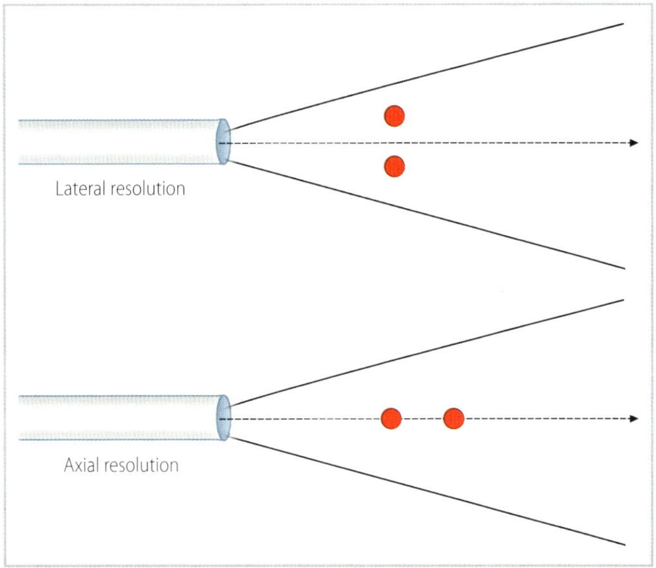

Figure 4.7 Lateral and axial resolution.

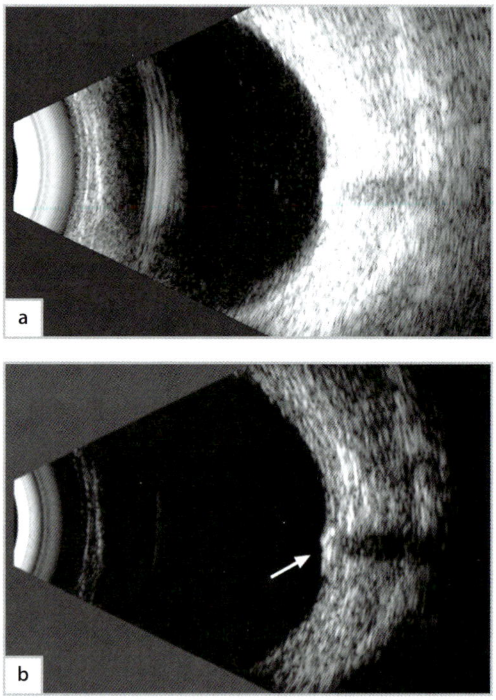

Figure 4.8 Decibel gain setting. (a) High gain setting. (b) Low gain setting. At low gain, a calcified lesion with shadowing (arrow) is better identified.

Indications for ocular echography

Ultrasound enjoys two unique properties that distinguish it from other ocular imaging modalities. The first property is its ability to depict subsurface tissue and structures behind opaque media, e.g. dense cataract. The second property is its ability to display kinetic features in real time, e.g. retinal detachment's movement. Even in clear media, ultrasound can provide acoustic data that will help in tissue diagnosis and differentiation between various mass lesions. As the speed of sound in ocular structures is now well known (**Table 4.1**), numerous biometric measurements can be performed accurately. The best example is axial length calculation. Biometry, however, is not only restricted to axial eye length measurement but also extends to other applications such as measuring tumors' dimensions and chorioretinal layer thickness. The combination of the above features with the safety, accessibility, and low cost of ultrasound makes this imaging method very useful in the diagnosis of many ocular disorders.

An important application of ultrasound is in the investigation of children with leukocoria. Children can be examined in most cases without anesthesia, but ultrasound can also be introduced as part of the examination under anesthesia. Ultrasound is very sensitive in detecting calcification, an important diagnostic finding in retinoblastoma.

Table 4.2 lists the indications for ocular ultrasound. Biometry of axial eye length and intraocular lens (IOL) calculation are not included as they are outwith the remit of this book. Many of the echographic diagnoses listed in the table are described in later sections, but the role of ultrasound in the clinical workup of dense cataract and VH, being the two most common indications after axial eye length, is given special attention in this section.

Screening of dense cataract

When ophthalmoscopy is impeded due to dense cataract, ultrasound is used to exclude important posterior segment abnormalities such as retinal detachment and ocular tumors. Additionally, the echographer needs to elicit other unexpected or subtle but clinically important findings such as small macular elevation, large disc cupping (Winder 1996), asteroid hyalosis (**Figure 4.10**), and posterior staphyloma (**Figure 4.11**); the latter two will also make axial length measurement difficult or inaccurate.

By definition, dense cataract will likely eliminate laser interferometry (IOL Master) as the method of choice for axial length measurement. In such cases, A-scan and immersion B-scan become the only practical means for measuring axial length. A well-centered immersion B-scan of a horizontal axial section of the eye (**Figure 4.12**) is an accurate and complimentary method of axial length measurement in cases where A-scan is difficult, such as in eyes filled with silicon oil and emulsified oil bubbles, also when there is posterior staphyloma or an undiagnosed macular lesion. A suggested protocol for cataract screening is illustrated in **Figure 4.13**.

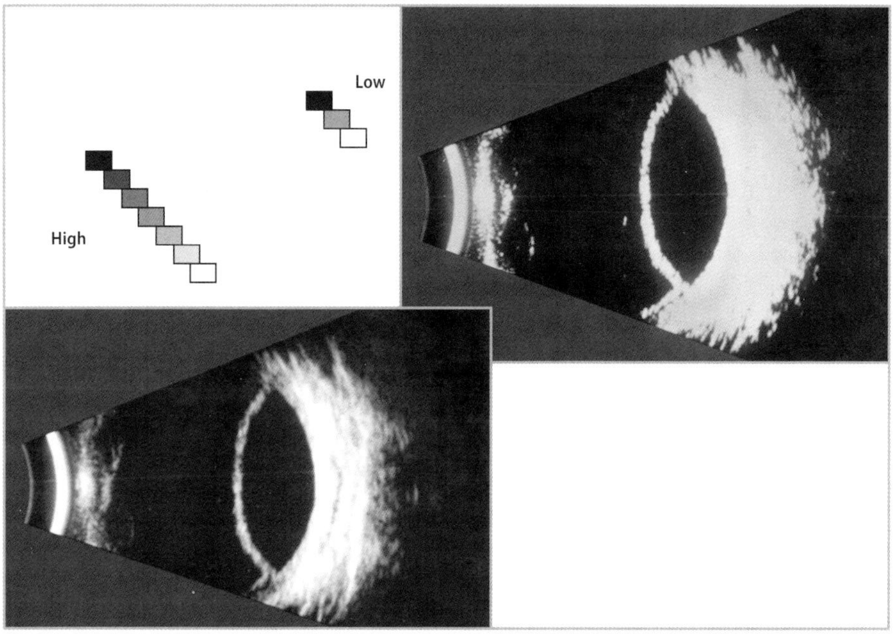

Figure 4.9 Gray scale setting. Top right is a low gray scale image; bottom left is a high gray scale image.

Table 4.2 Indications for ocular ultrasound

Indications	Echographic findings/functions
I. Opaque media	
Dense cataract	Posterior segment abnormality Macular lesion Large (pathological) cupping of the disc Abnormal globe wall/staphyloma B-scan axial length
Vitreous hemorrhage	Retinal tear and retinal detachment Proliferative diabetic retinopathy Bleeding disciform and eccentric disciform Bleeding retinal macroaneurysm
Corneal opacity, miosis, and pupillary membrane	Dense cataract Iris/ciliary body lesion Retrolenticular and cyclitic membrane Posterior segment abnormality
Hyphema	Vitreous hemorrhage Bleeding mass lesion Trauma/IOFB
Hypopyon	Vitreous cells Endophthalmitis Necrotizing tumor
II. Clear media	
Mass lesion	Choroidal melanoma Choroidal metastasis Choroidal hemangioma Other masses
Macular lesion	Disciform (calcified drusen) Osteoma (calcification)
Retinal detachment	Exclude exudative retinal detachment and subretinal mass
Posterior scleritis	Confirm diagnosis
Choroiditis	Chorioretinal layer thickness Choroidal nodules Vitreous cells
Choroidal folds	Orbital scan to exclude mass Globe wall flattening

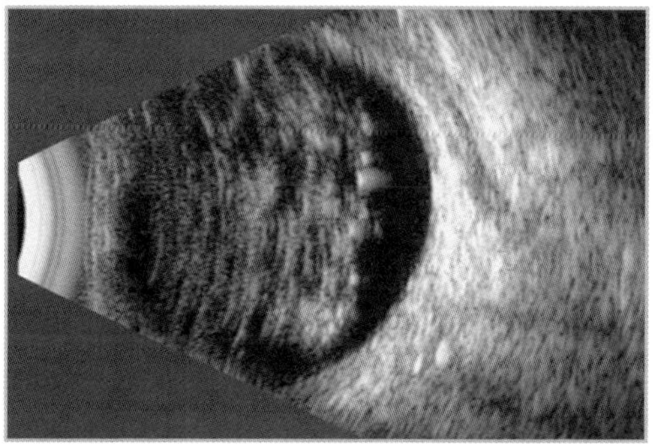

Figure 4.10 Asteroid hyalosis: a common finding at cataract screening.

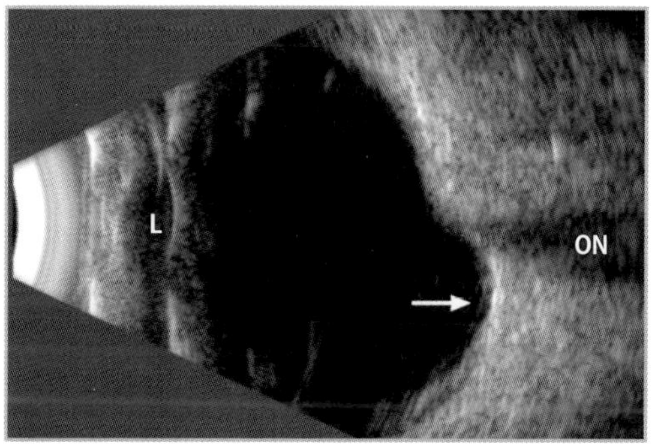

Figure 4.11 Posterior staphyloma. Vertical axial B-scan showing marked staphyloma below the optic nerve (arrow). L, lens; O, optic nerve.

Table 4.2 *Continued*

III. Leukocoria	Retinoblastoma ROP Coats' disease PHPV Other lesions
IV. Ocular trauma	IOFB (radiotranslucent) Posterior scleral rupture Choroidal hemorrhage/detachment Retinal detachment Lens rupture/dislocation

IOFB, intraocular foreign body; PHPV, persistent hyperplastic primary vitreous; ROP, retinopathy of prematurity.

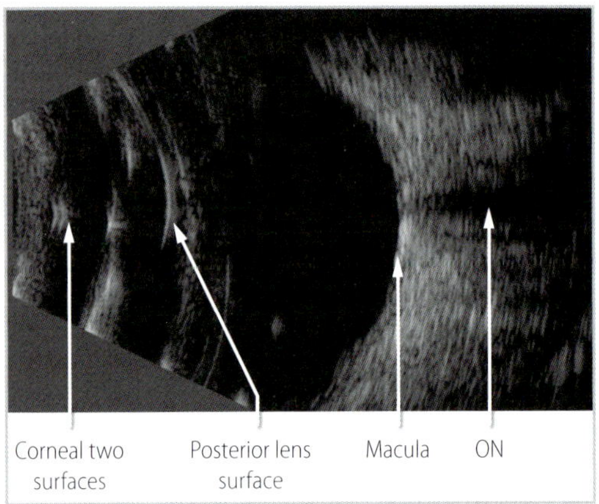

Figure 4.12 Immersion B-scan, horizontal axial section.

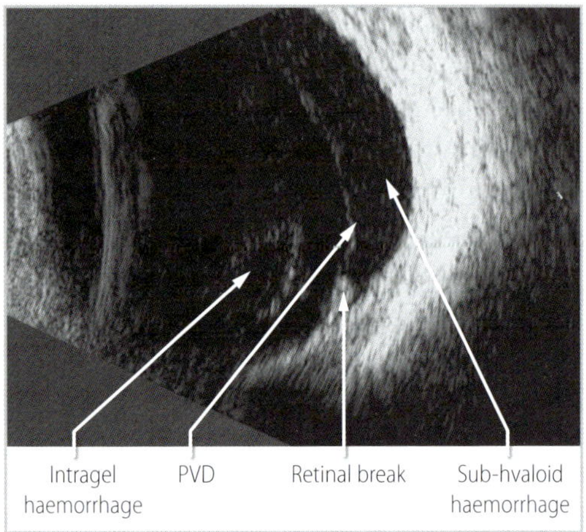

Figure 4.14 Retinal break and vitreous hemorrhage. PVD, posterior vitreous detachment.

Assessment of vitreous hemorrhage

The echographer needs to establish a protocol and a strategy of assessing VH with ultrasound. The aim is to:

1. Determine the topographic types of VH, namely intragel hemorrhage, subhyaloid hemorrhage (SHH), or mixed
2. Rule out retinal tears and retinal detachment
3. Search for other sources of bleeding
4. Arrange echographic follow-up

It is clinically valuable to determine the topographic type of VH. Intragel VH is likely to resolve quicker than SHH. In addition, and without history of retinopathy, a retinal break must be suspected in SHH. The primary function of ultrasound in VH must always be the detection of retinal break (**Figure 4.14**) or retinal detachment (**Figure 4.15**). If not detected during the first visit, serial ultrasound examinations on a weekly basis are indicated until ophthalmoscopy is possible and retinal detachment is excluded. Other common causes of VH, diabetic retinopathy, vitreoretinal traction, bleeding disciform, including eccentric disciform, and bleeding from retinal macroaneurysms can be detected using ultrasound.

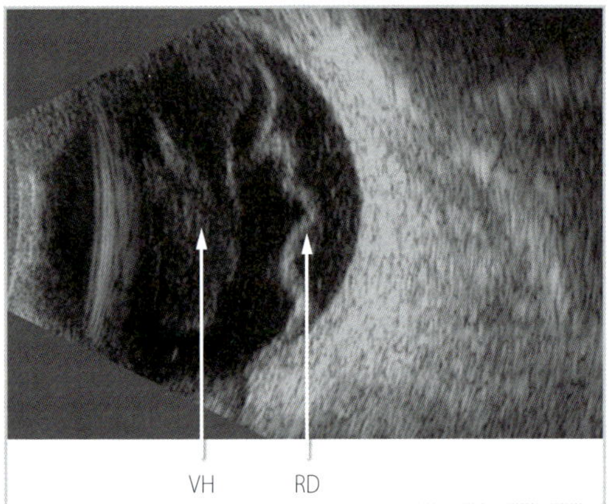

Figure 4.15 Vitreous hemorrhage harboring retinal detachment.

Figure 4.16 summarizes my findings, over a period of 2 years, of the causes of VH (excluding trauma) as identified on ultrasound. All the findings were confirmed either by ophthalmoscopy after clearance of VH or at the time of vitrectomy. It is worth noting that choroidal melanoma is a rare cause of VH, and in most cases it is the mushroom-shaped type that is liable to bleed (Byrne 2002). It is to be noted also that, in my series, in 18% of cases ultrasound was unable to identify a cause of VH. There was normal fundus examination after clearance of VH in these cases, and Valsalva maneuver or hemorrhagic posterior vitreous detachment (PVD) without retinal break is presumed to be the cause. This emphasizes the need for ultrasound follow-up in such cases to ensure that subtle retinal break or early retinal detachment is not present.

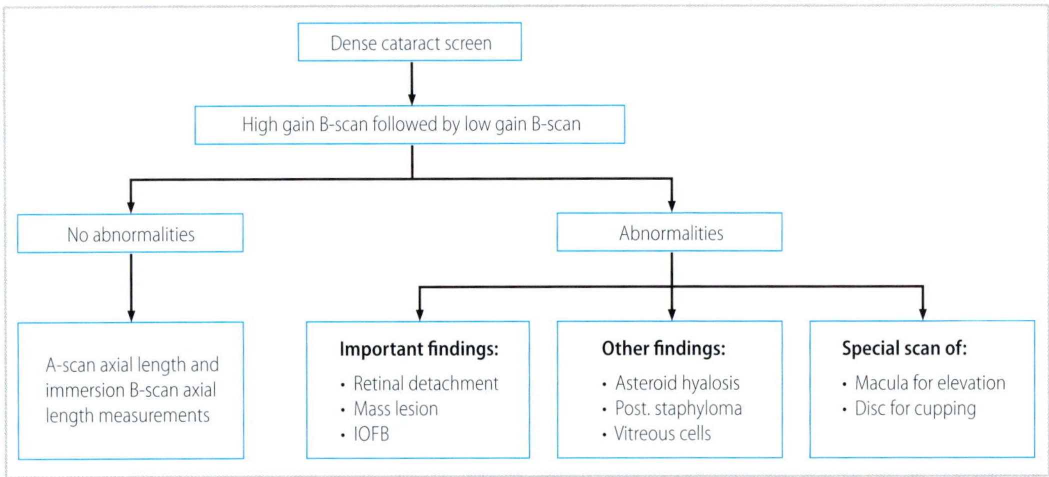

Figure 4.13 Suggested routine for cataract ultrasound screening.

	n	%	
Diabetic retinopathy	18	37	
Bleeding disciform (and eccentric)	7	14	
Tear and/or retinal detachment	6	12	
Retinal vein occlusion	3	6	
Terson's syndrome	3	6	
Bleeding retinal macro-aneurysm	2	4	
Choroidal melanoma (mushroom)	1	2	
Unconfirmed pathology	9	18	
TOTAL CASES	49	100	100%

Figure 4.16 Causes of vitreous hemorrhage as identified on ultrasound: 2 years consecutive observational series.

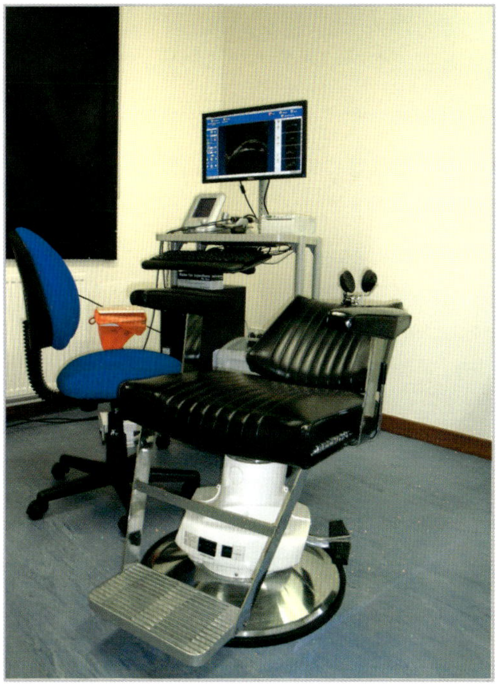

Figure 4.17 The patient's chair with the head as near as possible to the screen.

Examination techniques

General principles

Ultrasound examination is an operator-dependent investigation. This means that the operator scanning the patient will also be the individual responsible for interpreting the findings and making a diagnosis. This multitasking process is a unique feature that distinguishes ultrasound from other imaging modalities such as fluorescein angiography, optical coherence tomography, computed tomography (CT), and magnetic resonance imaging (MRI). In such methods, images may be obtained by one individual and interpreted by another. This is mainly because, in ultrasound, most of the important diagnostic (acoustic) data are gathered in real time during the dynamic scanning.

It follows that the best results are obtained when:

- The appropriate examination techniques are employed
- The maximum acoustic data are collected
- The correct echographic interpretation and diagnosis are made

To achieve the above, the echographer is required to master the technical ability to scan the eye, to be able to distinguish between normal and abnormal findings, and to discard irrelevant (rather common) artifacts. The examiner also needs to be familiar with the anatomy of the eye and have sufficient knowledge of the pathology and disease processes of the ocular disorders that are likely to require ultrasound examination. It is important for the examiner to be aware of the clinical findings and working diagnosis but not biased them, and to reach the echographic diagnosis solely from the acoustic data. In this regard, an ultrasound request form is best devised that clearly states the clinical findings and the precise reason for requesting ultrasound examination.

If possible, diagnostic ultrasound is best performed in a separate room with facilities for dim lighting and a reclining swivel chair for the patient. Scanners should be loaded on mobile trolleys or work surfaces for ease of access and to maneuver the instrument as close to the patient's head as possible. In this way, the operator will be able to easily conduct the examination while observing, in comfort, the images on the screen (**Figure 4.17**).

Many eye-dedicated scanners are now available with a wider range of choices of accessories. The examiner can choose only B-scanner, combined A-and B-scanner where A-scan should ideally be standardized for tissue diagnosis, and B-scanner with more than one probe offering different frequencies, including very high frequency (30–60 MHz) for anterior segment imaging. The determining factor, apart from the financial constraint, is the experience of the examiner and the needs of a given department and the subspecialty interests within it. Choosing a B-scanner for ophthalmic use requires a minimum suitability for obtaining enhanced resolution to image the episclera and the globe wall as separate layers from the orbit (**Figure 4.18**). It is important to accurately measure the height of the mass to diagnose posterior scleritis.

In ocular diagnosis, both A-scan and B-scan are utilized to gather the maximum acoustic data that are required to differentiate lesions and reach echographic tissue diagnosis (**Table 4.3**).

These acoustic data fall into three main categories:

1. Topographic data (mainly collected by B-scan):
   a. Shape
   b. Borders
   c. Location
   d. Extension
   e. Dimension
2. Kinetic data:
   f. Movement (mainly collected by B-scan)
   g. Vascularity (mainly collected by A-scan)
3. Quantitative data (mainly collected by A-scan):
   h. Reflectivity
   i. Internal structure
   j. Sound attenuation

Doppler ultrasound is used to detect vascularity and measure blood flow (kinetic data). However, it is not discussed further in this chapter because it has much more limited application in the globe than in the orbits.

A-Scan

As previously mentioned, A-scan is a one-dimensional display of returning echoes. In ophthalmology, unlike other medical disciplines, A-scan continues to be used frequently and is clinically employed for two purposes: first, to calculate axial eye length by measuring distance between echo spikes and, second, to obtain tissue diagnosis by measuring the amplitude and pattern of echo spikes (**Figure 4.19**).

Three types of A-scans are recognized in ophthalmic use:

1. Biometry A-scan

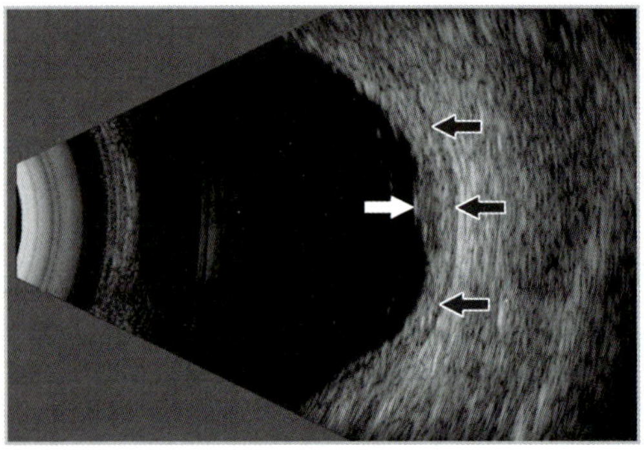

Figure 4.18 The minimum requirement of B-scan resolution is its ability to show the low reflective episclera (three black arrows) separating the globe wall from the orbit. A mass in the globe wall (white arrow) can then be accurately measured.

Table 4.3 Acoustic data in ocular ultrasound diagnosis and mode of choice

Topographic B > A	Kinetic B and A	Quantitative A > B
• Shape • Borders • Location • Extension • Dimension	• Motility • Vascularity	• Reflectivity • Internal structure • Sound attenuation

2. Vector A-scan
3. Standardized A-scan

It is important to distinguish between these three types of A-scan since accurate and reliable tissue diagnosis is only possible with standardized A-scan.

Biometry A-scan is used to measure axial eye length. It utilizes linear amplification to display signals. Linear amplification facilitates the display of highly reflective spikes of the familiar interfaces in the normal eye, namely the cornea, lens, and retina, which are required to measure the axial length. However, linear amplification has a small dynamic range and is limited in its ability to display and differentiate a large number of (abnormal) signals that is required for tissue diagnosis.

Vector A-scan is produced as a sample of the B-scan and both are often displayed simultaneously on the screen (**Figure 4.20**). Although useful for reference and B-scan correlation, vector A-scan is limited for tissue differentiation, since its amplification is logarithmic as it follows the B-scan. Logarithmic amplification has a large dynamic range but low sensitivity that is not optimum for detecting small differences in echo strength. Both biometry and vector A-scans also incorporate a focused sound beam, a feature that is not suitable for determining perpendicularity. This is a function best attained with a parallel sound beam (**Figure 4.21**).

Standardized A-scan

To address the needs for tissue diagnosis, a specifically designed A-scan was developed by Ossoinig (1974, 1979) who incorporated S-shaped amplification that combines dynamic range and sensitivity features of both linear and logarithmic amplifiers for optimum tissue differentiation (**Figure 4.22**). Another important specification of standardized A-scan includes nonfocused parallel beam and sound frequency of 8 MHz. The use of tissue model for external calibration of the dB gain and the setting of 'T-sensitivity' is also an important feature of standardized A-scan (**Figure 4.23**), as it ensures the same appearance of similar tissues in different scanners. The combination of the above feature allows the harmonization of all standardized A-scan instruments and limits the variables in external factors that influence the strength of echoes so that only tissue types will determine the amplitude of the echo spikes.

Examination steps of A-scan

Systematic examination steps are recommended to maximize the standardization of A-scan:

1. The instrument is set at 'T-sensitivity' (**Figure 4.23**)

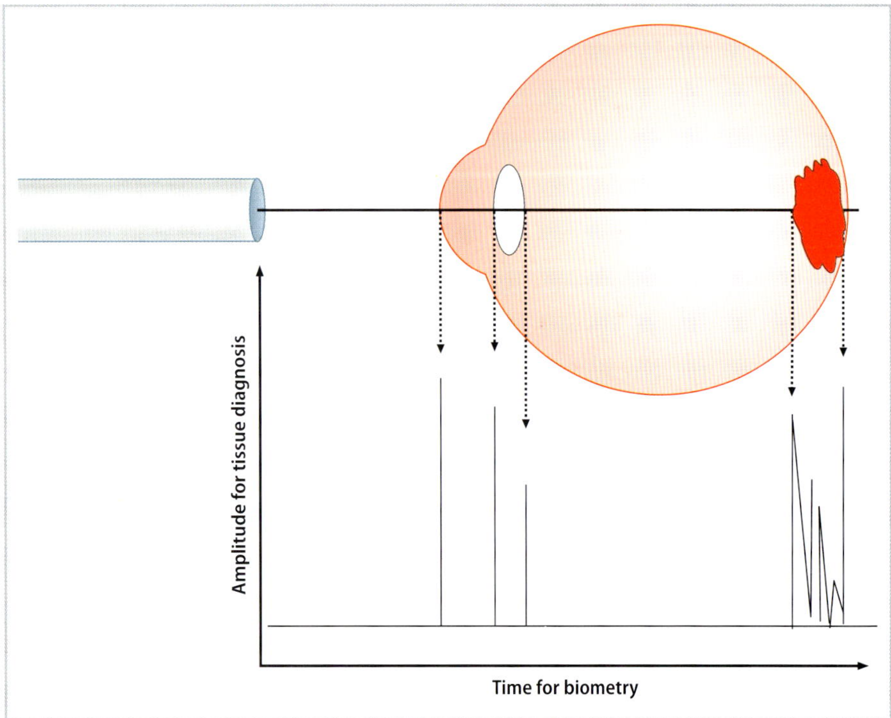

Figure 4.19 Function of A-scan. Vertical axis for amplitude (the basis of tissue diagnosis); horizontal axis for time (the basis of biometry).

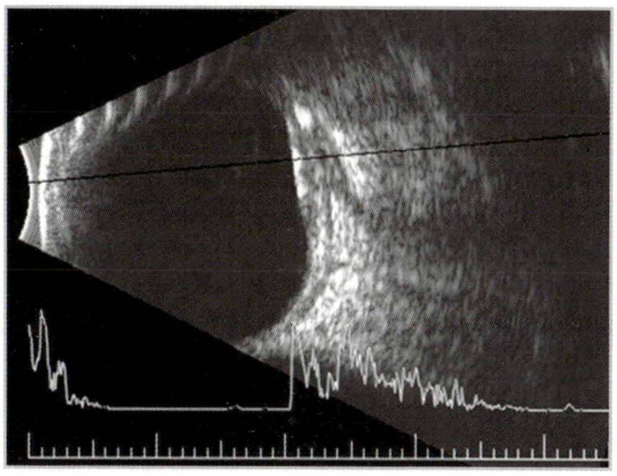

Figure 4.20 Vector A- and B-scan display.

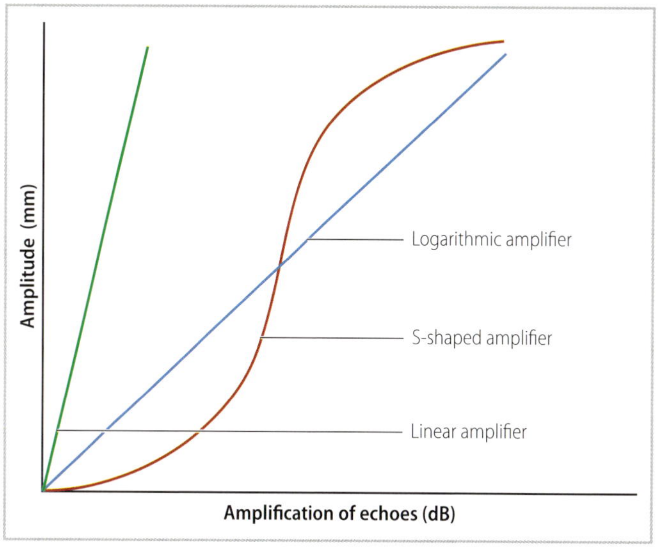

Figure 4.22 Types of amplification curves. The S-shaped curve represents optimum amplification for ophthalmic tissue diagnosis.

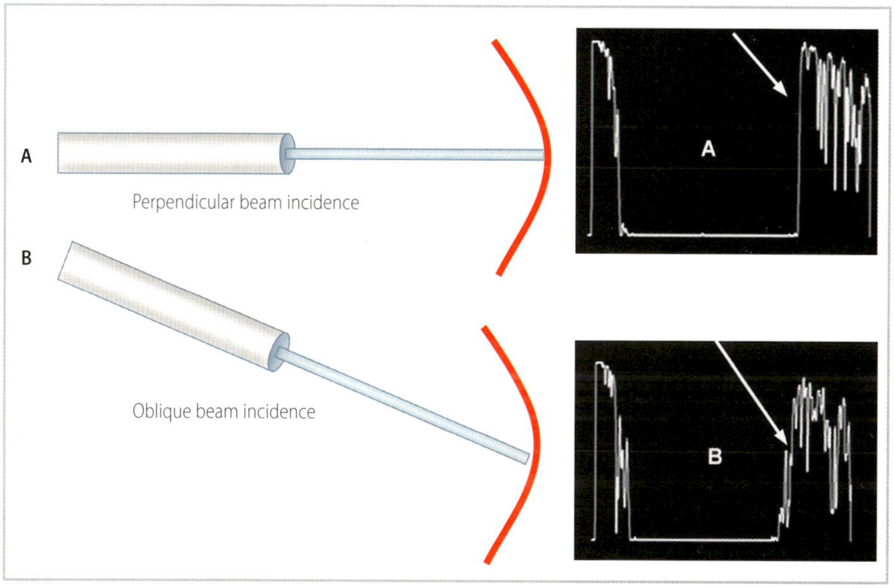

Figure 4.21 Parallel sound beam determining perpendicularity. (a) Smooth tall retinal spike (arrow) when the beam is perpendicular on the globe wall. (b) Serrated short retinal spikes (arrow) when the beam is oblique on the globe wall.

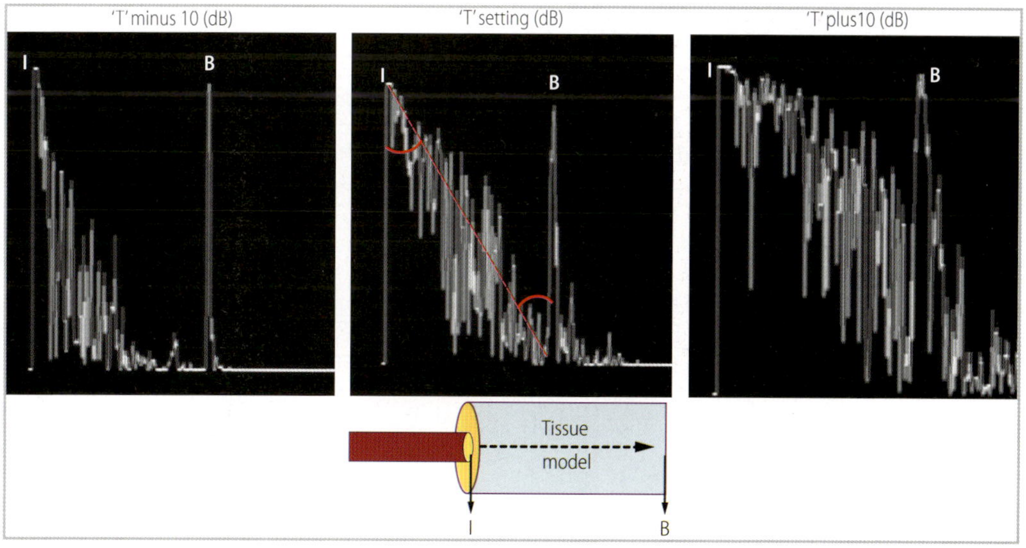

Figure 4.23 Setting of T-sensitivity. A probe is placed on a tissue model and the echo trace is observed. The left trace shows low spikes from a weak decibel (dB) level. The right trace shows high spikes from a strong dB level. The middle trace shows N-shaped pattern indicating correct T-sensitivity dB level. B, bottom of tissue model; I, initial contact between probe and tissue model.

2. The patient is positioned with the head near the screen
3. Topical anesthetic drops are instilled into the eye
4. The probe is placed on the globe. No coupling jelly is required, as the tear film is adequate for sound transmission. For biometry, an axial scan is obtained by placing the probe on the cornea with the patient gazing at the primary position (**Figure 4.24**, left). For diagnosis utilizing A-scan, the lens is better avoided and the probe is placed on the sclera near the limbus (posterior scan) with the patient gazing at the opposite meridian to that of the probe (**Figure 4.24**, right)
5. Eight meridians are scanned (**Figure 4.25**) by shifting and tilting the probe in a single, smooth arc movement in an anterior–posterior direction, from the limbus to the fornix; the globe wall is scanned posterior–anteriorly. In all scans, perpendicularity of the beam incidence is maintained and verified by observing a smooth, steeply rising, tall retinal spike (**Figure 4.21**). A degree of operator skill is required, during the dynamic scanning, to alter the probe position to achieve and maintain perpendicularity.
6. For reference, comparison, and follow-up, a system of labeling of scans is required. A suggested system is to name the scans according to the clock hour and the anterior–posterior location of the beam on the globe wall (**Figure 4.25**). In 12E, the scan beam is located at 12 o'clock equator and the probe is placed at 6 o'clock halfway between the limbus and the fornix. In 3P, the scan beam is at 3 o'clock posterior to equator and the probe is at 9 o'clock limbus. In 9A, the beam is at 9 o'clock anterior to equator and the probe is at 3 o'clock fornix.

Interpretation of diagnostic A-scans

A diagnostic A-scan mainly provides quantitative data and to a lesser degree kinetic data (Ossoinig 1974). This is in comparison to B-scan, which, mainly provides topographic and kinetic data (see **Table 4.3**). The quantitative data include reflectivity, internal structure, and sound attenuation.

Reflectivity is the measurement of spike amplitude. This can be an absolute value in dB or a percentage comparison between the initial spike (100% tall) and the spike in question. The sclera, for example, is the most highly reflective structure with a 95–100% tall spike. Retinal detachment, when scanned perpendicularly, normally produces a 90–100% tall spike. PVD usually displays a spike < 80% tall (**Figure 4.26**). These results, however, depend largely on the examiner's skill in scanning perpendicularly in order to maximize the spike height. Also in some cases, a low retinal spike is encountered if the retina is very folded and a high spike is encountered in long-standing, thick inferior PVD, commonly seen in diabetic retinopathy with chronic VH.

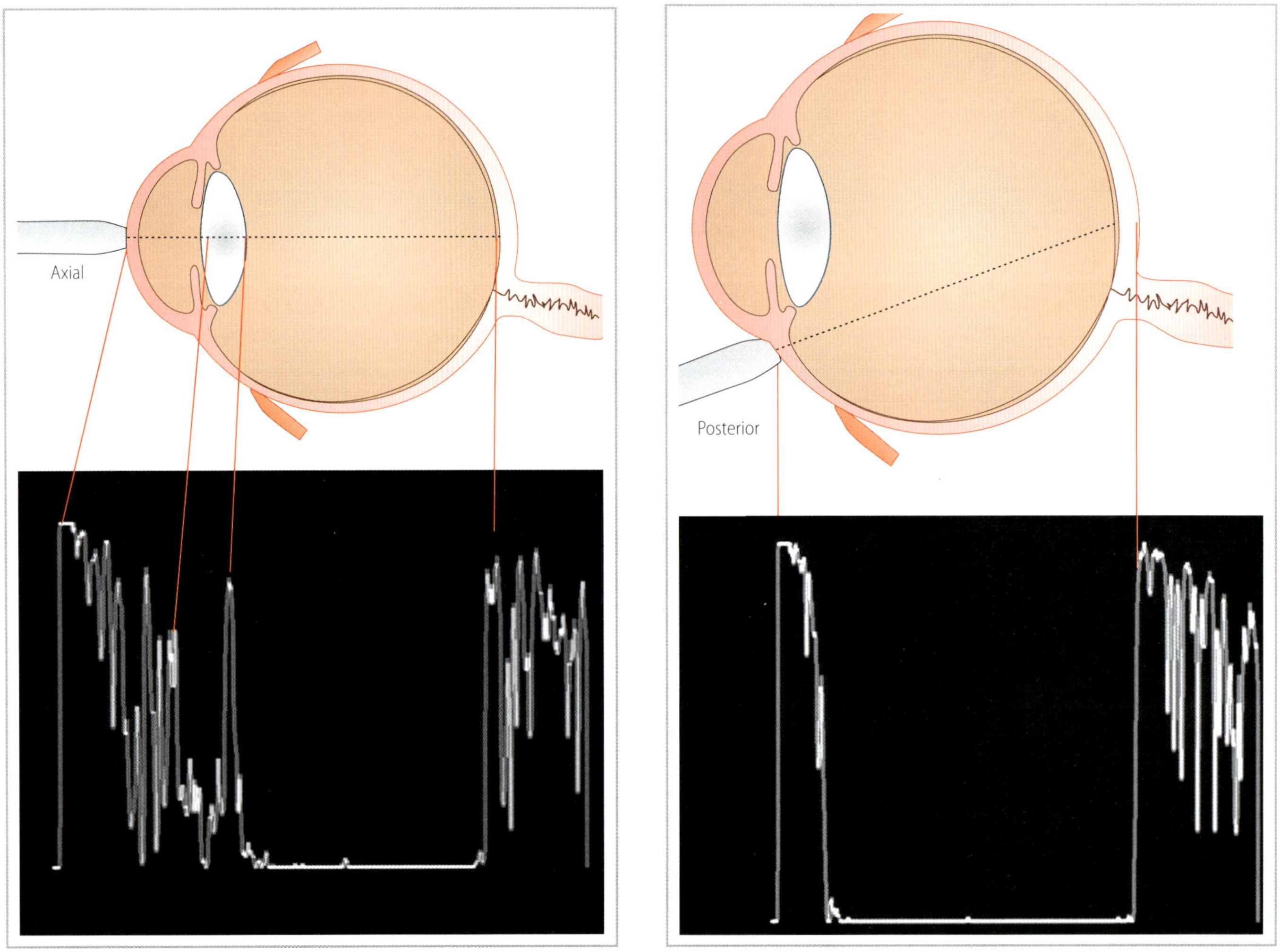

Figure 4.24 Axial A-scan (left) for biometry. Posterior A-scan (right) for tissue diagnosis.

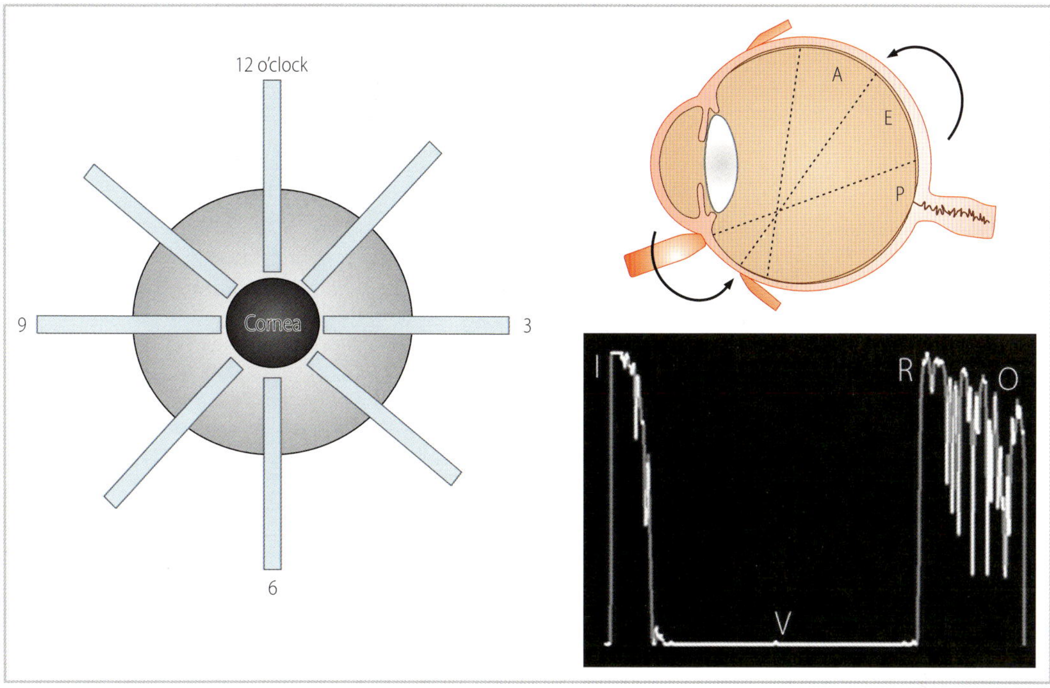

Figure 4.25 Technique for screening the globe for tissue diagnosis. A, anterior; E, equator; P, posterior; I, initial spike; O, orbital spikes; P R, retinal spike; V, vitreous baseline.

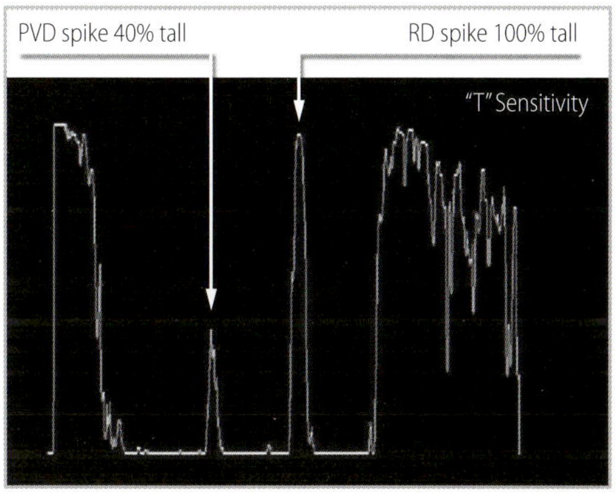

Figure 4.26 A-scan in a case of combined RD and PVD. PVD, posterior vitreous detachment; RD, retinal detachment.

Internal structure describes the regularity of height and interval of a group of spikes representing a mass lesion. Regularly structured spikes tend to originate from a regular (small or large) histological unit, giving rise to homogeneous acoustic interfaces, e.g. choroidal melanoma and choroidal hemangioma. The opposite applies to irregularly structured lesions such as choroidal metastasis and disciform macular lesion.

Sound attenuation is the angle of decline in the height of spikes (the so-called angle kappa) along the beam path, produced by factors such as sound absorption. Normally, choroidal melanoma produces strong sound attenuation, while choroidal hemangioma produces weak sound attenuation. **Figure 4.27** illustrates the above functions and shows the typical A-scan characteristics of choroidal melanoma, choroidal hemangioma, and choroidal metastasis. However, reading the trace of A-scan requires a degree of experience akin to that required to read a electroretinogram. The skill of pattern recognition of A-scans is eventually gained with the experience of scanning a critical number of lesions.

Normal and abnormal A-scan results

In diagnostic A-scan, a posterior scan is performed to avoid scanning through the lens. The A-scan trace is read from left to right.

In the normal eye, the first spike is that of the initial (100% tall) spike where the probe meets the globe, followed by the flat, echo silent vitreous line, followed by the retinal spike (100% tall), and then ending with a series of high reflective spikes, decreasing in amplitude from left to right, which represents the echoes from the orbital fat. **Figure 4.25** demonstrates the appearance of normal A-scan.

Globe lesions that produce abnormal A-scan can be summarized into three categories:

1. *Membrane lesion*
   Retinal detachment, choroidal detachment, and PVD. In these cases, a single spike arises from the vitreous line. The amplitude and mobility of the spike depend on the lesion. Retinal detachment produces a high amplitude and mobile spike. PVD produces a low amplitude and very mobile spike. Choroidal detachment produces a very high, thick (double peaked), and immobile spike (**Figure 4.26**)
2. *Mass lesion*
   Malignant melanoma, metastasis, hemangioma, and macular disciform (**Figure 4.27**). All solid mass lesions demonstrate an immobile surface spike, and the appearance of the echoes between the surface spike and scleral spike is determined largely by the histological structure of the lesion (**Figure 4.27**). In a well-centered scan (showing high surface and scleral spikes), an accurate measurement of the height or thickness of the lesion is also obtained
3. *Discreet opacities*
   VH, asteroid hyalosis, and vitreous cells (**Figure 4.28**). The vitreous line in these cases contains numerous small (low amplitude) and tightly packed spikes. The number and height of spikes depend on the density and size of the units producing the echoes (asteroid hyalosis producing the highest amplitude and inflammatory cells the lowest)

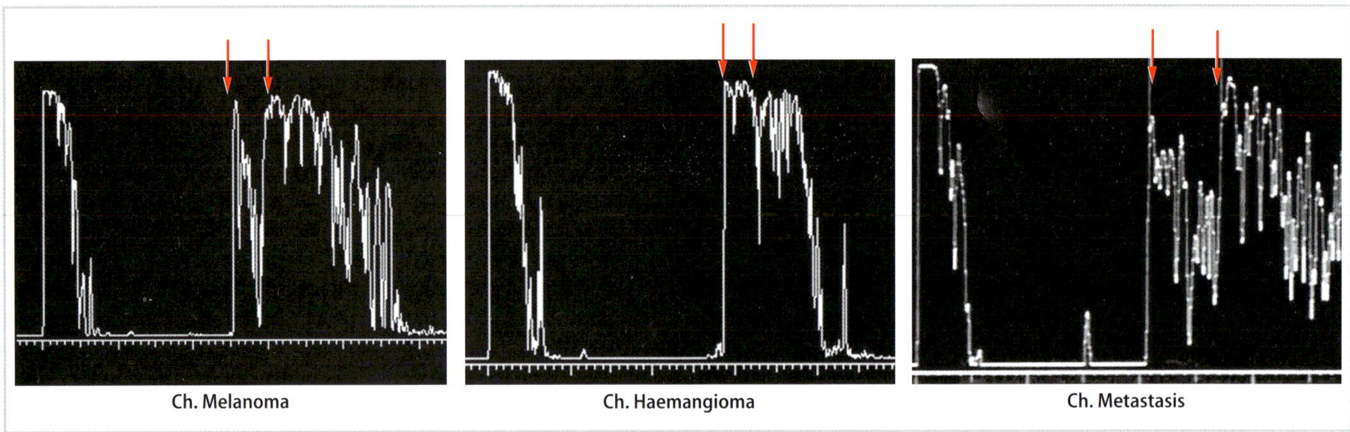

Figure 4.27 Standardized A-scans of ocular mass lesions Ch, choroidal.

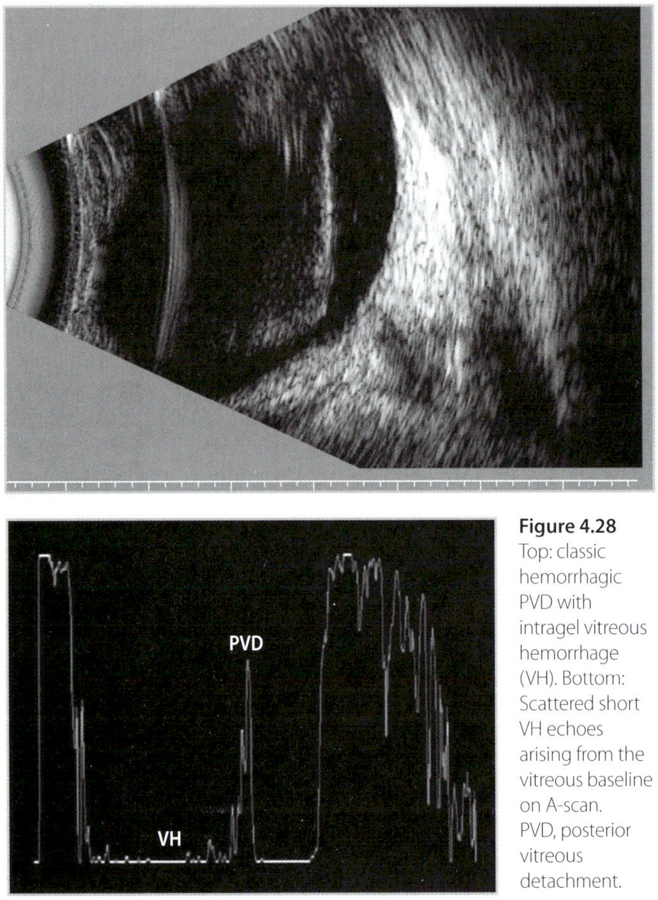

Figure 4.28 Top: classic hemorrhagic PVD with intragel vitreous hemorrhage (VH). Bottom: Scattered short VH echoes arising from the vitreous baseline on A-scan. PVD, posterior vitreous detachment.

B-Scan

General principles

In contrast to the one-dimensional images produced by A-scan, B-scan produces two-dimensional images. The probe emits a focused sound beam, similar to a slit lamp light. Eye-dedicated scanners emit a sound beam with a focal zone that coincides with the posterior globe wall and anterior orbit. At the focal zone, the beam is at its most focused point and images are at their sharpest (**Figure 4.29**). Also in an axial scan, the lateral sweep of the beam will only scan adequately from the equator to equator, offering the advantage of image magnification. Scanning of the periphery, therefore, necessitates shifting the probe and the patient's gaze to bring lesions into the central, most sensitive part of the beam path to produce best echograms (**Figure 4.30**). This important maneuver is greatly facilitated by applying the probe directly on the globe through open lids. Placing lesions in the center of the echogram is therefore an important objective and requires a degree of skill on the part of the examiner. As well as allowing the patient to direct their gaze to the desired position, scanning through open lids also improves the resolution and quality of images by minimizing sound attenuation from the lids. The majority of patients do not object to scanning directly on the anesthetized globe. Only in a few circumstances is scanning carried out on closed lids, such as in some cases of traumatized eyes and in children.

B-scan orientation and sections

The conversion of real two-dimensional images into virtual three-dimensional interpretations by the examiner is an essential mental exercise that is required to scan the entire globe, locate and measure lesions accurately, and finally produce the best images. It is often the most demanding aspect for trainee echographers to learn.

To facilitate this task and provide agreement and consistency between examiners, the following points should be taken into account:

- The orientation of the beam and realization of the section of the globe being scanned are helped by a marker placed near the probe face (**Figure 4.31**). The marker determines the axis of the beam on the fundus (**Figure 4.32**), and it also indicates the upper end of the echogram on the display screen
- The optic nerve, with its familiar landmark, is used as an echographic center of the globe and as a reference for the three B-scan sections (described below)
- The globe is divided concentrically into three equal zones: posterior (P), equator (E), and anterior (A)
- The globe is further divided radially into clock hour meridians
- When there is a choice of placing the probe marker at the nasal or temporal location or at the up or down location, the nasal and up locations are selected

The following three sections are recommended and are widely used by workers in this field. Some examiners may adopt other systems but, regardless of the system used, it must be consistent and allow

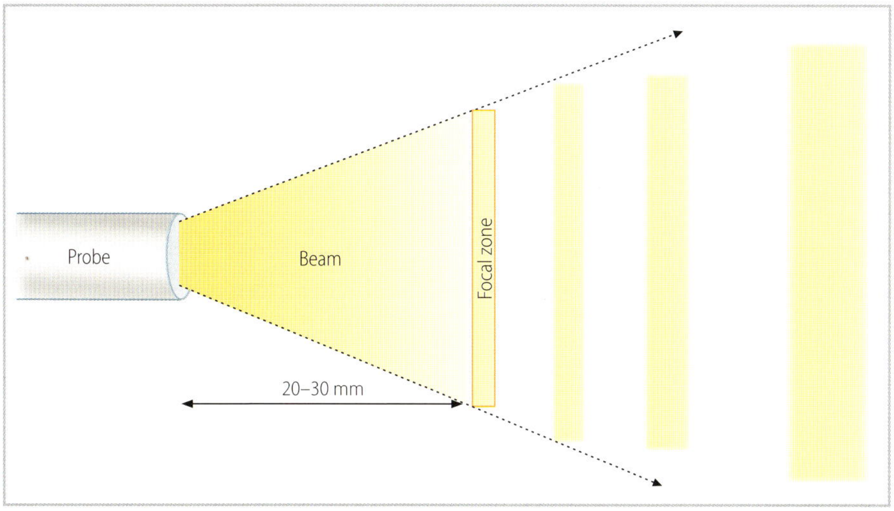

Figure 4.29 B-scan beam profiles. The beam diverges, widens, and becomes less focused beyond the focal zone.

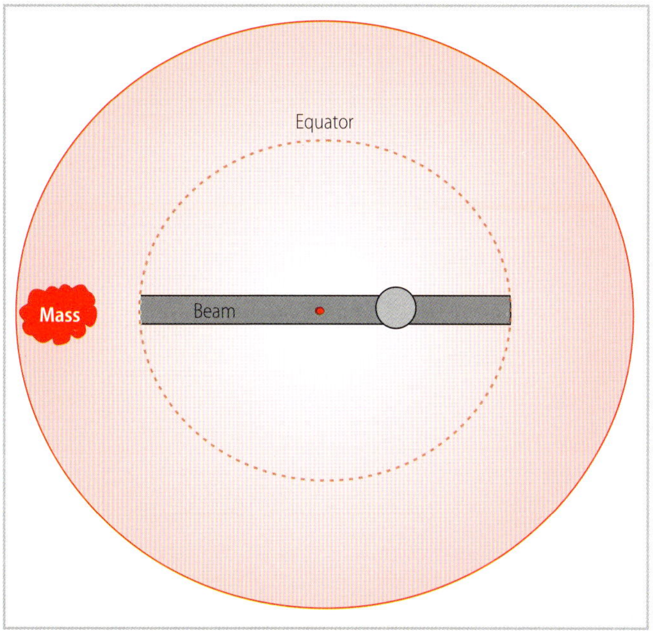

Figure 4.30 Extent of B-scan beam equator-to-equator. An axial B-scan will not detect a peripheral mass lesion.

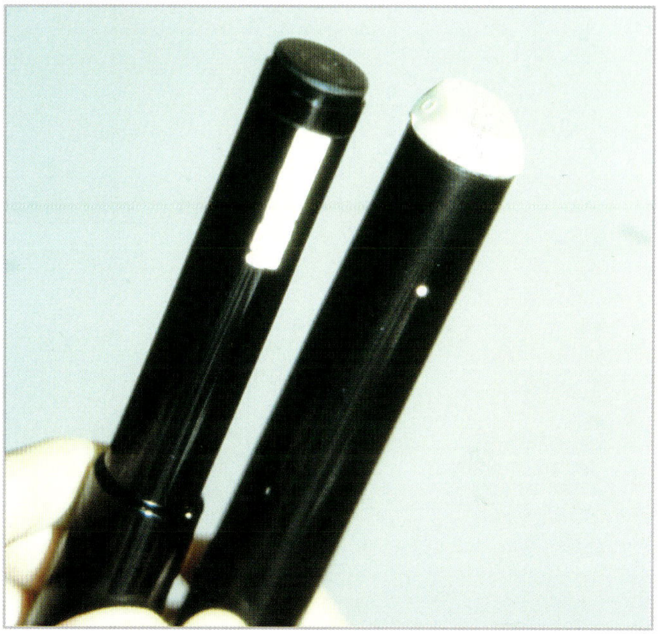

Figure 4.31 B-scan probe markers (white line and white dot).

scanning of the entire globe from the posterior pole to the ciliary body and in all the clock hours.

1. **Axial section** – In this section, the patient fixates at the primary gaze and the probe is placed on the cornea and directed axially. Sections of all the clock hours can be performed by rotating the probe on its axis, and the echograms are labeled after the location and orientation of the beam on the fundus, e.g. horizontal axial, vertical axial, 1.30 axial, and 10.30 axial (**Figure 4.33**). In all well-centered axial sections, the posterior lens surface and optic nerve head are placed in the center of the echogram (**Figure 4.34**).

   Axial section is used to display posterior pole lesions and attachment of membranes to the optic nerve head. A horizontal axial section will display the macula below the disc and, when an immersion technique is used, B-scan axial eye length measurement can be accurately calculated (**Figure 4.12**). However, in axial sections, because of the scatter and strong sound attenuation created by the lens, higher dB gain levels are usually needed to show structures at the expense of resolution. Also in pseudophakic eyes, strong, unwanted artifacts are produced by the lens implant. Another disadvantage of axial scan is that peripheral lesions such as ciliary body mass, retinoschisis, and retinal breaks are likely to be missed or partially displayed (**Figure 4.34**).
2. **Longitudinal section** – This section produces an image of the globe wall along one meridian only, from the optic nerve (lower portion of the echogram) to the ciliary body (upper portion of the echogram) (**Figure 4.35**). A longitudinal section is created by placing the probe on the sclera near the limbus with the marker radially placed at its corneal side, thus avoiding scanning through the lens. The periphery and ciliary body are brought into view by directing the patient's gaze 180° away from the probe marker (i.e. toward the meridian to be scanned). The echograms are labeled after the clock hour location of the beam (not the probe and marker). For

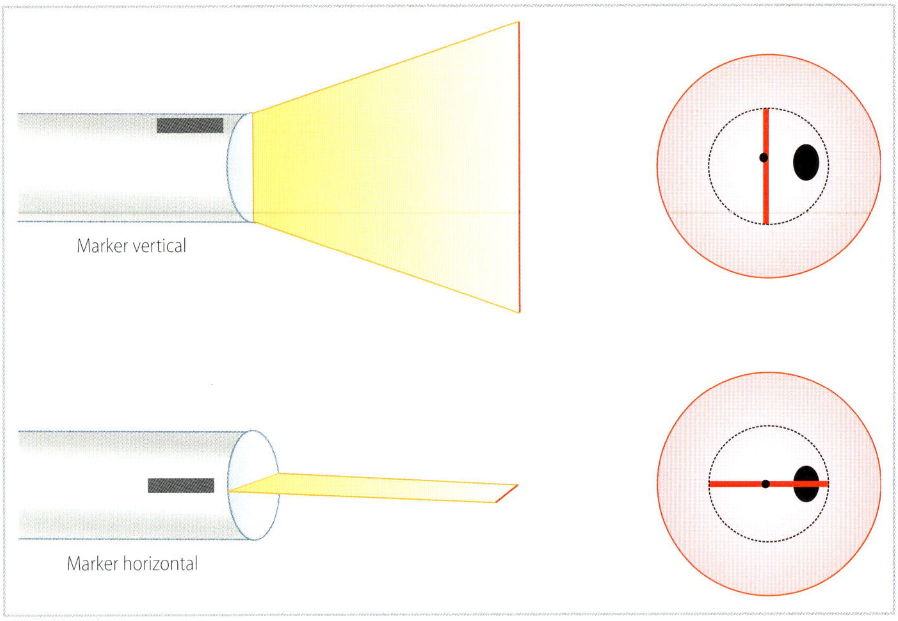

Figure 4.32 The probe marker indicates beam orientation on globe wall.

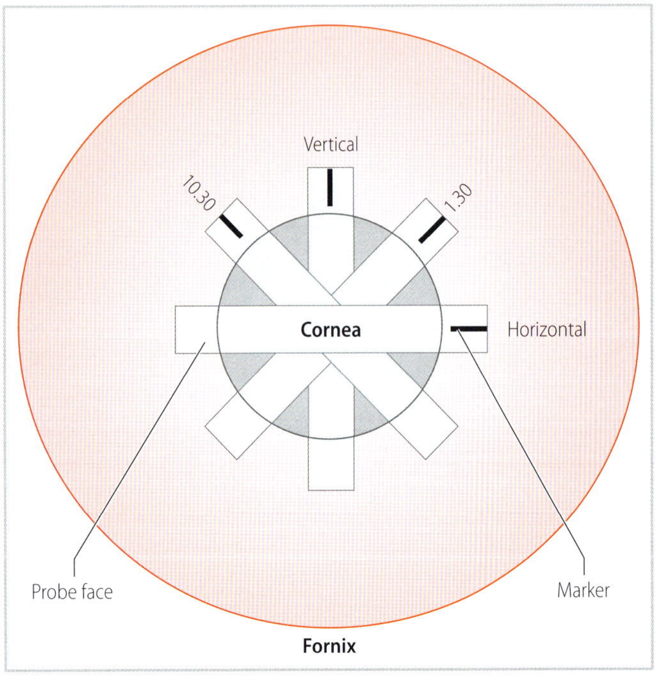

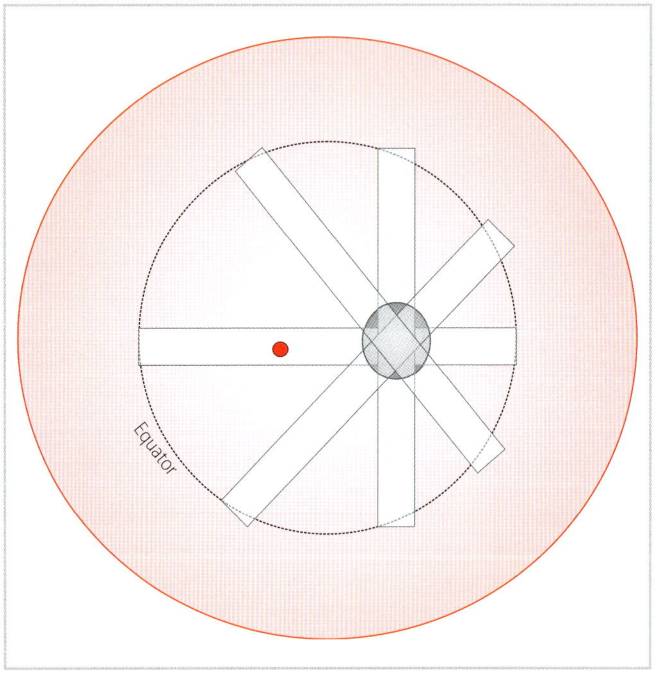

Figure 4.33 Left: axial right eye probe on the globe. Right: axial right eye beam on the fundus.

example: L12 section is created by a probe and marker placed at 6 o'clock (**Figure 4.36**) and L1:30 by a probe and marker placed at 7:30 (**Figure 4.37**).

Longitudinal scans are suitable for displaying the anterior–posterior limits of lesions and the attachment of membranes to the optic nerve head. By avoiding the lens, better resolution and fewer artifacts are achieved. Well-placed horizontal longitudinal sections produce good images of the macular area. In the right eye, it is L9 (**Figure 4.38**) and in the left eye it is L3 (**Figure 4.39**).

3. **Transverse section** – In this section, the beam traverses many meridians (unlike a longitudinal section that scans along one meridian), and in a well-centered transverse section the (clock hour) meridian of lesions can be quickly verified. A better resolution of the globe wall and the detection of weak reflecting echoes are achieved by placing the probe on the sclera (**Figure 4.40**).

In transverse sections, the probe is placed on the scleral side of the limbus and directed posteriorly. In a single smooth arc movement (following the curvature of the globe) it is shifted and rotated anterior–posteriorly, from the limbus to the fornix, scanning the opposite globe wall posterior–anteriorly. Perpendicularity is helped by directing the patient's gaze 180° away from the probe. The echograms are labeled according to the clock hour at the center

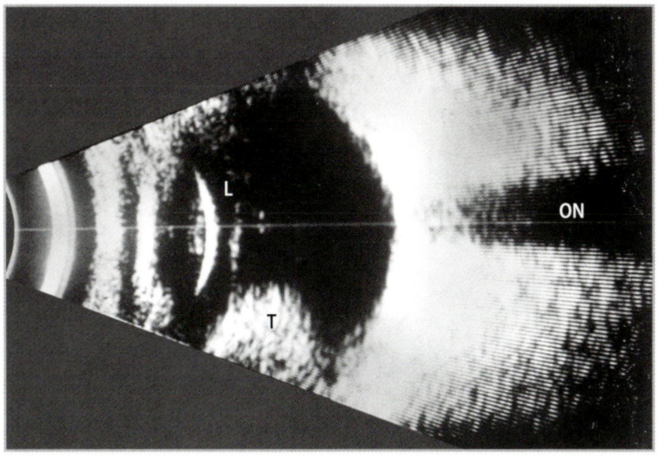

Figure 4.34 Axial B-scan echogram. The lens (L) and the optic nerve (ON) are well centered. The peripheral tumor (T) is incompletely visualized at the bottom.

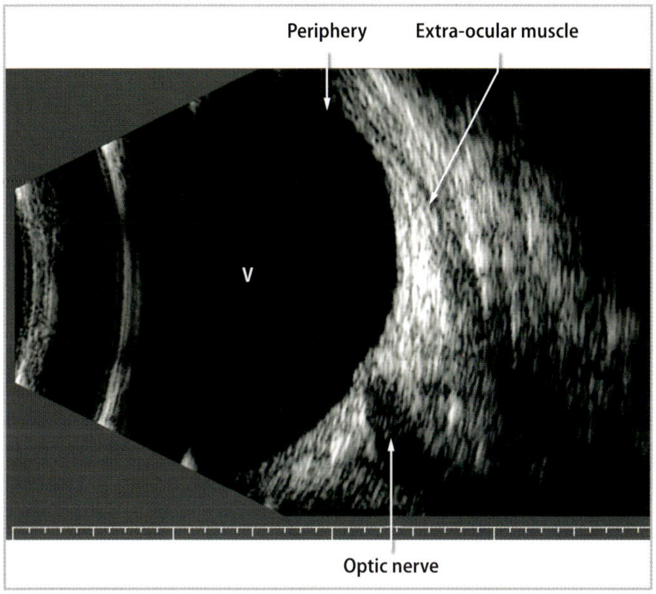

Figure 4.35 Longitudinal section: normal echogram. V, vitreous (echo silent).

of the beam, and also to the beam's anterior–posterior location. For example, a section labeled transverse 12 posterior (12P) is produced by a probe located at 6 o'clock limbus (**Figure 4.41**) and transverse 7:30 posterior (P), equator (E), anterior (A) sections are produced by placing the probe at 1:30 limbus, mid distance, and fornix respectively (**Figure 4.42**). As mentioned, in transverse sections, it is conventional to place the probe marker nasally instead of temporally, and up instead of down.

Protocol for screening of the globe with B-scan

Regardless of which protocol and B-scan sections are used, these should provide consistency and repeatability and must ensure scanning of the entire globe anterior–posteriorly and in all meridians. The following routine is suggested, but examiners may develop their own steps and protocols. Placing lesions in the center of echograms is an important objective in order to display the best quality images:

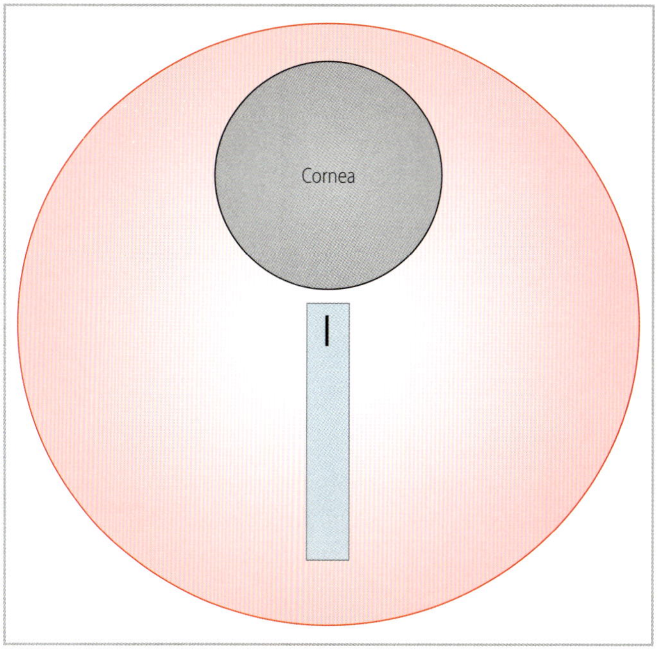

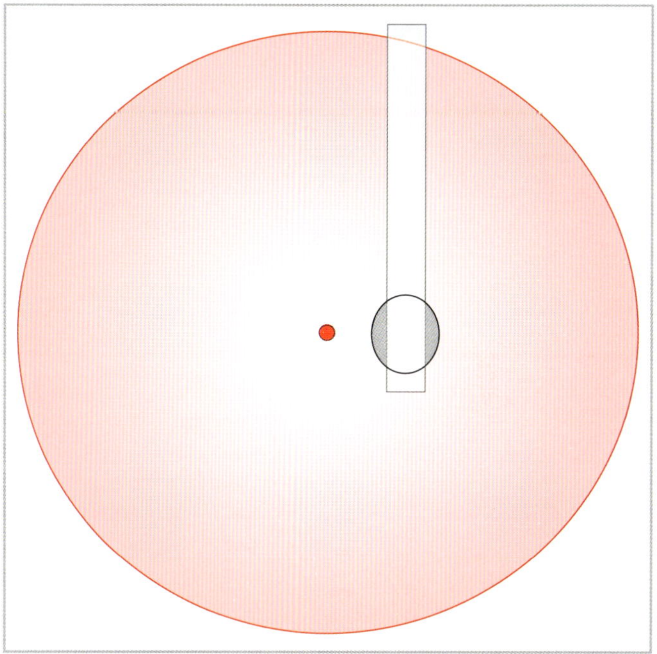

Figure 4.36 Top: longitudinal L 12 probe on globe. Bottom: longitudinal L 12 beam on fundus.

1. Topical anesthetic is instilled into the eye. Examination is conducted through open lids, directly on the globe
2. Coupling jelly, e.g. methylcellulose, is applied onto the tip of the probe
3. Four transverse sections (**Figure 4.43**) are performed as follows:
   - **a.** Transverse 12 – The patient looks up. The probe is placed at the 6 o'clock limbus with its marker nasally. Shifting and rotating the probe from limbus to fornix and scanning the superior retina posterior–anteriorly
   - **b.** Transverse 3 – The patient looks toward 3 o'clock and the probe is placed at the 9 o'clock limbus with its marker up. The probe is shifted and rotated from limbus to fornix, scanning

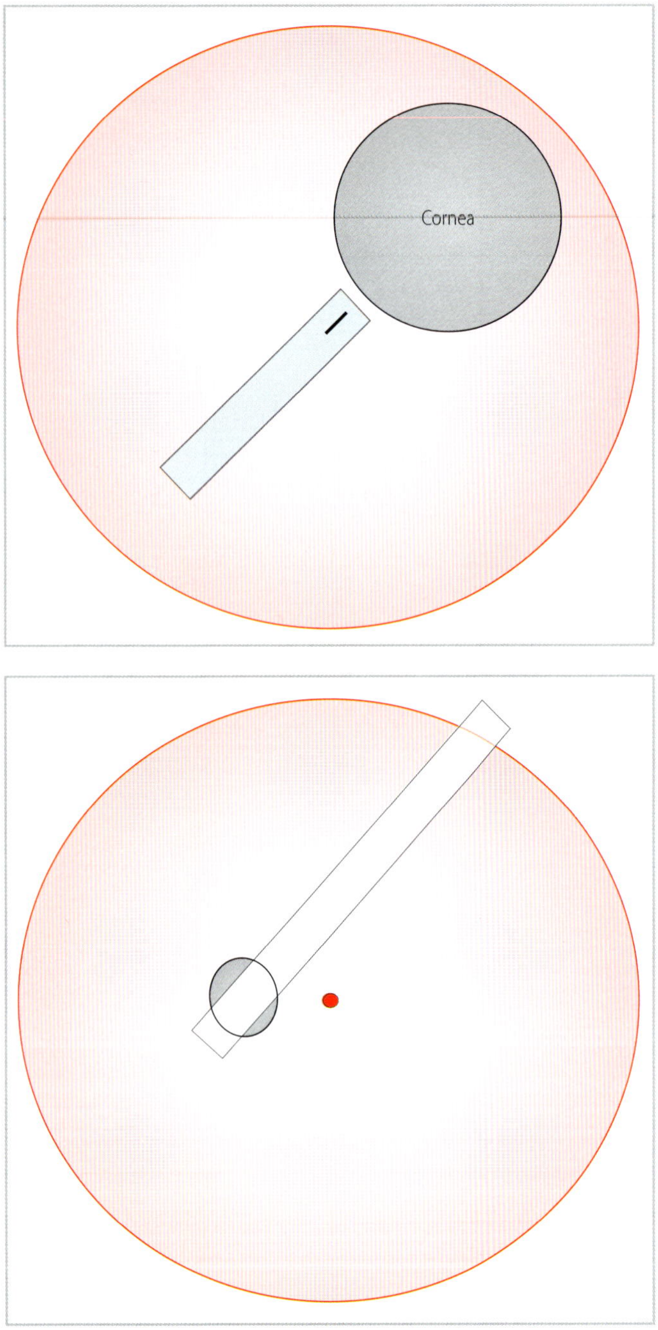

Figure 4.37 Top: longitudinal L1.30 probe on the globe. Bottom: longitudinal L1.30 beam on the fundus.

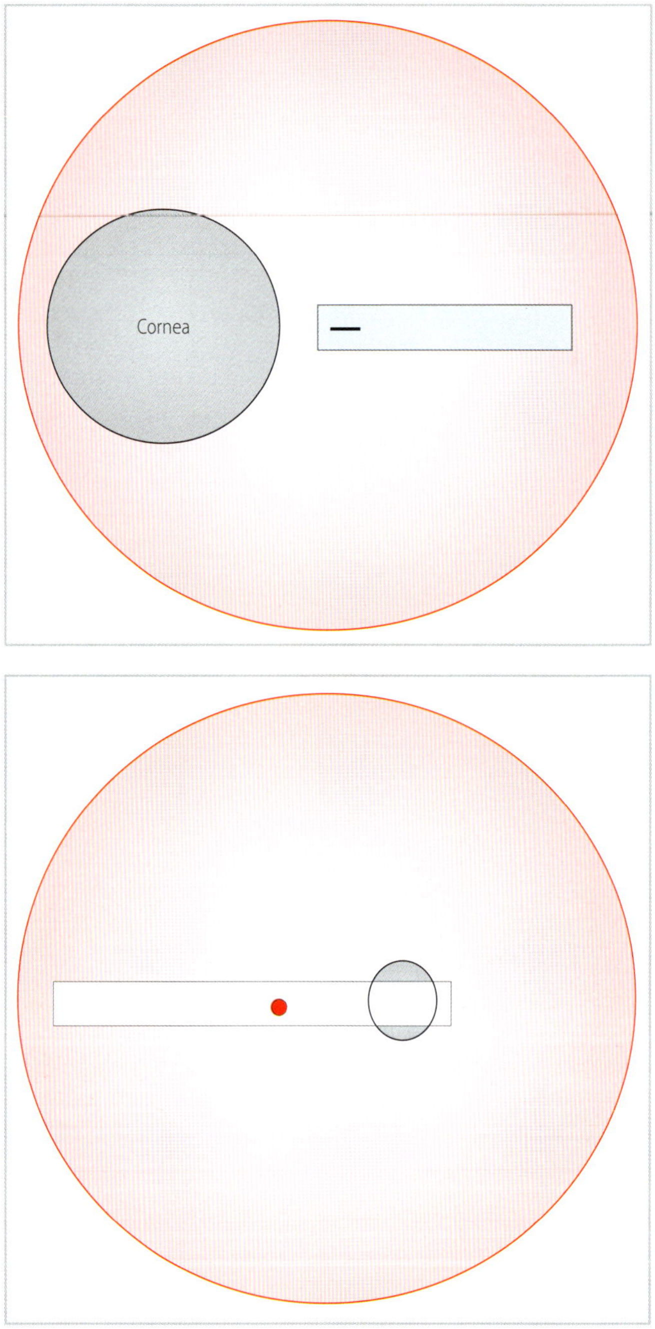

Figure 4.38 Top: longitudinal L9 right eye probe on the globe. Bottom: longitudinal L9 right eye beam on the fundus.

the nasal retina in the right eye and temporal retina in the left eye posterior–anteriorly

c. Transverse 6 – The patient looks down. The probe is placed at the 12 o'clock limbus with its marker nasally. Shifting and rotating the probe from limbus to fornix and scanning the inferior retina posterior–anteriorly

d. Transverse 9 – The patient looks toward 9 o'clock and the probe is placed at the 3 o'clock limbus, with its marker up. The probe is shifted and rotated from limbus to fornix, scanning the temporal retina in the right eye and nasal retina in the left eye posterior–anteriorly

These sections will overlap four quadrants of the globe wall; e.g. T12 and T3 sections will overlap the supranasal quadrant in the right eye and supratemporal quadrant in the left eye, thus ensuring that lesions are not missed. In addition, scanning of the periphery will ensure the detection of important lesions that are only located at the peripheral fundus, e.g. retinal breaks retinoschisis, ciliary body detachment, and ciliary body mass

4. Additional transverse scans of any of the other clock hour meridians, e.g. 1:30, 4:30, 7:30, and 10:30, may be performed in a similar fashion, if an abnormality is suspected at the given meridian. The aim is always to place lesions in the center of the echogram

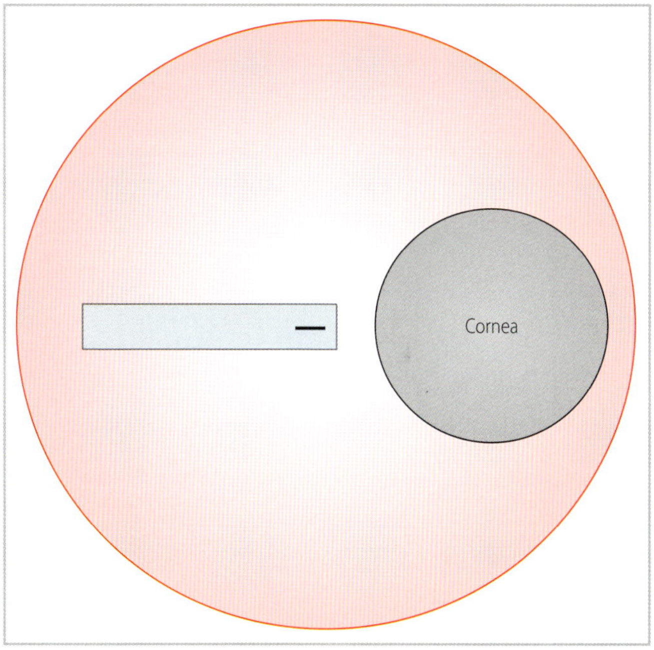

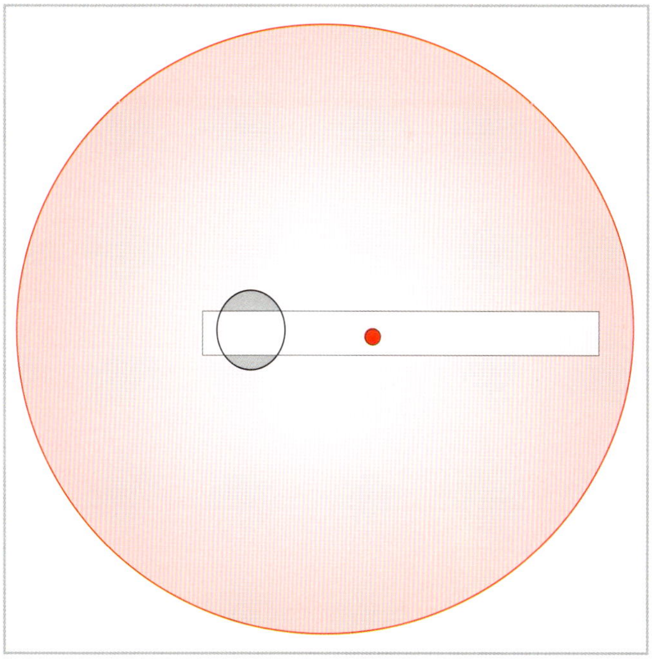

Figure 4.39 Top: longitudinal L3 left eye probe on the globe. Bottom: longitudinal L3 left eye beam on the fundus.

5. Scans are performed first with a high dB gain to detect low reflective echoes, e.g. fine vitreous opacities, and then repeated with a lower gain to achieve higher resolution, e.g. for better definition of layers of the globe wall and accurate measurement of mass dimensions. Experienced examiners tend to alter the dB gain setting a number of times during the dynamic scanning to produce the best images and gather the maximum information required for a given case
6. If no abnormalities are found after employing the above protocol, no further examination is usually required. If a lesion is detected, longitudinal and axial sections are additionally performed. Multiple sections are helpful for viewing lesions at different angles, locating their clock hour meridian and anterior–posterior position and creating the three-dimensional impression

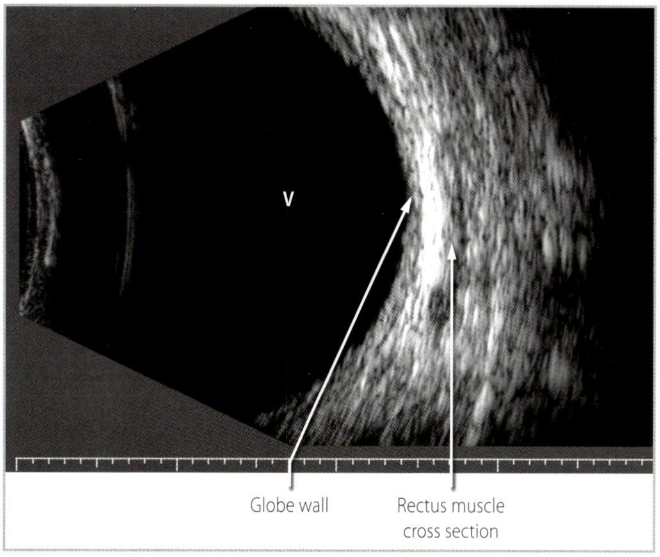

Figure 4.40 Transverse scan: normal echogram. V, vitreous (echo silent).

Normal and abnormal B-scan results

In eye-dedicated scanners, B-scan echograms are read from left (probe contact with globe) to right (orbital echoes). In some other scanners, it is read from top to bottom of the echogram. In axial scans, the lens and optic nerve are displayed. The optic nerve produces a characteristic V-shaped dark shadow in an otherwise bright (high reflective) homogeneous orbital pattern (**Figure 4.34**).

In a longitudinal scan, the optic nerve head and anterior portion of the retrobulbar optic nerve are displayed at the bottom of the echogram. At the top is the fundus periphery and ciliary body (**Figure 4.35**). In L12 and L6 sections, the dark shadow of the superior and inferior recti is displayed in the orbit pattern. In L3 and L9, the shadow of the medial and lateral recti is displayed.

In a transverse scan, the lens and optic nerve shadow are not normally displayed and cross section of a rectus muscle can be seen in its corresponding location (**Figure 4.40**). In normal globe scans no echoes are seen in the vitreous cavity, the normal globe contour is observed, and no membrane or mass lesion is encountered. Globe lesions that produce an abnormal B-scan can be summarized into four categories:

1. Membrane lesion – This includes retinal detachment (**Figure 4.15**), retinoschisis, choroidal detachment (**Figure 4.44**), PVD (**Figure 4.28**), and 'cord' as seen in persistent hyperplastic primary vitreous. **Table 4.4** displays the echographic features of common membrane lesions
2. Mass lesion – This includes melanoma (**Figure 4.45**), nevus, metastasis, hemangioma, macular disciform (**Figure 4.46**), and eccentric disciform lesions and other rarer masses such as tuberous sclerosis and inflammatory nodules. **Table 4.5** displays the echographic features of common mass lesions
3. Discreet opacities – This can be either multiple as in asteroid hyalosis (**Figure 4.10**) and VH (**Figure 4.47**) or single as in intraocular foreign body
4. Globe wall abnormalities – This includes globe deformities/staphyloma (**Figure 4.11**) and calcification of the globe wall as in idiopathic sclerochoroidal calcification, choroidal osteoma, disc drusen, and phithisis bulbi. Posterior scleritis is also included in

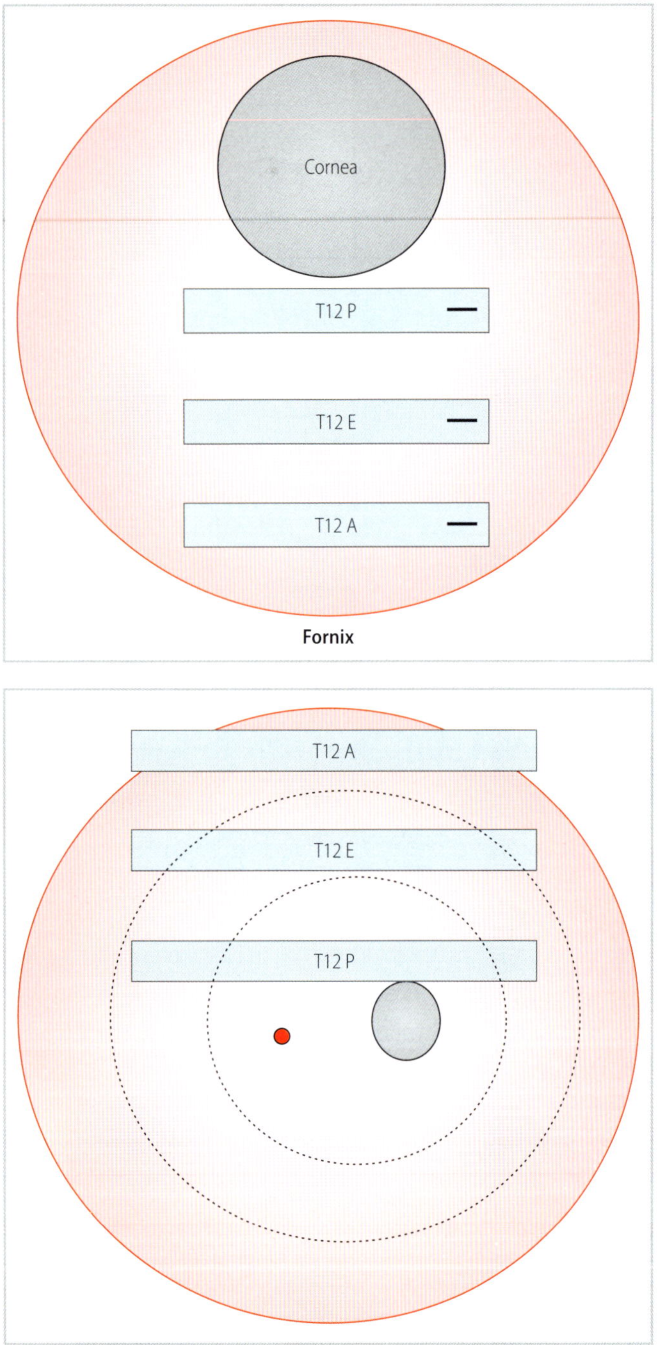

Figure 4.41 Top: transverse T12 right eye probe on the globe. Bottom: transverse T12 right eye beam on the fundus.

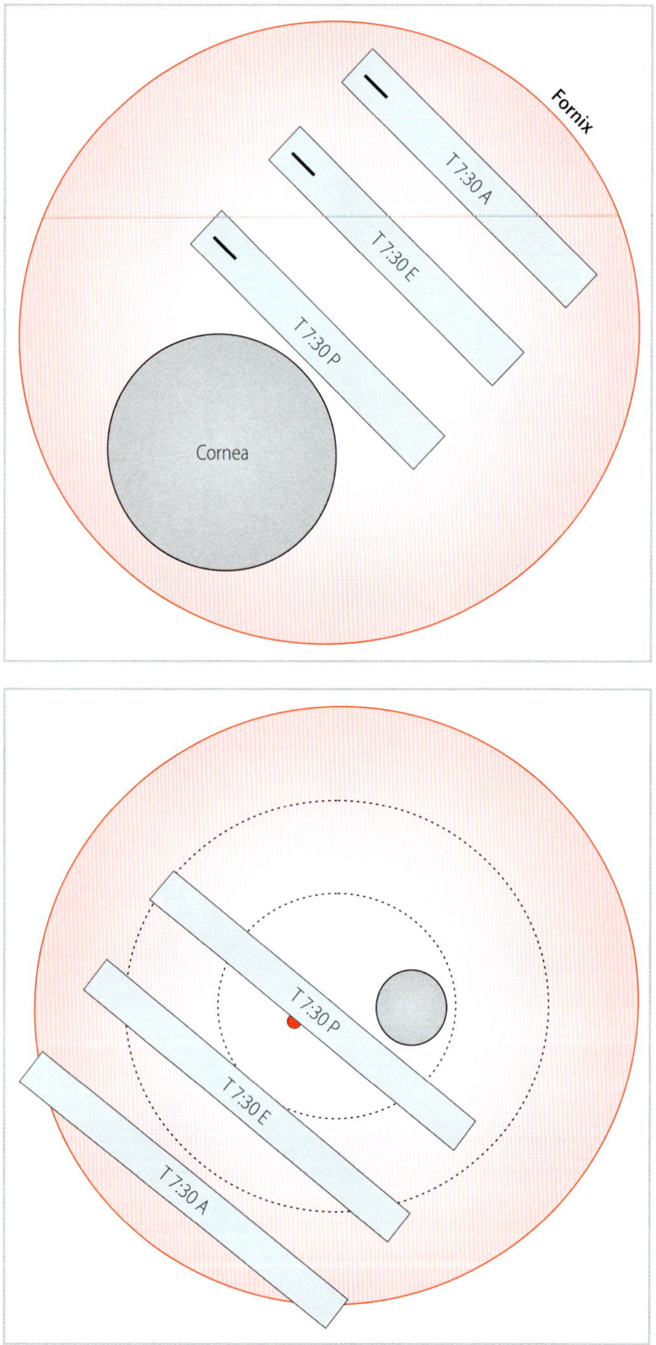

Figure 4.42 Top: transverse T7.30 right eye probe on the globe. Bottom: transverse T7.30 right eye beam on the fundus.

this category and is considered an important ultrasound function that provides positive diagnosis of a disease that otherwise would be diagnosed only by exclusion (**Figure 4.48**)

Artifacts

The examiner needs to be aware of artifacts that are commonly encountered during B-scanning. Some artifacts are undesirable and are caused by poor technique such as inadequate jell/weak contact between probe and globe (**Figure 4.49**), and reverberation from IOL implant when scanning axially. Other artifacts are desirable as they indicate specific abnormality and help make the diagnosis, e.g. shadowing from calcification, ringing and shadowing from intraocular foreign body, and retained oil bubbles (**Figure 4.50**).

DISORDERS

Macular degeneration

Ultrasound is a useful compliment to other modalities in the investigation of macular degeneration, particularly when fundoscopy and retinal imaging are hampered by media opacity. The most common

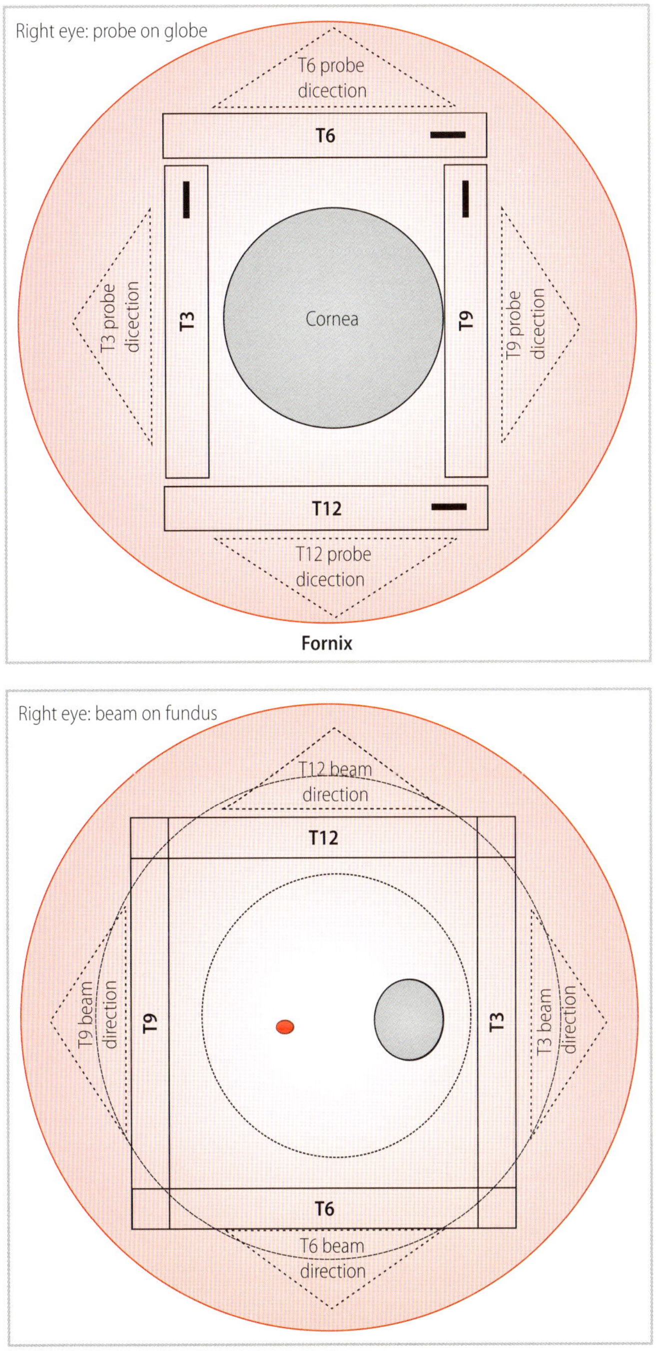

Figure 4.43 Screening of the globe with four overlapping B-scan sections.

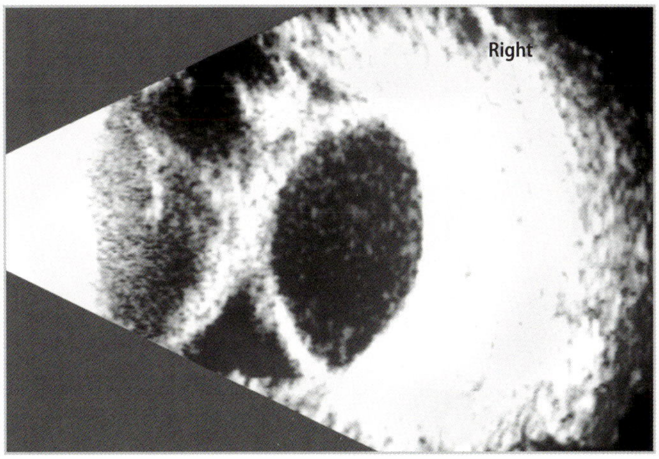

Figure 4.44 B-scan showing two high dome-shaped choroidal detachments producing the characteristic appearance of kissing choroids.

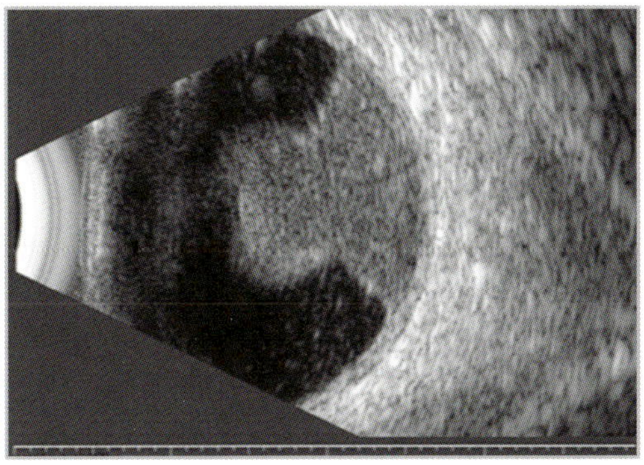

Figure 4.45 Characteristic mushroom-shaped choroidal melanoma.

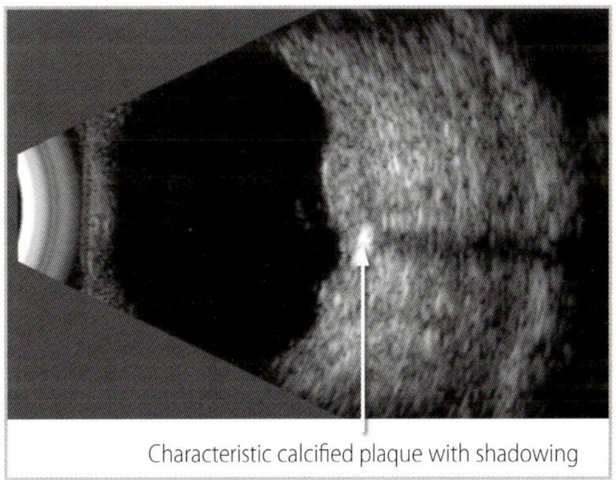

Figure 4.46 Disciform macular mass lesion.

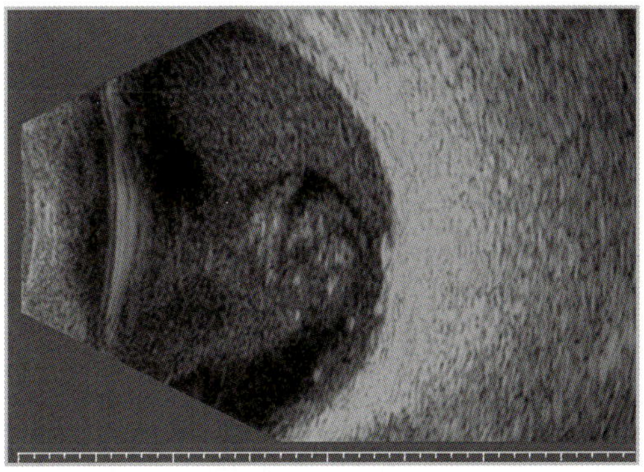

Figure 4.47 Dense, scattered echoes of vitreous hemorrhage.

clinical example is a bleeding disciform macular lesion resulting in dense VH (**Figure 4.51**). This may occasionally be the first presentation of otherwise asymptomatic macular disease, and ultrasound is the only method of detecting the preexisting macular disease. Another possible clinical scenario is the discovery of a macular mass lesion during ultrasound screening of a patient with dense cataract. A further application of ocular ultrasound is in the tissue diagnosis of disciform macular lesion and in differentiating it from other macular masses, even in clear media (Byrne 1984).

Ultrasound plays an important role in the detection of eccentric disciform or peripheral choroidal vascular tumors (PCVT). These lesions develop as a manifestation of age-related hemorrhagic and

Table 4.4 Echographic features of common membrane lesions

Data (scan mode)	Choroidal detachment	Retinal detachment	PVD
Topographic (B)			
Insertion into globe wall	Acute (dome shaped)	Gradual	Variable
Location	Peripheral	Variable	Variable
Attachment to optic nerve	No	Yes	Variable
Other	Kissing choroids Vortex vein	Folds Breaks	Thicker Inferiorly
Quantitative (A)			
Reflectivity	90–100%	80–100%	40–80%
Spike features	Double peaked, thick	Single peak, thick	Single peak, thin
Kinetic (B)			
Motility	Absent-minimal	Moderate	Marked

PVD, posterior vitreous detachment

Table 4.5 Echographic features of common mass lesions

Data (scan mode)	Choroidal melanoma	Choroidal metastasis	Choroidal hemangioma
Topographic (B)			
Shape	Dome Mushroom (unique)	Dome/Bidome Irregular, focal	Dome Smooth, diffuse
Location	Variable	Near macula	Near disc or diffuse
Associated retinal detachment	Variable	Common	Rare
Growth	Variable	Rapid	Slow
Quantitative (A)			
Reflectivity	Low/medium	Variable	High
Internal structure	Regular	Irregular	Regular
Sound attenuation	Strong	Variable	Weak
Kinetic (A and B)			
Vascularity	Present	Absent	Absent

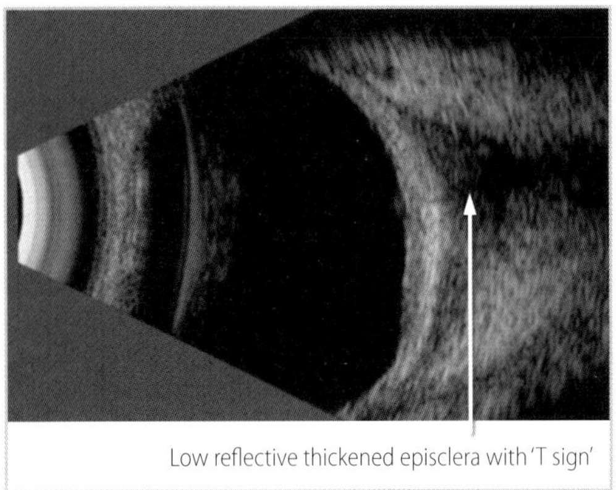

Figure 4.48 Posterior scleritis.

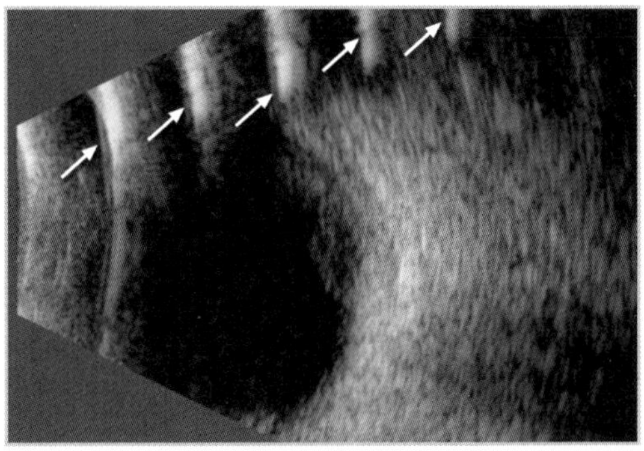

Figure 4.49 Artifacts (arrows) caused by poor probe globe contact.

exudative choroidal neovascularization, a disease process similar to macular disciform degeneration but with a peripheral location. By the nature of their peripheral location, often they remain asymptomatic until they bleed into the vitreous or are discovered incidentally during fundus examination. PCVT should therefore be included in the differential diagnosis of causes of VH, particularly in the elderly.

On B-scan ultrasound, a disciform lesion presents usually as an irregularly outlined mass with occasional one or more foci of calcification causing a shadowing effect (**Figure 4.46**). Calcification is frequently encountered in long-standing cases as it represents a healing process. The presence of calcification is a helpful diagnostic feature. Another characteristic finding is the detection of overlying pockets of sensory

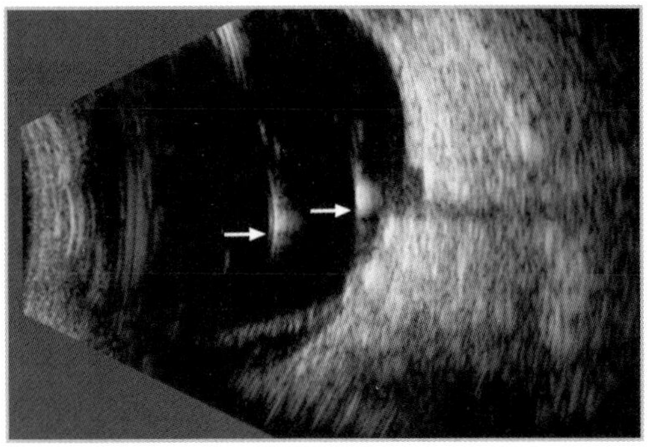

Figure 4.50 Artifacts: shadowing caused by silicone oil bubbles (arrows).

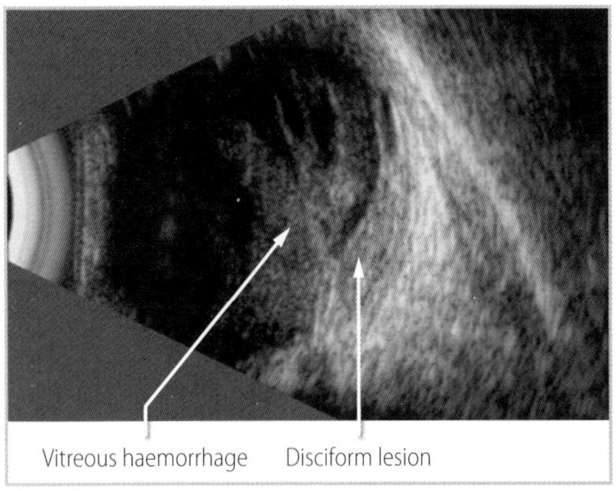

Figure 4.51 A bleeding disciform lesion.

retinal detachment. On A-scan examination, disciform lesions show variable reflectivity, irregular internal structure, and absent vascularity.

Purely on echographic findings, disciform lesions have features similar to choroidal metastasis with the exception of calcification. In such cases, a few weeks of observation should reveal rapid growth of metastasis and no growth or even regression of the size of disciform lesions. As described in the paragraph on B-scan techniques, the best sections to show the macula are T9 P and L9 on the right and T3 P and L3 on the left.

Choroidal disorders

Ultrasound is an important investigation in cases of choroidal folds. Its primary function is to rule out a retrobulbar orbital mass such as optic nerve swelling, an orbital mass such as hemangioma where folds are located at the posterior pole, and a lacrimal gland tumor where folds are normally discovered at a supratemporal fundus location. Posterior scleritis is a cause of choroidal folds and is easily diagnosed on ultrasound (**Figure 4.48**). In many cases, choroidal folds are idiopathic and ultrasound is helpful in ruling out orbital causes. It will often show flattening of the globe wall and reduction in axial eye length accompanied clinically by progressive hypermetropia over time (Atta 1988).

Optic nerve disorders

Ultrasound is a method of choice in the detection of optic nerve head drusen as it shows, very readily, the calcification at the nerve head with its characteristic shadowing effect (**Figure 4.52**). It is also a good method for eliciting buried nerve drusen. Generally, ultrasound is useful in cases of optic disc swelling in drusen or other causes of nerve head disorders (Atta 1988). On many occasions, an ultrasound may avert the need to subject the patient to more expensive investigations such as CT and MRI.

The best images of optic nerve head drusen are obtained at a relatively low dB gain setting to enhance the high reflective, calcified, nature of the drusen caused by the high calcium contents. Care must be taken not to confuse a bright disc papilla with drusen, and the diagnosis of disc drusen must only be made in cases where calcification and shadowing are clearly demonstrated.

Intraocular neoplasms

The ocular masses have already been briefly mentioned. The distinguishing quantitative A-scan features of three ocular neoplasms are illustrated in **Figure 4.27**, and a summary of all the echographic data is summarized in **Table 4.5**. In this section, a more detailed description is given of each of the three main ocular tumors, namely choroidal melanoma, choroidal metastasis, and choroidal hemangioma. The echographic appearance of choroidal osteoma is also presented.

Choroidal melanoma

Topographically, choroidal melanoma appears as a smooth dome or a mushroom-shaped solid mass on B-scan (**Figure 4.45**). The mass is a very diagnostic feature. Rarely, it presents as the diffuse melanoma type and appears as a slight irregular thickening of the choroidal layer extending over a wide area of the globe wall (Byrne 2002). A dome-shaped tumor centered in the beam path may produce the well-known choroidal excavation. Because of the low reflective nature of melanoma, the characteristic feature of acoustic hollowing has been described. Less commonly B-scan images can show irregular internal architecture in large tumors and, more rarely, ossification (Chan et al. 1995). Melanoma can occupy any part of the fundus and may be associated with retinal detachment, indicating initiation or acceleration of growth. Careful scanning of the entire tumor base is important to exclude extrascleral extension, a significant prognostic finding that is likely not to be detected on clinical examination and

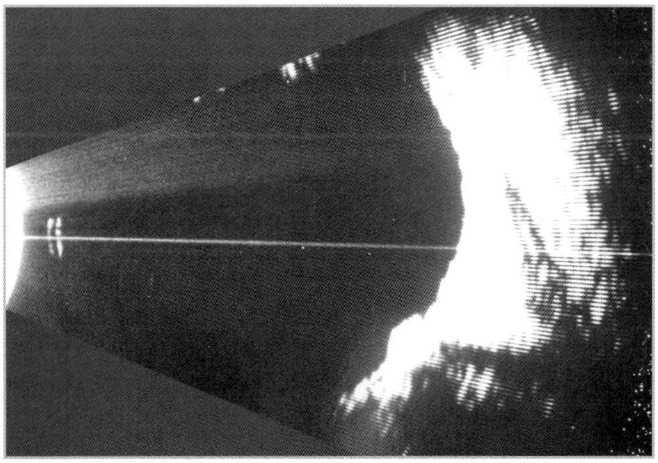

Figure 4.52 Calcified disc drusen with shadowing effect.

by using other retinal imaging techniques. Precise localization and measurement of the tumor are undertaken on B-scan by performing transverse, longitudinal, and occasional axial sections. The lateral (base) dimensions are obtained from B-scans, and measurement of the tumor height is performed on well-centered B-scan and more accurately on standardized A-scan. The precise localization and measurements of the tumor are required by the oncologist to accurately place the scleral plaque and deliver the correct dose of radiation treatment.

A quantitative examination involves A-scan assessment of reflectivity, internal structure, and sound attenuation. Malignant melanoma produces low-to-medium reflective, regularly structured lesion spikes, with medium-to-high sound attenuation. On kinetic echography, vascularity is common and is diagnostic. On A-scan this appears as fine, fast, vertical oscillation of echoes within the tumor mass. In very vascular, commonly mushroom-shaped lesions vascularity is also evident on B-scan. The A-scan appearance of choroidal melanoma is shown in **Figure 4.27** and also in **Figure 4.53**, which displays the average spike height of a tumor (25%), indicating low reflective lesion.

Choroidal metastasis

On topographic B-scan evaluation, choroidal metastases appear as dome-shaped lesions (**Figure 4.54**) but more characteristically as masses with an irregular outline. They are most frequently located in the posterior pole. Choroidal metastases tend to be associated with extensive retinal detachment, a manifestation of rapid growth (Byrne 2002). More than one lesion in the same eye and bilateral presentation are not uncommon, and follow-up studies usually illustrate rapid growth of the tumor over a relatively short period of time (few weeks).

A quantitative examination on A-scan shows a variable reflectivity depending on the primary lesion. The internal structure is irregular, and the sound attenuation is weak. Vascularity in metastasis is normally not detected, but it has been rarely reported in some cases of small cell carcinoma of the lung (Verbeek 1981). **Figure 4.54** illustrates the echographic appearance of choroidal metastasis from a primary carcinoma of the lung.

Choroidal hemangioma

Topographically, choroidal hemangioma appears either as a bright, solitary, dome-shaped, solid lesion located at the posterior pole and around the disc or macula or as a diffuse thickening of the choroidal layer that is commonly associated with Sturge-Weber syndrome (Byrne 2002). Hemangioma tends to remain static or grow very slowly and rarely produces retinal detachment, but localized focal cystic retinal changes may be seen in long-standing cases.

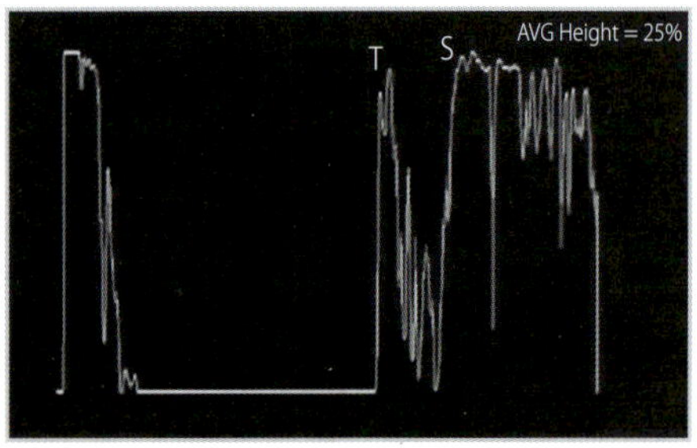

Figure 4.53 Typical A-scan appearance of choroidal melanoma. S, sclera; T, tumor surface.

Quantitative examination shows a very highly reflective, regularly structured tissue, producing weak sound attenuation. This appears to correlate well with the coarse, honeycomb histological structure of these lesions. On kinetic examination, although choroidal hemangiomas are classified as vascular hamartomas, they do not show the fast moving spikes on A-scan, as the large honeycomb spaces are filled with stagnant blood, with no significant blood flow. **Figure 4.55** illustrates the echographic appearance of choroidal hemangioma in A-and B-scans.

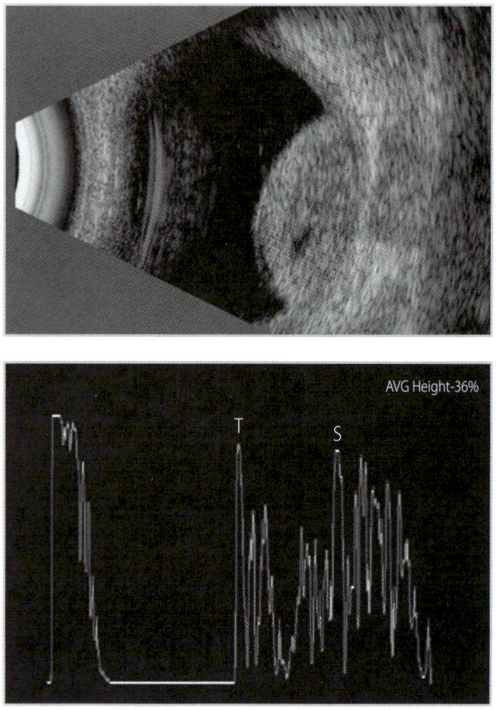

Figure 4.54 Top: large dome-shaped choroidal metastasis from lung carcinoma. Bottom: irregular A-scan pattern. S, sclera; T, tumor surface.

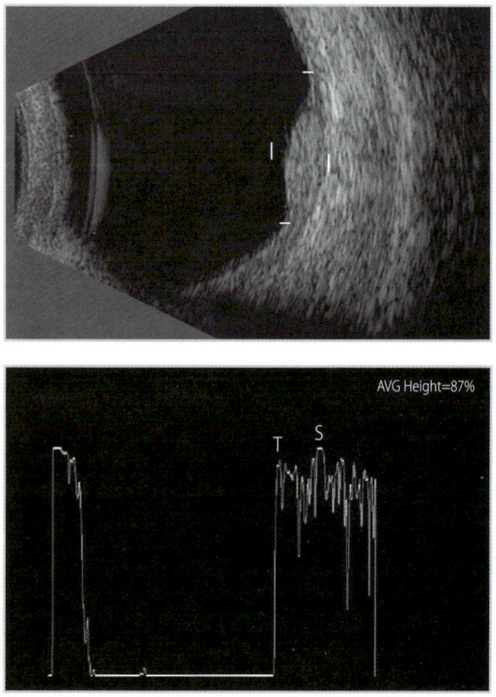

Figure 4.55 Top: solitary dome-shaped hemangioma (callipers are placed to measure the base and height of the lesion). Bottom: typical A-scan appearance (very height reflective lesion with an average spike height of 87%). S, sclera; T, tumor surface.

Choroidal osteoma

Ultrasound is a useful modality in the diagnosis of suspected choroidal osteoma because of the calcification and shadowing effect that is readily seen on B-scan, especially at low dB gain settings. Normally, choroidal osteomas are unilateral and are located at the posterior pole or at the macula. They are either flat (only showing a calcified but flat globe wall) or slightly elevated in an irregular pattern (**Figure 4.56**) (Gass 1997). Scanning of both eyes is recommended in such cases to rule out idiopathic sclerochoroidal calcification that looks similar to choroidal osteoma on ultrasound but presents more commonly as bilateral multiple lesions that are located more peripherally in the globe wall (Hanover et al. 2001).

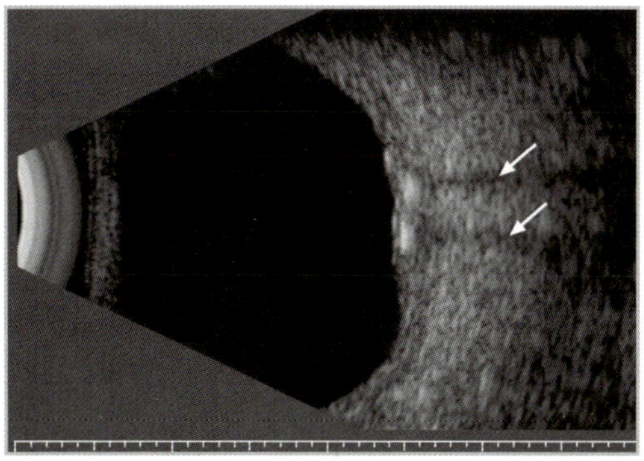

Figure 4.56 Choroidal osteoma presenting as an irregular calcified lesion with a shadowing effect (arrows).

REFERENCES

Atta HR. Ophthalmic ultrasound—a practical guide. Oxford: Butterworth Heinemann, 1996. ISBN 0443047731.

Atta HR. Imaging of the optic nerve with standardised echography. *Eye* 1988; **2**:358–366.

Atta HR, Byrne SF. The findings of standardized echography for choroidal folds. *Arch Ophthalmol* 1988; **106**:1234–1241.

Baum G, Greenwood I. The application of ultrasonic locating techniques to ophthalmology: theoretic considerations and acoustic properties of ocular media: part 1. Reflective properties. *Am J Ophthalmol* 1958; **46**:319–329.

Bronson NR, Turner FT. A simple B-scan ultrasonoscope. *Arch Ophthalmol* 1973; **90**:237–238.

Byrne SF. Differential diagnosis of disciform lesions using standardized echography. In: Hillman JS, LeMay MM (eds.), Ophthalmic echography. Dordrecht: Dr W Junk, 1984:149.

Byrne SF, Green RL. Ultrasound of the eye and orbit, 2nd edn. St Louis: Mosby, 2002. ISBN 0323 012078.

Chan TKJ, Atta HR, Scott GB. Ossification in choroidal melanoma. *Br J Ophthalmol* 1995; **79**:705.

Coleman DJ, Lizzi FL, Jack RL. Ultrasonography of the eye and orbit. Philadelphia: Lea & Febiger, 1977.

Fish PJ. Physics and instrumentation of diagnostic medical ultrasound. Chichester: Wiley, 1990. ISBN 0471926515.

Gass JDM. Stereoscopic atlas of macular diseases – diagnosis and treatment. 4th edn. St Louis: Mosby, 1997.

Gernet H. Biometrie des Auges mit Ultraschall. *Klin Monatsbl Augenheilkd* 1965; **146**:863–874.

Hanover SG, Shields CL, Demirci H, et al. Sclerochoroidal calcification. *Arch Ophthalmol* 2001; **119**:833.

Lerski RA. Practical ultrasound. Oxford: Iris Press, 1988. ISBN 1852210680.

Mundt GH, Hughes WE. Ultrasonics in ocular diagnosis. *Am J Ophthalmol* 1956; **41**:488–498.

Oksala A, Lehtinen A. Diagnostic value of ultrasonics in ophthalmology. *Ophthalmologica* 1957; **134**:387–395 (In German).

Ossoinig KC. Quantitative echography – the basis of tissue differentiation. *J Clin Ultrasound* 1974; **2**:33–46.

Ossoinig KC. Standardized echography: basic principles, clinical applications and results. *Int Ophthalmol Clin* 1979; **19**:127–210.

Pavlin CJ, Sherar MD, Harasiewicz K, et al. Clinical use of ultrasound biomicroscopy. *Ophthalmology* 1991; **98**:287–295.

Purnell EW. B-mode orbital ultrasonography. *Int Ophthalmol Clin* 1969; **9**:643–665.

Verbeek AM. A choroidal oat-cell carcinoma metastasis mimicking a choroidal melanoma. In: Thijssen JM, Verbeek AM (eds.), Ultrasonography in ophthalmology. Dordrecht: Dr W Junk, 1981:131.

Winder S, Atta HR. Ultrasonography of the optic disc cup in discs of various sizes. *Eye* 1996; **10**:732–736.

Chapter 5 Autofluorescence imaging

Victor Chong

INTRODUCTION

Fundus autofluorescence (AF) is defined as the signal detected when the fundus is illuminated with light. It was first observed with optic nerve drusen (**Figure 5.1**). These lesions can be seen before the injection of the dye while performing fluorescein angiography with conventional film-based camera. With the advance of scanning laser ophthalmoscopy, small and more subtle changes can be detected.

It is widely believed that the key component of the autofluorescent material is lipofuscin. At the retinal pigment epithelium (RPE) level, accumulation of lipofuscin occurs as a result of aging (Feeney 1978, Wing et al. 1978) and also linked to retinal diseases (Dorey et al. 1989). Lipofuscin accumulates in post-mitotic cells, such as those in the skin, brain, heart, and liver, as a result of degradation of organelles and macromolecules in lysosomes. However, in the RPE, lipofuscin is also produced during incomplete breakdown of photoreceptors' outer segment discs. Melanin granules accumulate in the apical portion of the RPE; lipofuscin granules are found in central and basal parts of the cell.

Imaging techniques

In 1995 von Ruckmann and colleagues published the first fundus AF images, which were obtained using a modified Zeiss confocal scanning laser ophthalmoscope (cSLO) with a blue excitation light filter of 488 nm and a barrier filter at 521 nm (von Ruckmann et al. 1995). The signals were collected on a videotape. The images were obtained by summation software overlaying the weak signals and eliminating the noise in a process based on the assumption that the signal is constant but noise is random. This process had to be carried out in the laboratory, limiting its use in clinical practice (**Figure 5.2**).

Fundus AF gained popularity throughout the world when imaging became practical using a commercially available Heidelberg HRA. This uses cSLO technology instead of using videotape, multiple images are obtained, and the summation is carried out by the same machine in real time. So an AF image can be viewed almost immediately after it has been taken.

AF imaging was further gaining acceptance when Spaide (2003) suggested that images can be obtained by modifying a Topcon fundus camera. This flash-based technique is slightly different, as multiple flashes are uncomfortable for patients, and summation software is not present on the camera, so the AF images are obtained by increasing the sensitivity of the digital camera by adjusting the gain (**Figure 5.3 a, b**).

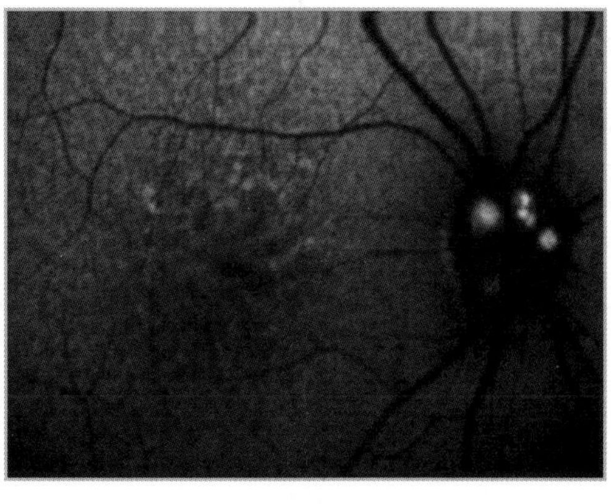

Figure 5.1 Autofluorescence (AF) imaging of the optic nerve head shows brightly fluorescent lobular drusen. The underlying AF signals from the retinal pigment epithelium cells are less intense.

Piccolino and colleagues reported the occurrence of AF in the near-infrared range when acquiring images of the fundus prior to the injection of indocyanine green (ICG) (Piccolino et al. 1996) while using the HRA setting for ICG angiography; this technique is now referred to as near-infrared autofluorescence (NIA). The NIA signals most likely emanates from melanin and melanin compounds in the RPE. A contribution from choroidal melanin appeared evident, with (**Figure 5.4 a, b**) an increased signal at the site of choroidal nevi and choroidal vessels (Keilhauer & Delori 2006). As NIA is relatively new and it is difficult to obtain good quality images in many patients, it remains mostly a research tool and is not discussed further in this chapter.

Differences between imaging machines

There are two main classes of machine available for obtaining AF images: one is confocal against non-confocal and the other is SLO against flash based. By using different wavelengths (color) for the emitting light and filters, the AF images appear different. Understanding these differences is important in arriving at the diagnosis.

For instance, NIA is a good example of using different emitting light/filter based on the cSLO technology. The other main reason for using different emitting light is to reduce the impact of macular pigment in the foveal area. The conventional shorter wavelength (blue) blocks the underlying AF signals from RPE, but a longer wavelength (green) lets transmission through the RPE.

At the time of writing (2013), a number of machines can acquire AF images; the details were collected by Professor Giovanni Staurenghi from Milan (**Table 5.1**). As companies change specifications on a regular basis, readers should check their machine's specification before using it for diagnosis.

Comparing SLO and flash-based images, the SLO images are more clearly defined due to the use of summation. In addition, a cataract can increase light scattering in a flash-based system, making the AF images hazy; this limits the use of the flash-based system in those with a cataract. In young patients with a clear lens or in those who are pseudophakic, the light scattering effect is minimal. The main and probably only reason for choosing a flash-based system is cost, as it is usually a relatively low-cost option, using an otherwise standard flash-based fundus camera.

In terms of confocal versus non-confocal, the confocal system can pick up AF materials from different level of the retina; for instance, when there are an AF signal from RPE and an AF signal from materials in the subretinal space, a confocal system can distinguish the two. It is currently unclear how important this is in a clinical setting using SLO-based machines. In particular, the current non-confocal SLO has a different emitting light/filter, making direct comparison difficult.

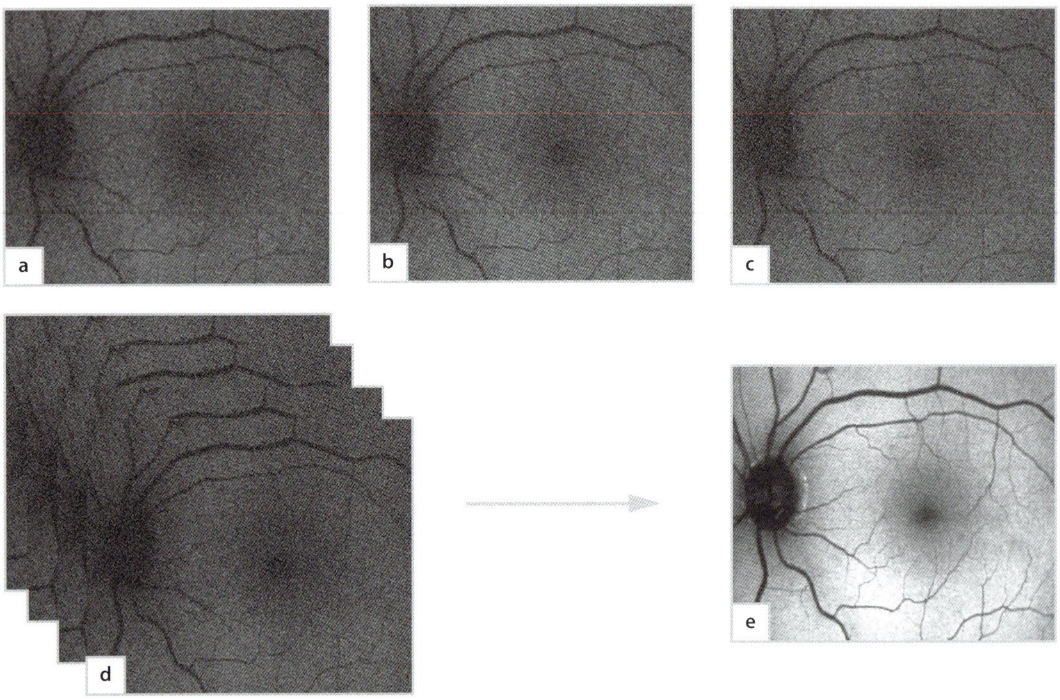

Figure 5.2 (a–e) The images were obtained by using summation software overlaying the weak signals and eliminating the noise based on the assumption that signal is constant while noise is random.

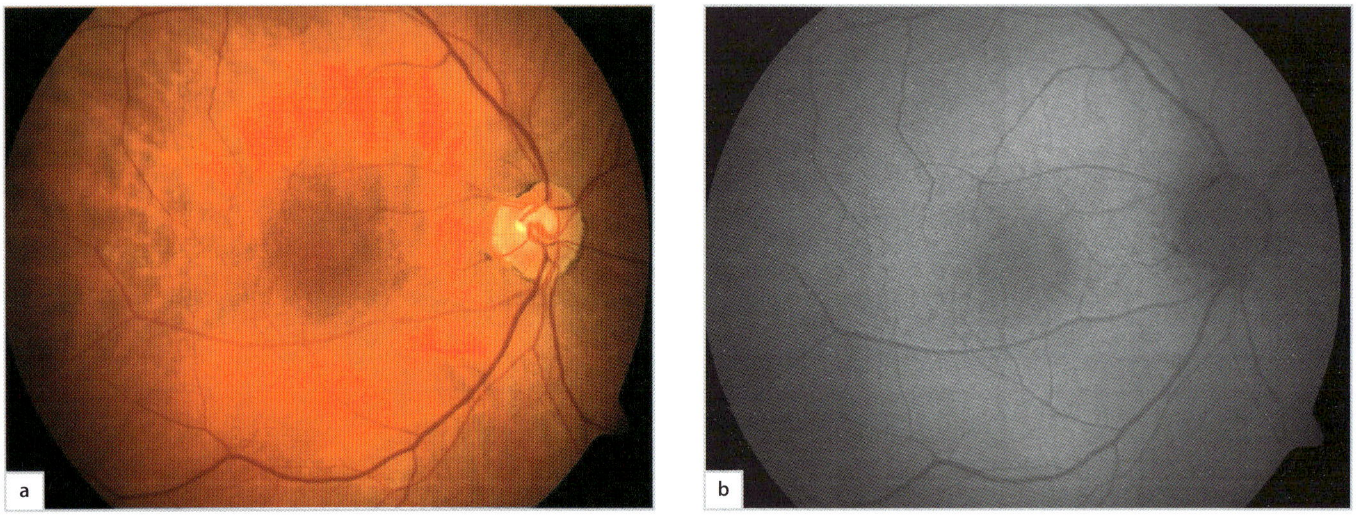

Figure 5.3 (a) The right eye shows normal fundus architecture. (b) The same eye showing autofluorescence acquired through a flash-based camera system.

Table 5.1 Comparison of the specifications of different autofluorescence machines

Machine	SLO	Confocal	Excitation wavelength (nm)	Barrier wavelength (nm)
Heidelberg HRA	Yes	Yes	488	495
Nidek F10	Yes	Yes	490	510
Optos Optomap	Yes	No	532	>600
Topcon	No	No	535–585	605–715
Zeiss 450	No	No	510–580	695–755
Canon CX-1	No	No	514–596	640
Kowa VX-20	No	No	490–610	630–750
Heidelberg HRA (NIA)	Yes	Yes	790	810

PRINCIPLES OF IMAGE INTERPRETATION

Normal distribution of fundus autofluorescence

The normal distribution of fundus AF is shown in **Figure 5.3** and **Figure 5.4**. Bearing in mind that the main AF signal comes from the RPE cells, anything that blocks the RPE, either totally or partially, would appear black or hypofluorescent, respectively. The optic nerve appears dark due to the absence of the lipofuscin-laden cells responsible for the AF signal.

Retinal vessels appear dark due to blood blocking the signal from the underlying RPE cells. The foveal area demonstrates a reduced AF signal (hypofluorescence) due to light absorption by the macular luteal pigment. A homogeneous AF signal is observed elsewhere.

As a general rule, the presence of a normal AF signal indicates a normal turnover of the outer segment photoreceptors and a healthy RPE supporting a normal retinoid cycle. However, one has to remember that with current imaging techniques, quantitative measurement is not possible; in other words, an increased AF signal of an area in a particular patient is that this area has increased signal as compared to the surrounding areas. However, a diffuse increase in AF signals, as seen for instance in some patients with age-related macular degeneration (AMD), cannot be detected.

Main causes of abnormal autofluorescence (Figure 5.5)

The main causes of increased AF signal (hyperfluorescence) are:

- Reduced clearance of lipofuscin by the RPE
- Increased turnover of photoreceptor outer segments
- Other cells, such as microglia or macrophages, contain lipofuscin
- Window defects, such as loss of retinal tissue in a full thickness macular hole

The main causes of decrease AF signal (hypofluorescence) are:

- Reduced turnover of photoreceptor outer segments
- RPE inactivity
- RPE loss
- Any material blocking the signal, such as blood and exudates

CLINICAL APPLICATIONS

The key advantages of AF imaging over angiogram are the noninvasiveness and simple method of acquiring the images. Some of the early clinical uses of AF imaging, for instance in distinguishing full thickness macular hole from pseudohole, have been succeeded by

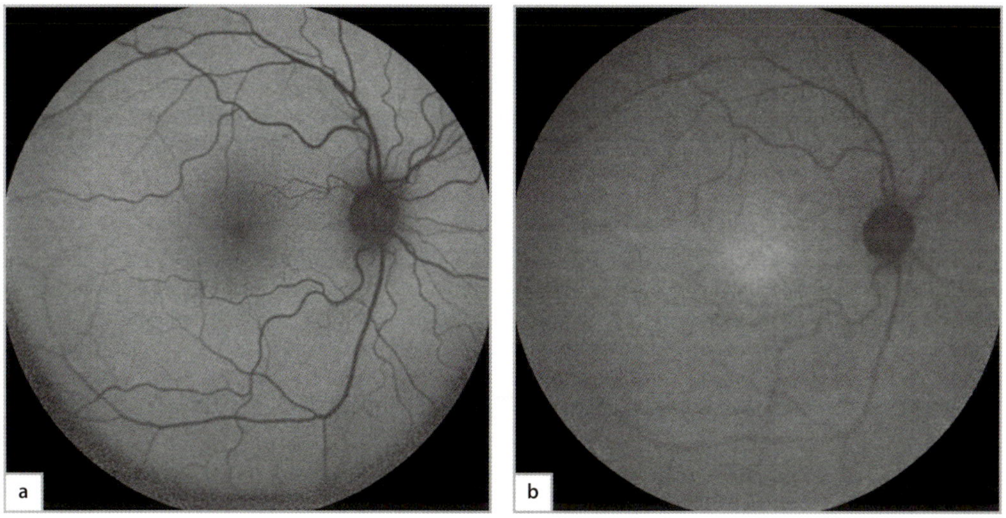

Figure 5.4 (a) Fundus image of the right eye acquired through confocal scanning laser ophthalmoscope (cSLO)-based system shows autofluorescence. (b) The right fundus shows autofluorescence through near-infrared fundus acquired by cSLO system.

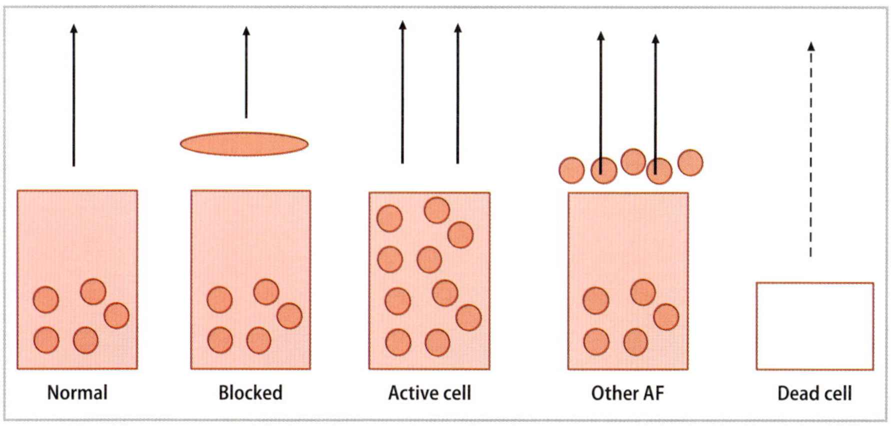

Figure 5.5 Basic principles of abnormal autofluorescence. The figure illustrates the normal, blocked, active cells, dead cells, and other causes.

spectral domain optical coherent tomography (SD-OCT). However, current SD-OCT can only show structural changes, while AF imaging can provide functional information on the RPE cells. The combination of the two techniques allows the retinal specialist to establish the diagnosis in difficult cases and in some circumstances provide important prognostic information. The use of fundus AF in clinical practice is still expanding.

Age-related macular degeneration

Early AMD

An attempt was made to classify AF patterns in early AMD (Bindewald et al. 2005). The following patterns have been described:

- Normal
- Minimal change
- Focal increase
- Patchy
- Linear
- Lacelike
- Reticular
- Speckled

The linear and lacelike patterns are associated with pigmentary changes of the RPE cells, so they carry the same risk of progression to end-staged diseases based on the age-related eye disease study (Ferris et al. 2005). AF imaging can identify these changes better than color fundus photograph (Delori et al. 2000).

The speckled pattern is similar to the pattern seen in some patients with Stargardt's disease, and many of these patients carry the at-risk ABCA4 polymorphisms. And hence has a higher risk of developing geographic atrophy (GA).

The reticular pattern is probably the same as reticular pseudodrusen (RPD); the presence of this particular type of drusen has a high risk of progressing to end-staged macular degeneration in both choroidal neovascularization and GA. Fundus AF can be used to identify RPD much more easily than slit-lamp biomicroscopy. There is an increasing interest in RPD; the ability to identify people who have this phenotype might allow targeted treatment in the prevention of end-staged AMD. These drusen can also be readily seen with infrared imaging (**Figure 5.6**).

The relationships of drusen, pigment, and focally increased autofluorescence (FIAF) have been assessed in early, atrophic and high-risk fellow eyes of neovascular AMD (nAMD) patients. A clear relationship between AF patterns and clinical AMD status has been found. In early AMD, FIAF colocalization with large, soft drusen and hyperpigmentation is several times greater than would occur by chance, suggesting a link with the disease processes (**Figure 5.7**). In advanced atrophic AMD, FIAF is mostly found adjacent to drusen and GA, suggesting that dispersal of drusen-associated lipofuscin is a marker of atrophic disease progression. In neovascular AMD, a large group of fellow eyes have no FIAF abnormalities, suggesting that lipofuscin is not a major determinant of CNV (Smith et al. 2006).

Neovascular AMD

The treatment of nAMD has been revolutionized by intravitreal injection of anti-vascular endothelial growth factor agents. In the pivotal trials, 10% of patients lost three lines of vision. Rosenfeld and colleagues evaluated the color fundus photographs of eyes that lose three lines or more of vision: there were an increased area of RPE abnormality. In the CATT (Comparison of Age-related macular degeneration Treatment Trials) study comparing Lucentis and Avastin for the treatment of nAMD, at the end of 2 years, the rate of GA was highest in the Lucentis monthly group based on the examination of color fundus photographs. None of these studies have included AF imaging at baseline, so it is unclear whether the atrophy noted at the end of the study is a function of treatment or progression of atrophy. It is also unclear whether AF imaging can predict visual outcome.

A continuous and predominantly preserved AF pattern at the macula correlates with better visual acuity in patients with nAMD (Vaclavik et al. 2008) and seems to predict a better visual outcome following anti-vascular endothelial growth factor therapies (Heimes et al. 2008). Conversely, in patients with nAMD, confluent absence of AF, a measure of retinal pigment epithelial cell loss, is a significant predictor of poor visual acuity both at baseline and at follow-up (Kumar et al. 2013) (**Figure 5.8**).

It is, however, unclear how useful AF imaging would be in practice in terms of management decision making. For instance, when a patient does not have preserved AF, should the clinician elect not to treat the patient? It is true that one can give a guarded prognosis for the treatment, but it is unclear whether this group of patients might sustain more severe visual loss if left untreated. It is also unclear whether this group of patients might need more or less intensive therapy as compared with those with preserved AF.

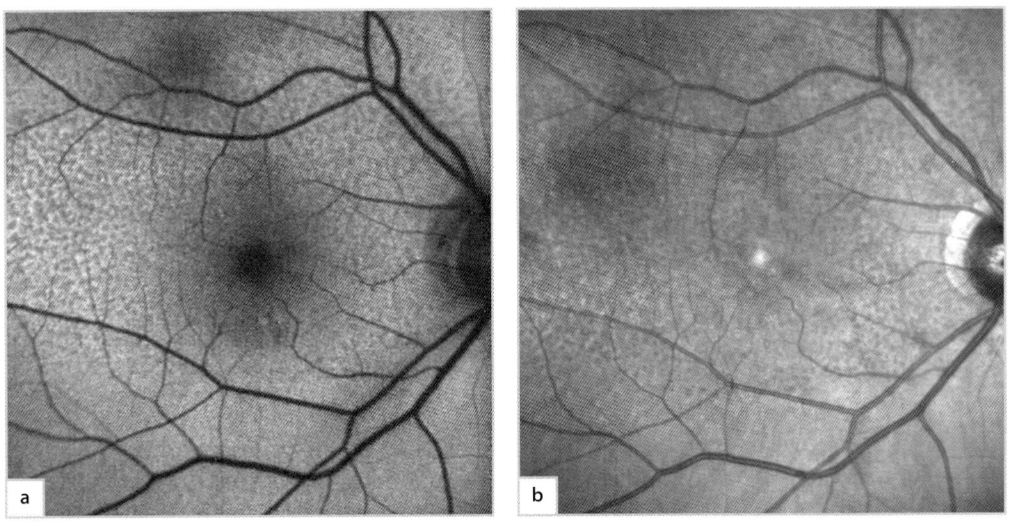

Figure 5.6 Reticular pseudodrusen. (a) Autofluorescence imaging shows reticular pseudodrusen may be an early indication of age-related macular degeneration (AMD). (b) Infrared imaging shows reticular pseudodrusen with possible AMD.

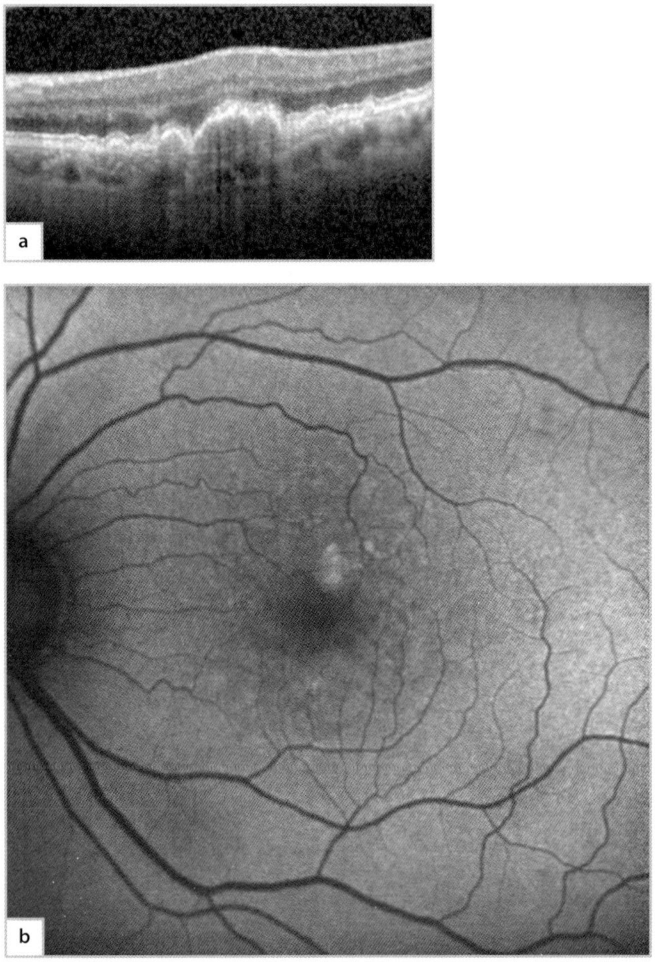

Figure 5.7 (a) Optical coherence tomography (OCT) shows large soft drusen with retinal pigment epithelium hypertrophy. (b) Autofluorescence (AF) imaging shows increased AF signal from the same area of the large soft drusen seen in the OCT.

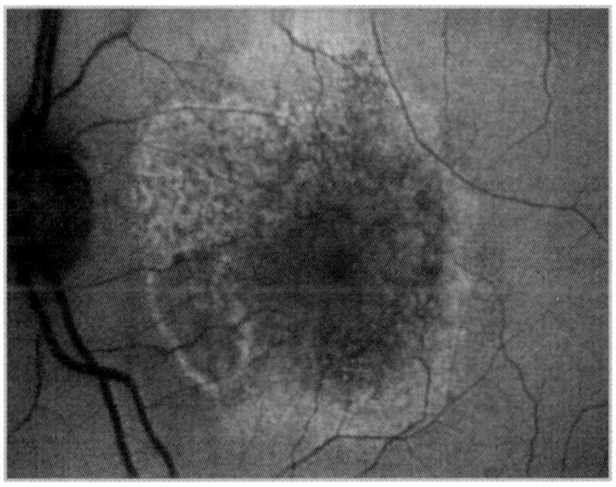

Figure 5.8 The left fundus shows large area of confluent absence of autofluorescence signals in neovascular age-related macular degeneration, an indication of poor visual acuity.

In eyes with polypoidal choroidal vasculopathy (PCV), the polypoidal lesions and the branching choroidal vascular networks appear to affect the RPE and induce peculiar AF changes. When compared with the patients with typical nAMD, widespread RPE damage was more frequently observed in the patients with PCV, both in the affected eyes and in the unaffected fellow eyes (Yamagishi et al. 2012). The clinical significance of this remains unclear.

Geographic atrophy

AF imaging is the current gold standard in measuring the presence and rate of enlargement of areas of RPE atrophy in patients with GA. There is software to aid the measurement of the area of atrophy, and hence to measure the rate of enlargement in a reliable fashion. However, SD-OCT is catching up fast, and foveal changes might be easier to see in SD-OCT than with AF imaging.

In patients with GA, AF changes might have prognostic implications. It has been shown that the pattern of fundus AF surrounding areas of GA may be used to predict the speed of progression of atrophy (Holz et al. 2007). Thus, in patients with a homogenous pattern of AF, the area of GA tends to progress more slowly than those with widespread AF changes. However, this might be related to the fact that patients with homogenous pattern tend to have smaller area of atrophy (**Figure 5.9**). The size of the atrophy at baseline appears to be more important. Significance of statistical correlation between the original and advancing growth of the GA area can be markedly minimized by computing the square root of the affected area (Feuer et al 2013).

Generalized retinal degeneration

Retinitis pigmentosa

Patients with retinitis pigmentosa (RP) have decreased AF signal in the midperiphery in the bone spicules pigmentation area (**Figure 5.10**). This is not unexpected, due to loss of photoreceptor cells and corresponding RPE loss. However, parafoveal rings of increased AF are also observed which are not visible with slit-lamp biomicroscopy (**Figure 5.11**). Robson and colleagues have shown that in patients with RP and good visual acuity there is only preserved cone sensitivity inside the ring of increased AF, with reduced cone sensitivity outside this ring and reduced rod sensitivity inside and outside it, despite the relatively normal distribution of AF in these areas (Robson et al. 2004, 2006).

Leber congenital amaurosis

Patients with Leber congenital amaurosis (LCA) may have a normal distribution of AF throughout the fundus, demonstrate parafoveal rings of increased AF, and/or have moderately reduced AF signal at and anterior to the vascular arcades (Scholl et al. 2004).

Patients with LCA due to mutations in the RPE65 gene, for which genetic treatment is currently under investigation, characteristically present much reduced AF signal in the midperipheral retina (Lorenz et al. 2004). At the macula, the signal is low at the fovea but, around it, a relatively spared AF signal may be seen. These findings can be used clinically to guide genetic testing and, thus, to help in the identification of patients who may be suitable for genetic therapy.

Choroideremia

Fundus AF can be helpful in the diagnosis of early choroideremia in young patients with only minimal RPE mottling in the midperipheral retina, often difficult to detect on slit-lamp biomicroscopy (Renner et al. 2006). AF demonstrates mottled increased and decreased AF signal in the midperipheral retina and extending to the macula but sparing the fovea, where it remains normal until the late stages of the disease.

Macular dystrophies

Pattern dystrophy

Patients with pattern dystrophy demonstrate a variety of patterns of accumulation of yellow-white material in the deeper retinal layers. A strong AF signal is observed at the site of accumulation of the

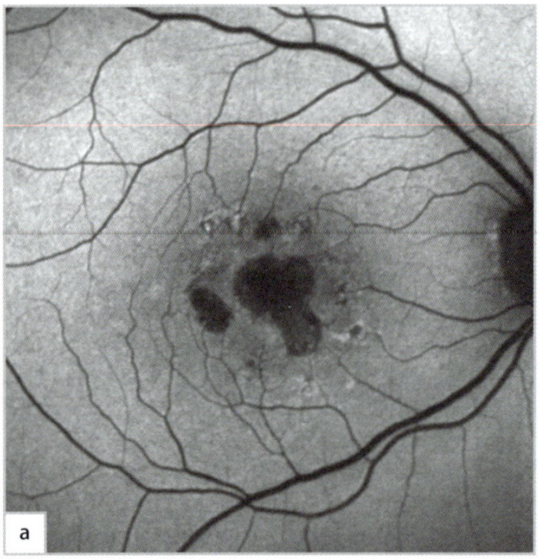

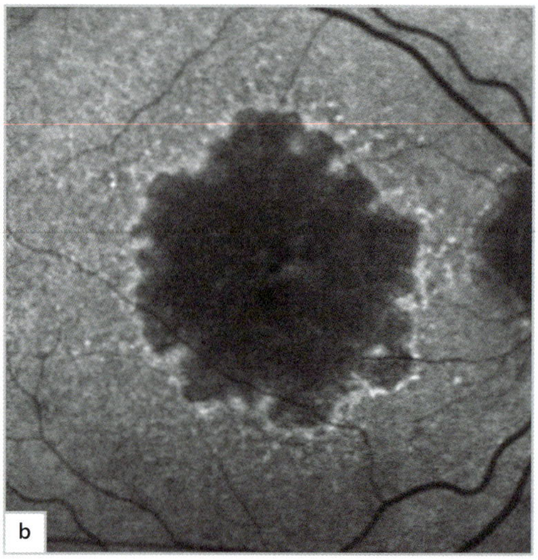

Figure 5.9 (a) Autofluorescence (AF) imaging shows several small areas of retinal pigment epithelial atrophy. (b) AF imaging shows a large area of geographic atrophy of the retinal pigment epithelium with increased AF signal surrounding the edges of atrophy.

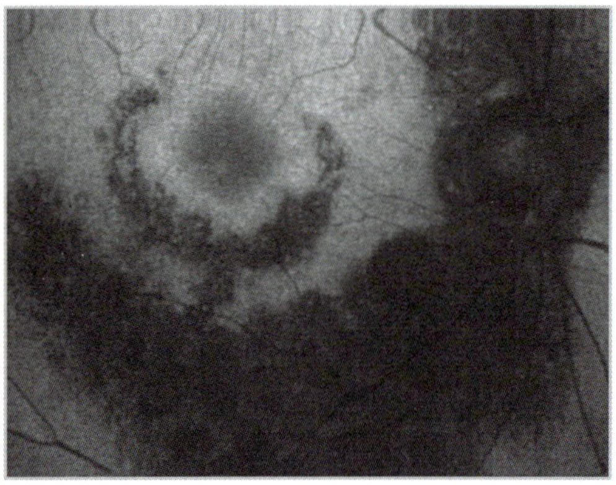

Figure 5.10 The right fundus of a patient with rhodopsin mutation and inferior retinitis pigmentosa involving the inferior midperiphery shows reduced autofluorescence signals with foveal sparing.

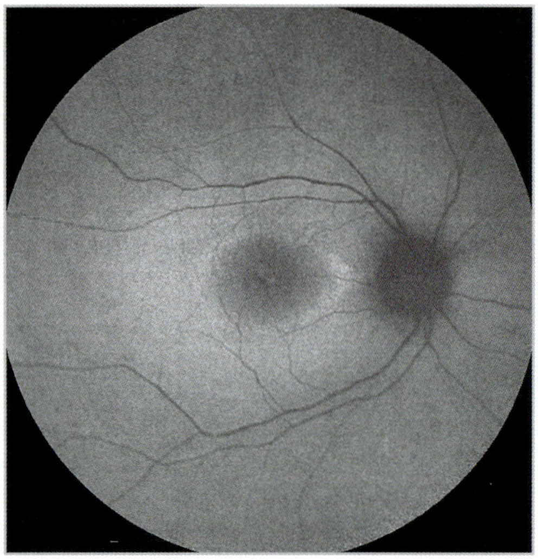

Figure 5.11 The left fundus shows increased autofluorescence parafoveal ring in a patient with retinitis pigmentosa.

yellow-white material. This strong AF signal is highly suspicious of a diagnosis of pattern dystrophy and is extremely helpful to differentiate this inherited retinal disease from other conditions such as drusen, which can have an increased AF signal but not as strong as that in pattern dystrophy (**Figure 5.12**).

Stargardt's disease

Many patients with Stargardt's disease can be diagnosed on the basis of findings on slit-lamp biomicroscopy of yellow-white fleck and depigmentation at the macula and midperipheral retina associated with the foveal atrophy. However, if only resorbed flecks are present, as seen in patients with more advanced stage of disease, the diagnosis becomes a challenge. Under these circumstances, fundus AF is extremely useful by demonstrating a characteristic pattern of small foci or reduced AF signal in the macula and, in some cases, also in the midperipheral retina (Lois et al. 2001, 2004). The characteristic of peripapillary sparing can be readily seen in AF imaging. AF imaging allows the evaluation of areas of atrophy at the macula and midperipheral retina; the latter have been linked to a more severe phenotype with reduced generalized cone and rod function (Lois et al. 2001) (**Figure 5.13**). It can also monitor the progression of the disease by disclosing enlargement of areas of atrophy, the development of new areas of atrophy, and the appearance and disappearance of flecks over time.

Maternally inherited diabetes and deafness

In patients with maternally inherited diabetes and deafness, a typical pattern of AF can be found that is characterized by multiple semiconfluent parafoveal areas of atrophy with foveal sparing combining with multiple focal changes of AF signals on the rest of the retina (Rath et al. 2008) (**Figure 5.14**). The defect is in the mitochondria. Not all patients are diabetic or deaf, but the AF findings are very typical and the genetic test can confirm the diagnosis.

Best's disease

In the previtelliform stage, there is no abnormality in the distribution of AF and, thus, fundus AF does not help in the detection of affected individuals at this stage of the disease. In the vitelliform, pseudohypopyon and vitelliruptive stages increased AF is present at the site where accumulation of yellow material is observed on slit-lamp biomicroscopy. In the fibrotic stage, there is a predominantly low AF signal at the center of the macula, at the site previously occupied by the yellow material (**Figure 5.15**). The role of AF imaging in Best's disease is uncertain, but the low AF signal is commonly associated with reduced vision and hence can help to explain the visual loss.

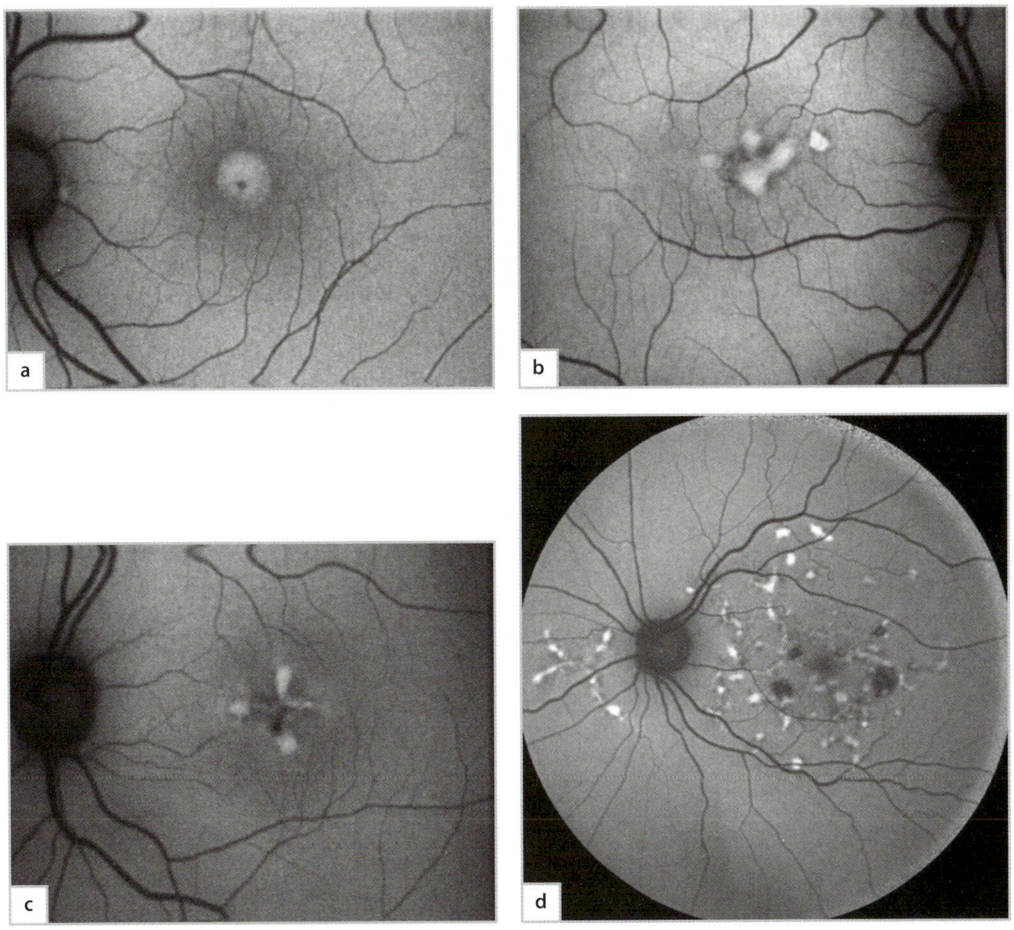

Figure 5.12 Autofluorescence (AF) imaging of pattern dystrophy. (a) Adult vitelliform macular dystrophy shows increased localized AF from the foveal changes. (b, c, and d) Patients with pattern dystrophy demonstrate a variety of patterns of accumulation of yellow-white material in the deep retina/retinal pigment epithelium. A strong AF signal is observed at the site of accumulation of the yellow-white material.

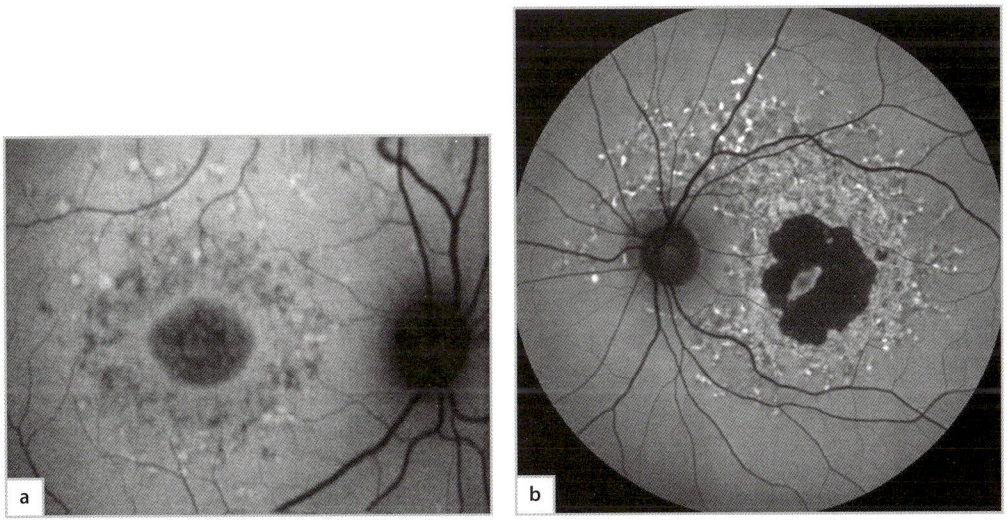

Figure 5.13 Autofluorescence (AF) imaging of Stargardt's macular dystrophy. (a) A patient with only macular involvement with central foveal atrophy and parafoveal flecks shows increased AF signals and some with decreased AF signals. (b) More extensive involvement showing peripapillary sparing and foveal sparing.

X-Linked retinoschisis

Historically, early cases of X-linked retinoschisis could be difficult to detect. AF imaging can visualize the cystic changes due to the displacement of the macular pigment and the cystic space creating a shadow and hence reducing the AF signals. The early detection of X-linked retinoschisis is now best carried out with SD-OCT (**Figure 5.16**).

Central serous chorioretinopathy

Fundus AF can be used and may be helpful for evaluating patients with acute central serous chorioretinopathy (CSC). This imaging technique is particularly useful in establishing the diagnosis of chronic CSC. In chronic CSC, AF imaging discloses multiple areas of increased AF signal, not always visualized by slit-lamp biomicros-

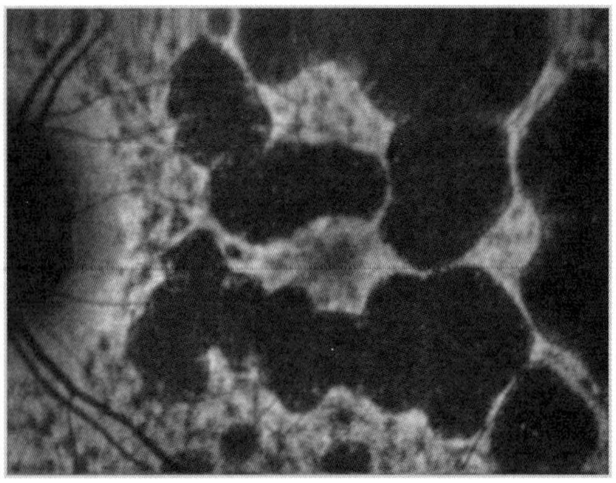

Figure 5.14 Autofluorescence imaging of a maternally inherited case of diabetes and deafness shows typical parafoveal atrophy.

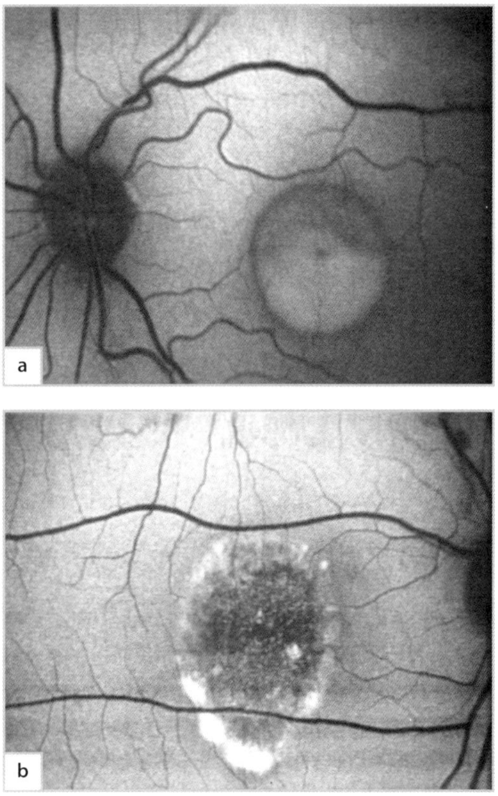

Figure 5.15 Autofluorescence (AF) imaging of Best's disease. (a) Vitelliform stage shows a fluid level. (b) Fibrotic stage showing central atrophy shows reduced AF signal.

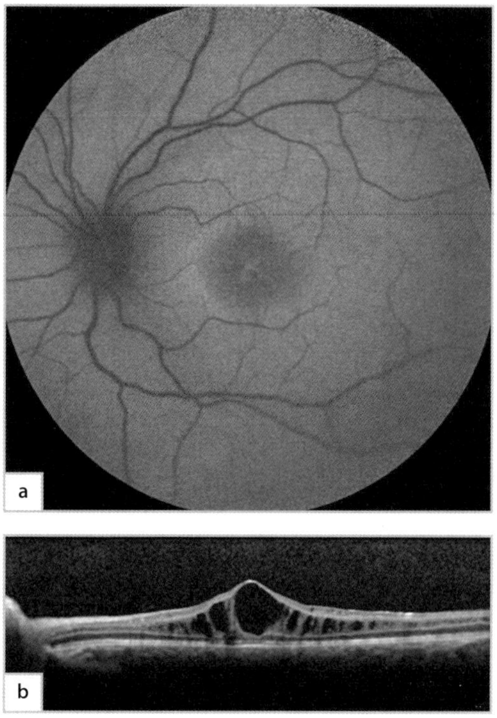

Figure 5.16 X-Linked retinoschisis. (a) In central retinoschisis there is strong autofluorescence at the macular area. (b) Optical coherence tomography image shows cystic spaces.

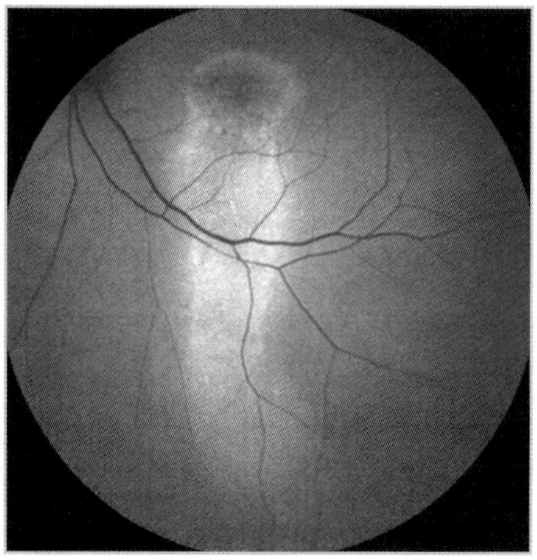

Figure 5.17 Chronic central serous retinopathy. Autofluorescence imaging shows the snail's track pattern due to tracking of serous fluid during the active stage of the disease.

copy. In patients with multiple episodes and more extensive damage, areas of reduced AF can also be detected. The classical gravity dependent tract of AF changes is seen frequently (**Figure 5.17**).

NEW DEVELOPMENTS

There are several new developments in AF imaging. As mentioned, current AF imaging is based on the changes in comparison between the affected and the surrounding area. So a diffuse increase in AF signal in some AMD patients cannot be detected. However, quantitative AF imaging is now possible at least in mice (Sparrow et al. 2013), and human prototype is currently under testing.

Wide-field AF imaging is now commercially available with the Optos system, combining the wide-field imaging system and non-confocal SLO imaging. Tan and colleagues have recently reported that among patients with nAMD, nearly 70% have peripheral AF abnormalities (Tan et al. 2013). This is not totally surprising as peripheral lesions in the form of drusen and reticular changes are commonly seen. The clinical significance of these AF abnormalities is unknown.

CONCLUSIONS

Fundus AF imaging is a noninvasive tool for the evaluation of patients with posterior segment disorders. In many scenarios, as described above, these imaging techniques are extremely helpful in providing clinicians with clues that assist in establishing a diagnosis and providing a prognosis for their patients.

REFERENCES

Bindewald A, Bird AC, Dandekar S, et al. Classification of fundus autofluorescence patterns in early age-related macular disease. *Invest Ophthalmol Vis Sci* 2005; **46**:3309–3314.

Delori FC, Fleckner MR, Goger DG, et al. Autofluorescence distribution associated with drusen in age-related macular degeneration. *Invest Ophthalmol Vis Sci* 2000; **41**:496–504.

Dorey CK, Wu G, Ebenstein D, et al. Cell loss in the aging retina: relationship to lipofuscin accumulation and macular degeneration. *Invest Ophthalmol Vis Sci* 1989; **30**:1691–1699.

Feeney L. Lipofuscin and melanin of human retinal pigment epithelium: fluorescence, enzyme cytochemical, and ultrastructural studies. *Invest Ophthalmol Vis Sci* 1978; **17**:195–200.

Ferris FL, Davis MD, Clemons TE, et al. Age-related eye disease study (AREDS) research group. A simplified severity scale for age-related macular degeneration: AREDS Report No. 18. *Arch Ophthalmol* 2005; **123**:1570–1574.

Feuer WJ, Yehoshua Z, Gregori G, et al. Square root transformation of geographic atrophy area measurements to eliminate dependence of growth rates on baseline lesion measurements: a reanalysis of age-related eye disease study report no. 26. JAMA Ophthalmol 2013; **131**:11.

Heimes B, Lommatzsch A, Zeimer M, et al. Foveal RPE autofluorescence as a prognostic factor for anti-VEGF therapy in exudative AMD. *Graefes Arch Clin Exp Ophthalmol* 2008; **246**:1229–1234.

Holz FG, Bindewald-Wittich A, Fleckenstein M, et al. Progression of geographic atrophy and impact of fundus autofluorescence patterns in age-related macular degeneration. *Am J Ophthalmol* 2007; **143**:463–472.

Keilhauer CN, Delori FC. Near-infrared autofluorescence imaging of the fundus: visualization of ocular melanin. *Invest Ophthalmol Vis Sci* 2006; **47**:3556–3564.

Kumar N, Mrejen S, Fung AT, et al. Retinal pigment epithelial cell loss assessed by fundus autofluorescence imaging in neovascular age-related macular degeneration. *Ophthalmology* 2013; **120**:334–341.

Lois N, GE, Bunce C, Fitzke FW, Bird AC. Phenotypic subtypes of Stargardt macular dystrophy-fundus flavimaculatus. *Arch Ophthalmol* 2001; **119**:359–369.

Lois N, Halfyard AS, Bird AC, et al. Fundus autofluorescence in Stargardt macular dystrophy-fundus flavimaculatus. *Am J Ophthalmol* 2004; **138**:55–63.

Lorenz B, Wabbels B, Wegscheider E, et al. Lack of fundus autofluorescence to 488 nanometers from childhood on in patients with early-onset severe retinal dystrophy associated with mutations in RPE65. *Ophthalmology* 2004; **111**:1585–1594.

Piccolino FC, Borgia L, Zinicola E, et al. Pre-injection fluorescence in indocyanine green angiography. *Ophthalmology* 1996; **103**:1837-1845.

Rath PP, Jenkins S, Michaelides M, et al. Characterisation of the macular dystrophy in patients with the A3243G mitochondrial DNA point mutation with fundus autofluorescence. *Br J Ophthalmol* 2008; **92**:623–629.

Renner AB, Kellner U, Cropp E, et al. Choroideremia: variability of clinical and electrophysiological characteristics and first report of a negative electroretinogram. *Ophthalmology* 2006; **113**:2066–2073.

Robson AG, Michaelides M, Saihan Z, et al. Comparison of fundus autofluorescence with photopic and scotopic fine-matrix mapping in patients with retinitis pigmentosa and normal visual acuity. *Invest Ophthalmol Vis Sci* 2004; **45**:4119–4125.

Robson AG, Saihan Z, Jenkins SA, et al. Functional characterisation and serial imaging of abnormal fundus autofluorescence in patients with retinitis pigmentosa and normal visual acuity. *Br J Ophthalmol* 2006; **90**:472–479.

Scholl HP, Chong NH, Robson AG, et al. Fundus autofluorescence in patients with leber congenital amaurosis. *Invest Ophthalmol Vis Sci* 2004; **45**:2747–2752.

Smith RT, Chan JK, Busuoic M, et al. Autofluorescence characteristics of early, atrophic, and high-risk fellow eyes in age-related macular degeneration. *Invest Ophthalmol Vis Sci* 2006; **47**:5495–5504.

Spaide RF. Fundus autofluorescence and age-related macular degeneration. *Ophthalmology* 2003; **110**:392–399.

Sparrow JR, Blonska A, Flynn E, et al. Quantitative fundus autofluorescence in mice. Correlation with HPLC quantitation of RPE lipofuscin and measurement of retina outer nuclear layer. *Invest Ophthalmol Vis Sci* 2013; **54**:2812–2820.

Tan CS, Heussen F, Sadda SR. Peripheral autofluorescence and clinical findings in neovascular and non-neovascular age-related macular degeneration. *Ophthalmology* 2013; **120**:1271–1277.

Vaclavik V, Vujosevic S, Dandekar SS, et al. Autofluorescence imaging in age-related macular degeneration complicated by choroidal neovascularization: a prospective study. *Ophthalmology* 2008; **115**:342–346.

von Ruckmann A, Fitzke FW, Bird AC. Distribution of fundus autofluorescence with a scanning laser ophthalmoscope. *Br J Ophthalmol* 1995; **79**:407–412.

Wing GL, Blanchard GC, Weiter JJ. The topographic and age relationship of lipofuscin concentration in the retinal pigment epithelium. *Invest Ophthalmol Vis Sci* 1978; **17**:600.

Yamagishi T, Koizumi H, Yamazaki T, Kinoshita S. Fundus autofluorescence in polypoidal choroidal vasculopathy. *Ophthalmology* 2012; **119**:1650–1657.

Chapter 6 Optic nerve head imaging

Carol Y. Cheung, Yih-Chung Tham, Tin Aung

INTRODUCTION

Glaucoma is a progressive optic neuropathy characterized by gradual degeneration of retinal ganglion cells. In glaucoma, structural damage often occurs before detectable loss of visual function (Girkin 2004). Therefore, optic nerve head (ONH) evaluation is essential for the early diagnosis of glaucoma and for monitoring of glaucoma progression. The ONH can be clinically examined using a direct ophthalmoscope, using an indirect ophthalmoscope, or using a lens to examine the disc with a slit lamp. All these methods of clinical ophthalmoscopy involve subjective interpretation and have high inter-examiner variability; thus, alone, they are not ideal for monitoring progression of ONH changes. Fundus photography is the most common widely used and established method of ONH imaging for documentation of structural abnormalities and longitudinal changes in glaucomatous eyes.

Experiments in fundus photography originated with JD Wester in 1886. A half century of development culminated in the Carl Zeiss fundus camera, introduced in 1955. The introduction of the Carl Zeiss fundus camera laid a strong foundation for various ONH imaging modalities to be introduced in later years. With the development of the retinal fundus camera, the ONH became easily documented in a highly reproducible manner. As stereopsis provides better appreciation of the ONH structure, stereo photography of ONH was subsequently introduced. The standard monoscopic fundus camera can be used to obtain sequential optic nerve images from two different angles by changing the position of the camera. Photographs are taken in two positions to obtain dissimilar images and create a stereoscopic effect. Images obtained by this method are then simultaneously viewed with a mirrored, prismatic viewer. Nonetheless, images produced using this technique are merely 'near-stereoscopic.' It was not until 1964 that Donaldson first developed and successfully introduced simultaneous stereo photography using two sets of rhomboid prisms to split light from a single front lens and direct it toward two different frames of film. This technique has the advantage of a fixed stereo base and high reproducibility for ONH photography. The simultaneous paired images are then viewed using the stereo viewer.

Since the 1990s, digital fundus photography has become a standard technique. Digital fundus photography has replaced the use of film for easier storage and manipulation, as well as for great improvements from wide-ranging digital analysis of the ONH image.

Currently, subjective optic disc evaluation by observing the photograph pair with a stereo viewer remains the gold standard to assess structural glaucomatous appearance in clinical trials. Nevertheless, this method requires training for the graders and it is time consuming. Furthermore, intra- and interobserver variability in assessing ONH is relatively high even among glaucoma specialists. There are few computer-assisted programs to allow one to manually label disc and cup margins and consequently generate several disc parameters quantitatively. However, a fully automated ONH quantification method is still not available. **Figure 6.1** illustrates milestones in ONH imaging development.

Recent advances in retinal imaging technologies have provided opportunities for imaging and documenting ONH appearances (Lin et al. 2007, Sharma et al. 2008, Greenfield & Weinreb 2008). These include the optical coherence tomography (OCT), Heidelberg retinal tomography (HRT), and scanning laser polarimetry (GDx nerve fiber analyzer). Compared with these imaging devices, stereoscopic ONH photography is a low-cost method providing a three-dimensional full-color view of the ONH. Furthermore, an advantage of subjective assessment is that such comprehensive evaluation includes assessment of focal structural damage (e.g. disc hemorrhage and notching).

PRINCIPLES OF ONH IMAGING

A fundus camera is a specialized low-power microscope with an attached camera. Its optical design is similar to the indirect ophthalmoscopy that provides an aerial image of the fundus with

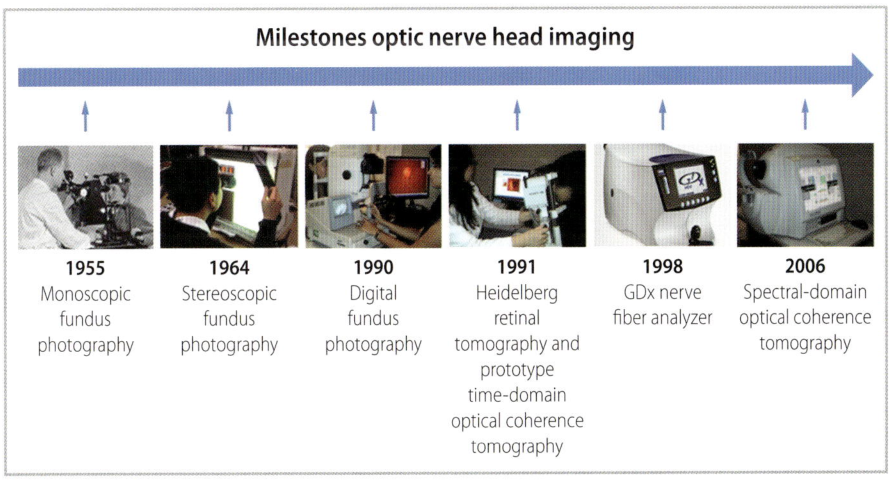

Figure 6.1 Milestones in optic nerve head imaging development.

magnification. Using a fundus camera, the retina can be photographed directly as the pupil is used as both an entrance and exit for the fundus camera's illuminating and imaging light rays. Fundus photography can also be performed with colored filters (e.g. green filter to enhance the contrast of the blood vessels) or with specialized dyes, including fluorescein and indocyanine green. The conventional fundus camera requires a pharmacological agent to dilate the patient's pupil (mydriatic fundus camera), while the latest non-mydriatic funds camera can permit retinal photography through the patient's natural pupil.

ONH IMAGING IN CLINICAL PRACTICE

Most fundus cameras are constructed similarly. It is advisable to read the camera manual and perform several trial attempts to become accustomed to the operations of a specific fundus camera.

Most fundus camera models are equipped with the following features:

- Ametropia correction: In certain camera models, there is a changer that places a lens in the observation system to select for the degree of ametropia, allowing settings for high myopes and high hyperopes
- Filters: For the purpose of image enhancement, certain cameras are also equipped with filter functions such as a red-free filter, a contrast filter, and a fluorescein exciter
- Field of view: Typical fundus camera models normally have fields of view ranging from 15 to 45°. Nonetheless, wide-angle fields of 50–60° can also be found in some models
- Focusing knob: This is generally on the side of the instrument
- Shutter release: This is normally located at the top of the joystick and is operated by the thumb or forefinger
- Light exposure setting: Exposure is normally controlled by the flash setting of respective cameras. There is little variation from patient to patient in the ideal exposure of retinas. Camera manuals normally give fairly accurate exposure settings. It is always advisable to follow the manufacturer's recommended settings and perform a few trial images

The recommended procedure for ONH imaging fundus camera is:

- Place the patient in a dim room in order to obtain sufficient natural dilatation
- For mydriatic cameras, dilate the patient's pupil using your routine regime
- Adjust the camera's flash setting and key in the patient's particulars accordingly
- Position the patient's chin comfortably in the chin rest of the instrument
- Line up the camera with the patient's pupil
- Instruct the patient to fixate at the fixation target
- Center the eye within the view screen by lateral and height adjustment using the camera joystick
- Focus on the retina until retinal features such as ONH and retinal vessels are clearly visible and well focused
- Continue manipulating the position of the camera to obtain proper alignment
- Once the retinal image is well focused and aligned, instruct the patient to maintain fixation and press/trigger the shutter button

CLINICAL APPEARANCE OF THE OPTIC NERVE HEAD

Normal appearance

The normal optic disc contains nerve fibers (the neuroretinal rim, which is pink owing to vascular perfusion), an area without nerve fibers (the optic cup, which is white generally), and branches of vessels from the central retinal artery and vein. Within the ONH, the central retinal artery is usually nasal to the vein (**Figure 6.2**). Age, gender, ethnicity, and refractive error influence the appearance of the normal ONH (Varma et al. 1994, Amerasinghe et al. 2008). These factors should be considered in distinguishing the normal ONH from glaucoma and other optic neuropathies.

Neuroretinal rim

The neuroretinal rim is the tissue between the outer edge of the cup and the disc margin. The color of a normal healthy rim is pink or orange appearance and shows a characteristic configuration. Usually, broadest neuroretinal rim is at the inferior disc region, followed by the superior, nasal, and, finally, temporal regions. This characteristic is coined as the 'ISNT rule' by Jonas et al. (1999) This neuroretinal rim structural feature is clinically important in the early detection of glaucomatous optic nerve damage.

Optic cup

The optic cup is normally devoid of nerve fascicles and normally appears as a round to oval depression of variable size, usually of a lighter color or pallid in appearance. However, accurate determination of the optic cup border should be evaluated by its contour and not by the appearance of pallor. The margin of the cup may not be clear and it is difficult to determine the border between the rim wall and the disc surface.

The normal optic cup may have one of the main appearances (**Figure 6.3**):

- A small dimple-like central cup

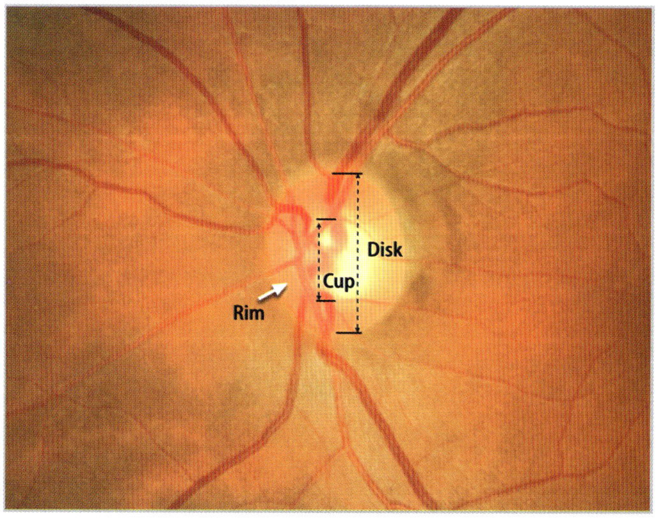

Figure 6.2 The normal optic nerve head.

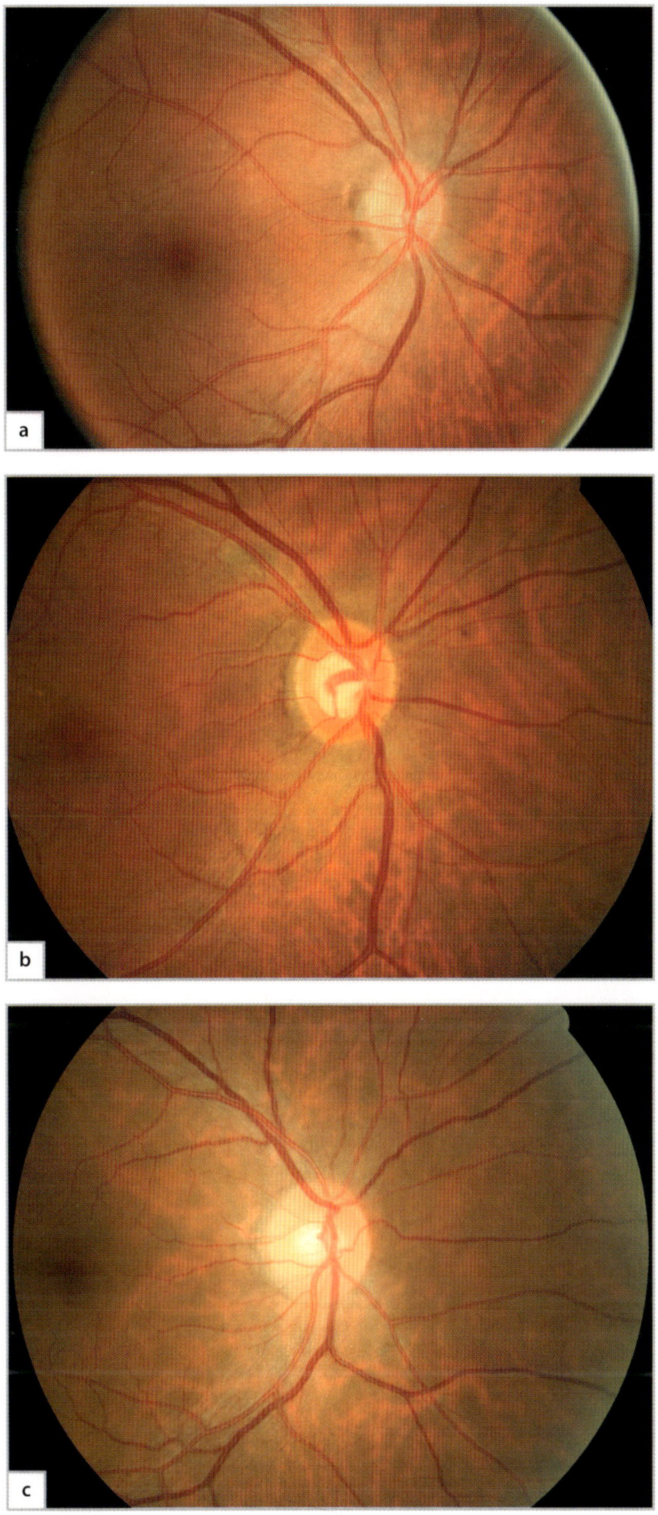

Figure 6.3 (a) Normal optic disc with a small dimple-like central cup. (b) Normal optic disc with a punched-out deep central cup. (c) Normal optic disc with a gently sloping temporal disc rim.

- A punched-out deep central cup
- A cup with a gentle temporal slope

Variations in the gradient of the cup walls may also influence assessment of the cup margin. For example, a more acute angle between the cup wall and the surface of the disc makes it easier to assess the cup margin. For accurate evaluation of the optic cup, stereoscopic examination would be ideal to appreciate the cup contour.

Tips: caveat for cup area judgment

- The pink/orange color of the rim often 'spills over' into the cup area. In these cases, cup area may be underestimated thus giving a smaller cup-to-disc ratio.
- In certain images, laminar openings at the floor of the cup may be visible, with a prominent whitish appearance. These should not be used as the sole information to estimate the size of the cup, which could be significantly larger.

Glaucomatous optic disc changes

In glaucoma, pathological cupping is caused by irreversible damage to nerve fibers, glial cells, and blood vessels, leading to thinning of the neuroretinal rim with excavation and enlargement of the optic cup. Increased cupping can be identified by increased vertical cup-to-disc ratio.

Notching

Notching can be likened to an 'erosion' of the optic nerve rim peripherally. It usually appears as focal vertical extension and produces excavation posteriorly. A notch indicates focal optic nerve rim damage and corresponds with visual field loss and retinal nerve fiber loss. Early notching may be very subtle; hence, careful evaluation of the ONH is crucial (**Figure 6.4**).

Concentric enlargement of optic disc cupping

Concentric enlargement of optic disc cupping is characterized by diffuse loss of neuroretinal rim, thinning equally along its circumference without notching (**Figure 6.5**). It is often associated with diffuse visual field loss. As optic disc cupping is usually symmetric and subtle at early stage, detection of this appearance may be challenging at early phases of glaucoma.

Disc hemorrhage

The prevalence of disc hemorrhages is about 4–7% of eyes with glaucoma. These hemorrhages are mostly splinter or flame shaped in appearance (**Figures 6.6a** and **b**). In early glaucoma, they are usually located in the inferotemporal or superotemporal disc regions. Subtle hemorrhages may also be found on the disc or touching the disc margin. In some instances, tiny hemorrhage can also be observed within the optic cup. Disc hemorrhages may resolve with time, leading to localized retinal nerve fiber layer (RNFL) defects, neuroretinal rim, and visual field losses. This may explain why the frequency of this sign is lesser at early and advanced stages of glaucoma but higher at moderate stage.

Tips: disc hemorrhage vs. retinal hemorrhage

Caution is required to differentiate between these, particularly when retinal hemorrhage occurs close to the optic disc in association with diabetic retinopathy or retinal vein occlusion.

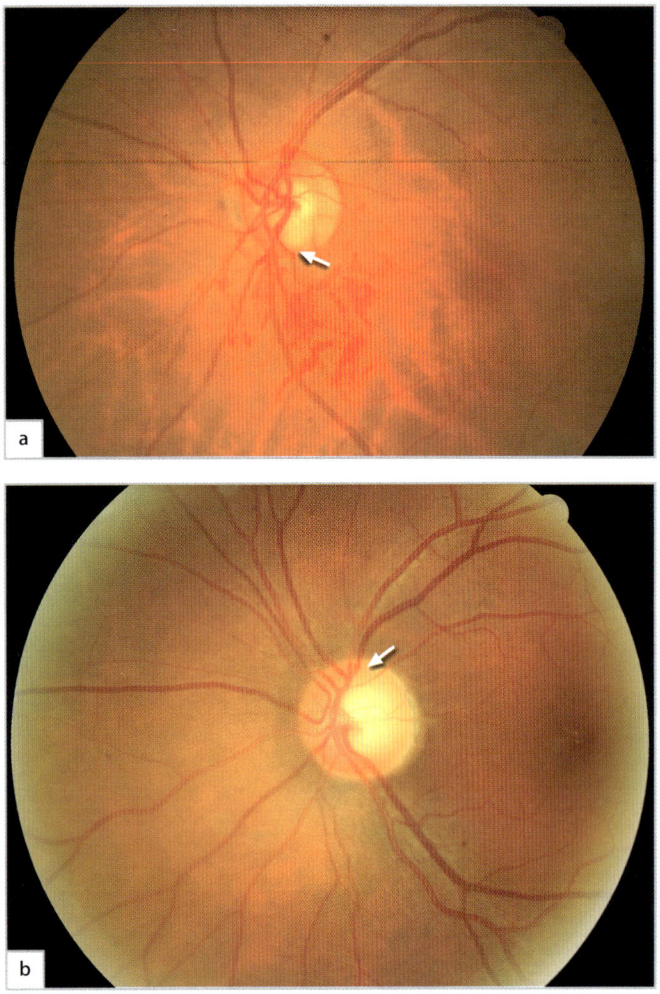

Figure 6.4 (a) Example of an optic disc with inferior rim notching. (b) Example of an optic disc with superior rim notching.

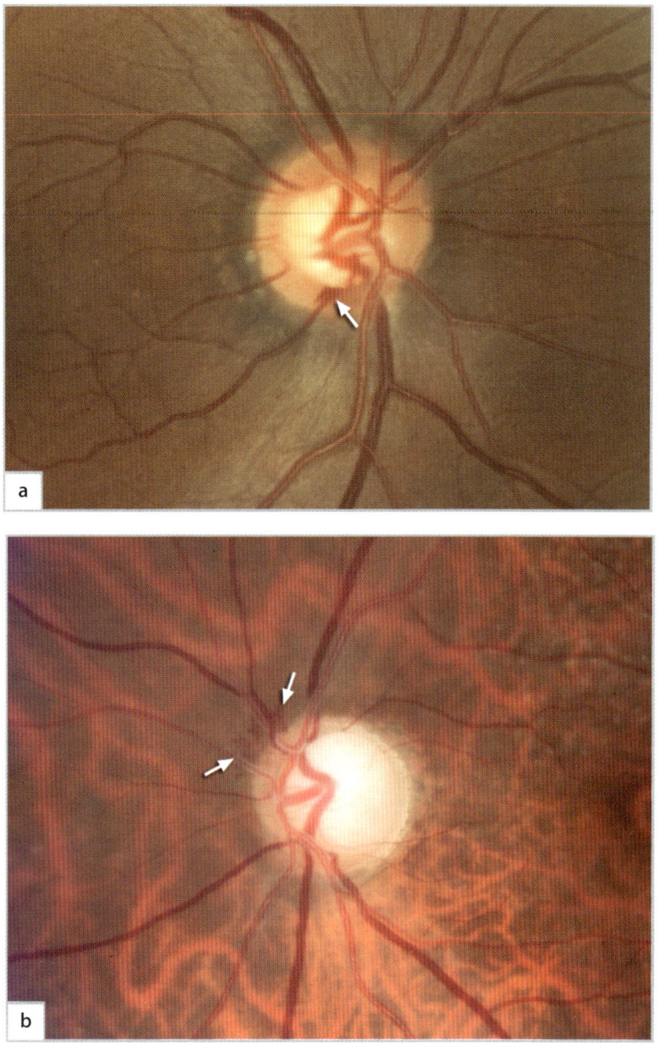

Figure 6.6 (a) Optic disc with disc hemorrhage located at the inferior rim region. (b) Optic disc with disc hemorrhage located at the superonasal disc margin.

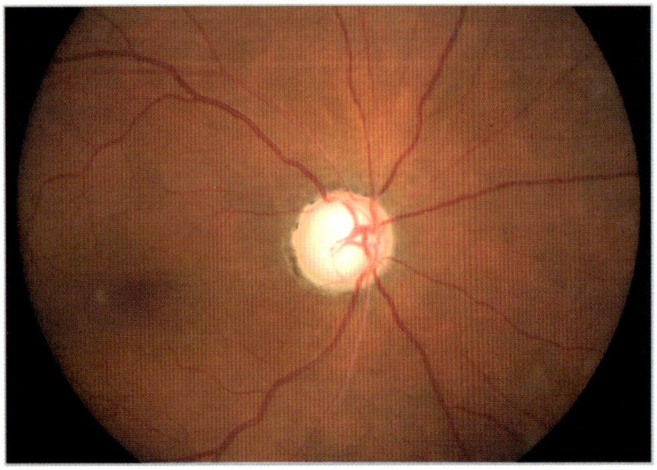

Figure 6.5 Concentric enlargement of optic disc cupping, characterized by equal thinning at the circumference the neuroretinal rim.

Peripapillary chorioretinal atrophy

Peripapillary chorioretinal atrophy can be classified into two types: the beta and the alpha type. In terms of location, the beta type is always closer to the disc than the alpha type. Beta is also known as inner beta zone and alpha as outer alpha zone (**Figure 6.7**). The outer alpha zone is always present in normal eyes characterized by irregular hypopigmentation and hyperpigmentation of the retinal pigment epithelium.

However, features of the inner beta zone are marked atrophy of the retinal pigment epithelium and choriocapillaris, good visibility of the large choroidal vessels and the sclera, and thinning of the chorioretinal tissues. The beta zone usually has smooth boundaries with the adjacent alpha zone and on its peripheral side and with the peripapillary sclera ring on its central side. The beta zone occurs more often in glaucomatous eyes than in normal eyes. The size of both zones and frequency of the beta zone are significantly correlated with a number of variables indicating the severity of the glaucoma damage, such as neuroretinal rim loss, reduced visibility of the RNFL bundles, and perimetric defects. Specifically, the location of peripapillary chorioretinal

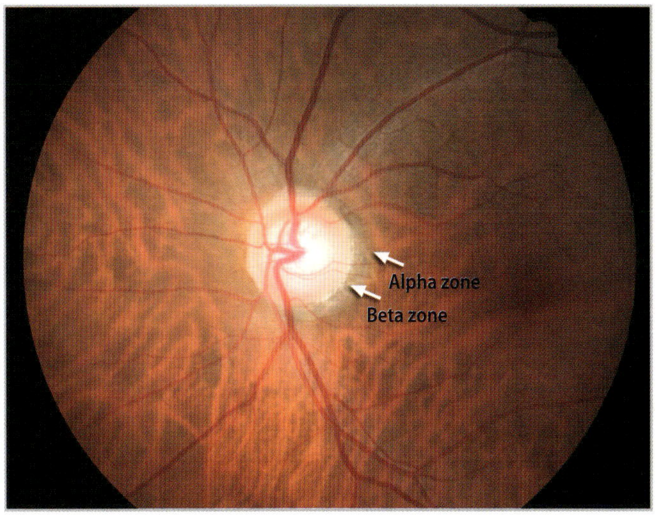

Figure 6.7 Optic disc with beta and alpha type peripapillary chorioretinal atrophy, located in the temporal region.

atrophy is spatially correlated with the neuroretinal rim loss in the intrapapillary region. The larger the peripapillary chorioretinal atrophy, the greater the neuroretinal rim loss.

Retinal nerve fiber layer defect

A RNFL defect may be localized or diffuse (**Figure 6.8**). Localized damage is characterized by slit defects in the RNFL that are best viewed with a red-free filter. As glaucoma advances, the RNFL defect may become more diffuse. Nonetheless, in eyes of high myopia, the RNFL is physiologically thin and localized defects are harder to detect in these cases.

Tips: RNFL defects in other diseases

RNFL defects are not specifically pathognomonic for glaucoma. They may also be observed in eyes with optic disc drusens, toxoplasmotic retinochoroidal scars, long-standing papilledema, or optic neuritis caused by multiple sclerosis.

Laminar dots

At the floor of the cup, the nerve fiber bundles pass through fenestrations in the lamina cribrosa. The floor of the cup and the lamina openings may not always be visible due to the size of the cup, the amount of tissue present, and the focus of the camera. Nonetheless, when the laminar dots can be seen, this is an indication of exposure of the lamina cribrosa due to loss of overlying neuroretinal tissue. The laminar dots normally appear as round or oval shadows or occasionally slit-like shadows, indicating stretching of the laminar floor (**Figure 6.9**). This appearance is more commonly observed in patients with advanced glaucoma.

Baring of a retinal vessel

Baring of a retinal vessel normally occurs near the margin of superior or inferior optic cup edge, indicating early thinning of superior or inferior neuroretinal rim. It is characterized by a space between the superficial (more anterior) blood vessel and the cup margin. In this

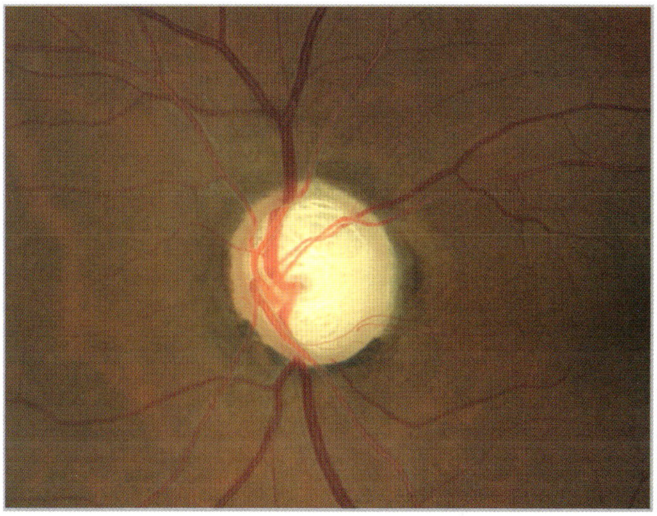

Figure 6.9 Severe glaucomatous disc with laminar dots indicating loss of overlying neuroretinal tissue.

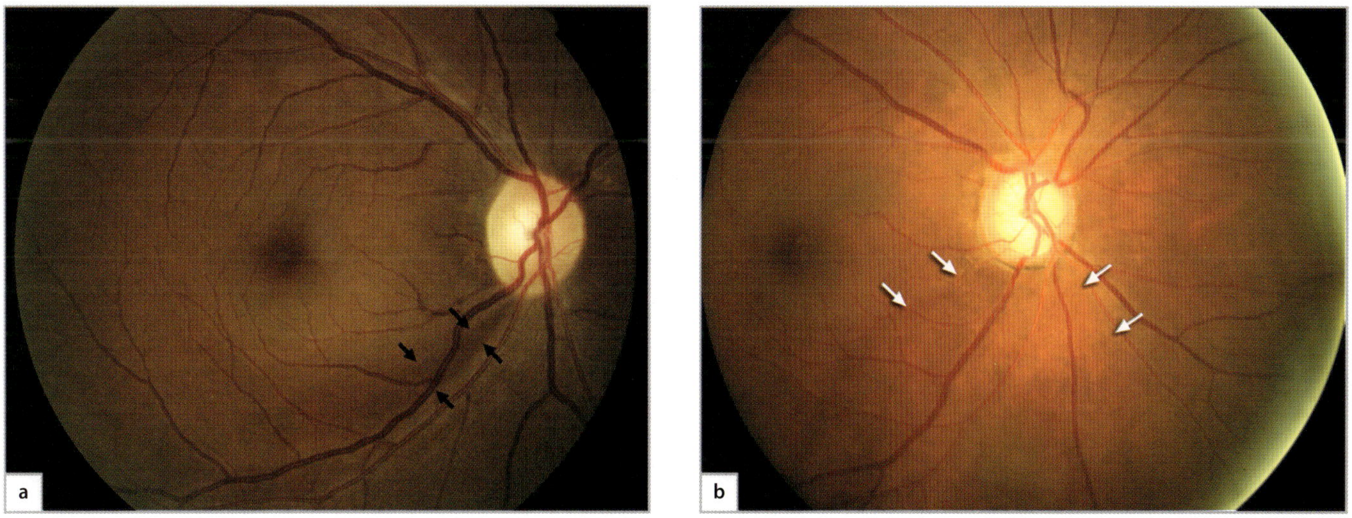

Figure 6.8 (a) A localized wedge-like retinal nerve fiber layer defect at the inferior temporal region. (b) A diffuse retinal nerve fiber layer defect at the inferior region.

instance, cup pallor can be visualized on both sides of the vessel. The vessel may appear like an overhanging bridge due to the loss of neuroretinal rim structural support (**Figure 6.10a**).

Tips: baring of retinal vessel vs. circumlinear retinal vessel

It is important to distinguish between the baring of a blood vessel and a circumlinear vessel. A circumlinear vessel is present in many normal ONHs that follow along the circumference of the cup margin until the vessel bends to pass over the rim of the disc and onto the disc surface (**Figure 6.10b**).

Bayoneting

Bayoneting may appear in the ONH with excavation of a steep wall. Bayoneting is characterized by double angulation of a blood vessel as it dives sharply backward and then turns along the excavation of the steep wall before angling again onto the floor of the disc (**Figure 6.11**).

Undercutting

Undercutting occurs in severe glaucoma where atrophy of the neuroretinal rim is so extensive that the walls of the cup disappear under a ledge of the rim tissue. As a result, the retinal vessels following the inner walls of the cup also disappear under the rim leaving visible only the vessels on the surface of the disc and the floor of the cup (**Figure 6.12**).

Large and small discs

The size of the optic disc is also clinically important. Eyes with a larger disc size have a relatively larger neuroretinal rim area, larger cup and cup-to-disc ratio, more optic nerve fibers, and less nerve fiber crowding. In contrast, small discs have lesser number of nerve fibers and are more crowded with nerve fiber bundles. This morphological structure suggests that small discs may be more susceptible to mechanical deformation or damage.

In normal eyes, the areas of the optic disc and optic cup are correlated with each other: the larger the optic disc, the larger the cup. Hence,

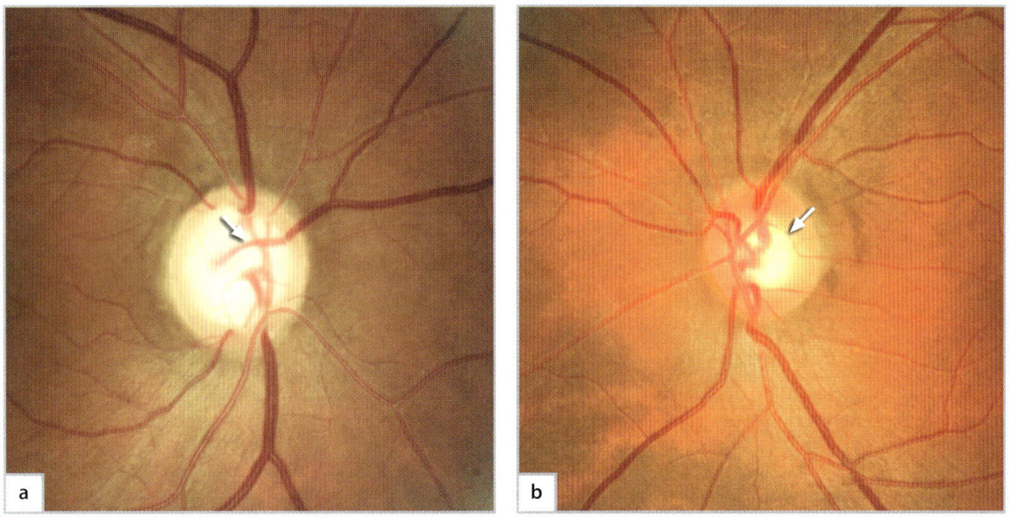

Figure 6.10 (a) Optic disc with a superior retinal vessel that exhibits baring. (b) Normal optic disc with a fine superior circumlinear blood vessel coursing along the superior cup margin.

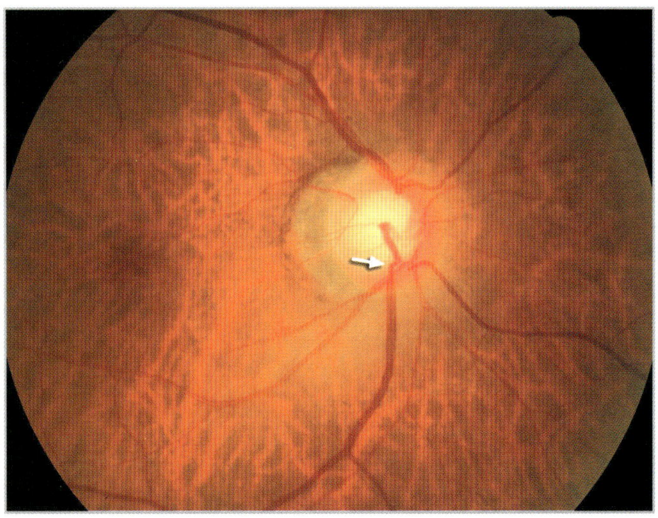

Figure 6.11 Optic disc with double angulation of the inferior branch retinal vein that displays bayoneting.

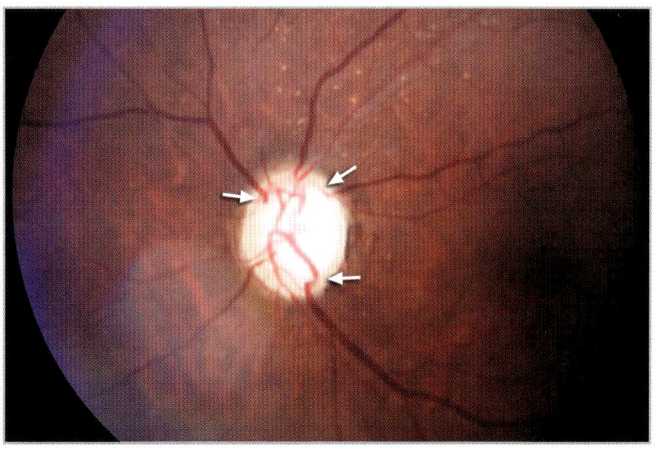

Figure 6.12 Severe glaucomatous disc with signs of undercutting, indicating extensive neuroretinal rim loss.

a large cup in a large disc may not necessarily indicate glaucomatous damage. In such instance, a holistic evaluation of other variables such as neuroretinal rim area and rim shape is needed (**Figure 6.13a**). In contrast, as small discs are more crowded, glaucomatous damage may occur even with relatively lower cup-to-disc ratio. Because of this reason, early and moderate glaucomatous damage in small discs may be easily overlooked. To overcome this challenge in cases with small discs, it is important to evaluate peripapillary abnormalities such as RNFL defect, focally reduced retinal arteriole diameter, and extensive peripapillary chorioretinal atrophy (**Figure 6.13b**) to complement the final diagnosis.

Tilted discs

The tilted disc is produced by an oblique insertion of the optic nerve into the globe, which produces relative prominence of the anterior pole and the impression of titling about an axis (**Figure 6.14**). A tilted disc is associated with myopia, astigmatism, and small optic disc area. The degree of optic disc tilt should be considered when interpreting the optic nerve.

Optic nerve head developmental malformations

Figure 6.15 shows ONH developmental malformations, including optic disc coloboma, optic disc pit, and staphyloma.

Other optic nerve conditions

Figure 6.16 shows other optic neuropathies, including a swollen disc and a pale optic disc (optic atrophy).

TECHNOLOGICAL CHALLENGES

Although standardized photographic protocols are available for the assessment of ONH, there are still different technological challenges in ONH imaging that may lead to misclassification or reduced precision of measurement. First, refractive error and axial length may affect the magnification and apparent dimensions of retinal structures on fundus photography. Other ocular factors including retinal pigmen-

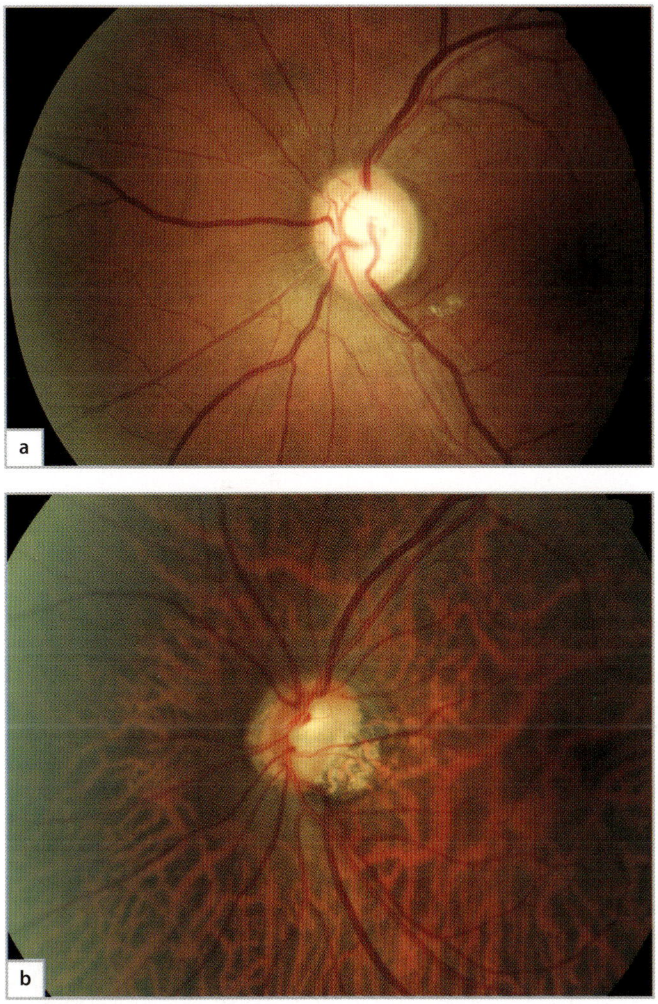

Figure 6.13 (a) Example of a normal disc with large physiological cup and large optic disc size. (b) Example of a small, myopic tilted disc with glaucoma.

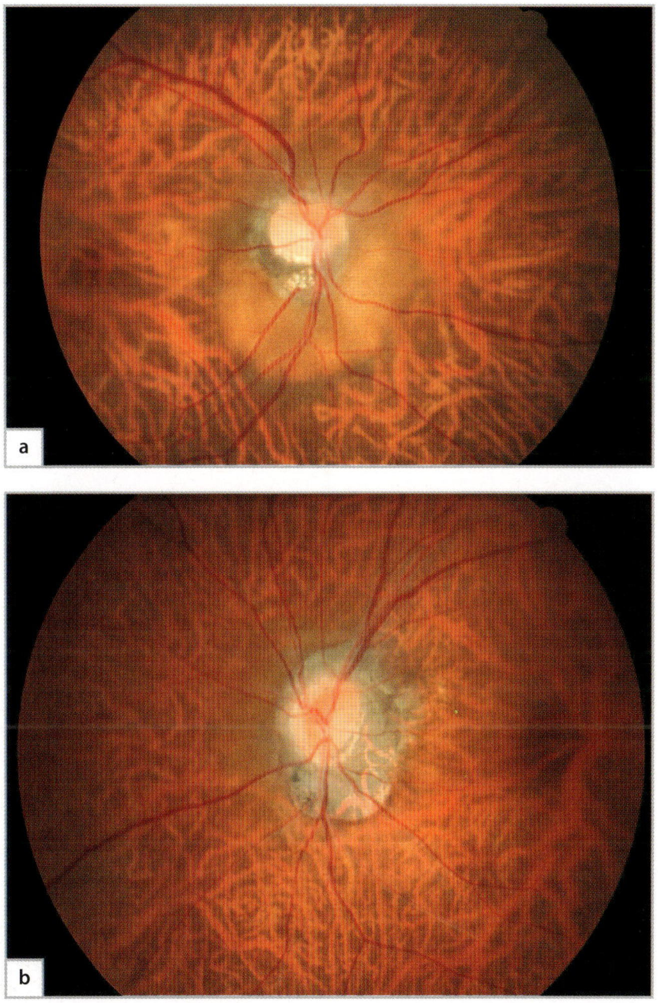

Figure 6.14 (a) Small and crowded myopic tilted disc. (b) Myopic tilted disc with extensive beta type peripapillary chorioretinal atrophy.

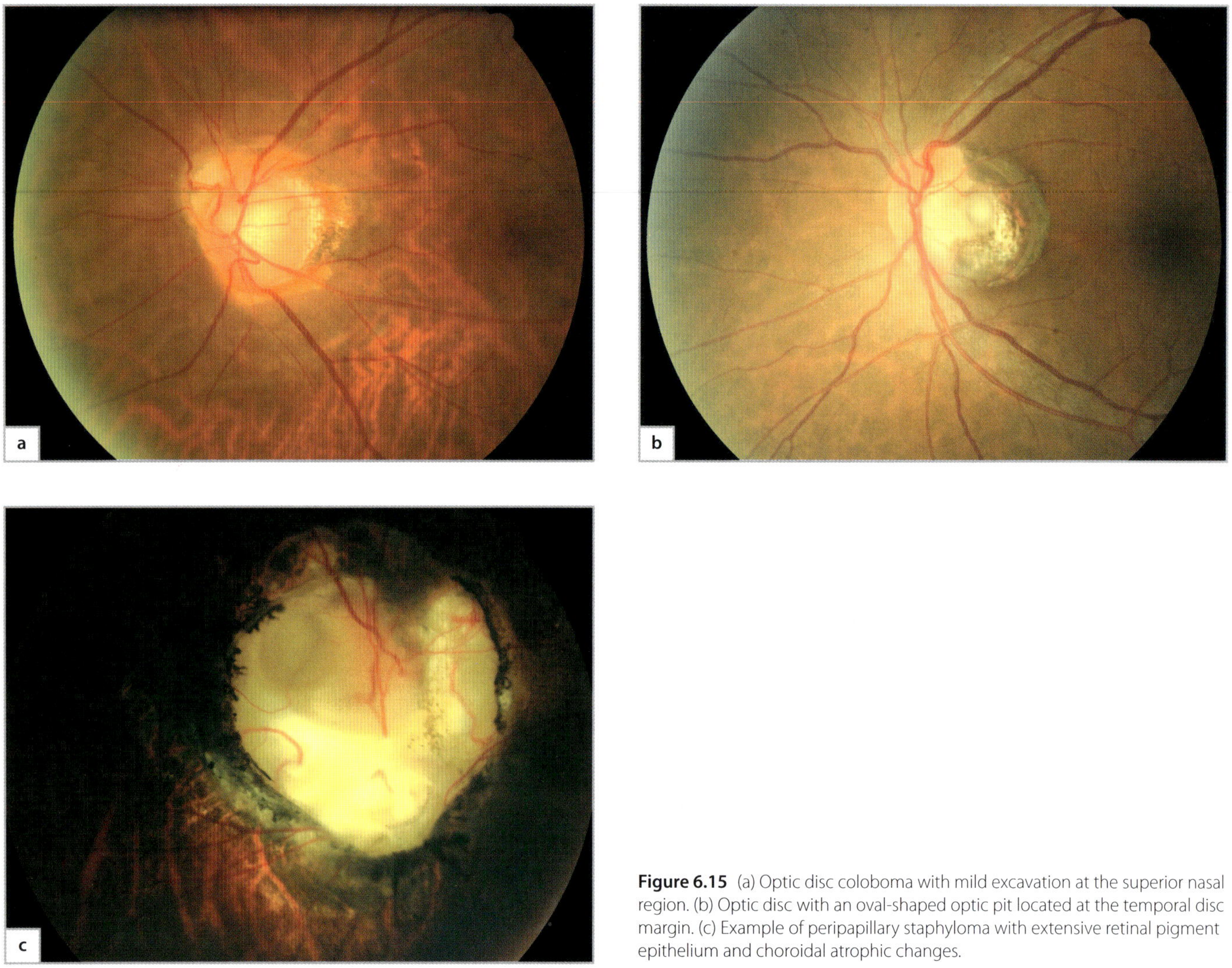

Figure 6.15 (a) Optic disc coloboma with mild excavation at the superior nasal region. (b) Optic disc with an oval-shaped optic pit located at the temporal disc margin. (c) Example of peripapillary staphyloma with extensive retinal pigment epithelium and choroidal atrophic changes.

tation, pupil dilation, presence of cataract, and other ocular media opacities may produce variations in image brightness, focus, and contrast that significantly affect the assessment of ONH. Furthermore, photographic technique and camera type may also affect the image quality for retinal fundus photography. Such possible ocular factors and confounders should be controlled for in the further development of retinal imaging technology.

Currently, ONH parameters (e.g. disc area and cup-to-disc ratio) from retinal fundus photographs are either manually or semiautomatically assessed with computer-assisted programs. The observer's manual input is still required and this may introduce additional variability in measurements. Further technical refinements are needed to minimize variability in measurements. Full automation in the measurement process and in detection of abnormalities is still underdeveloped.

OTHER NEW IMAGING TOOLS FOR OPTIC NERVE IMAGING AND ANALYSIS

Advanced ocular imaging tools, e.g. adaptive optics, confocal scanning laser ophthalmoscopy, swept source OCT, Doppler OCT, and OCT angiography, have recently been developed. These allow further measurement and analysis of the structure and function of the ONH, including the lamina cribrosa, choroidal vasculature, ONH blood flow, and perfusion. These new imaging tools have promise in the early evaluation of optic neuropathy. The clinical significance of these new technologies is yet to be evaluated.

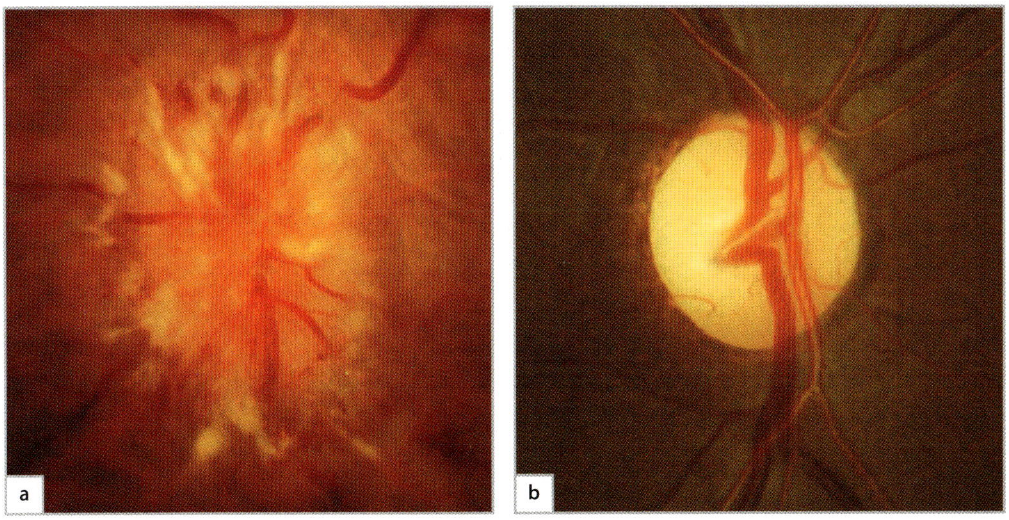

Figure 6.16 Other optic neuropathies: (a) Swollen disc. (b) Optic atrophy.

REFERENCES

Amerasinghe N, Wong TY, Wong WL, et al. SiMES Study Group. Determinants of the optic cup to disc ratio in an Asian population: the Singapore Malay Eye Study (SiMES). *Arch Ophthalmol* 2008; **126**:1101–1108.

Girkin CA. Relationship between structure of optic nerve/nerve fibre layer and functional measurements in glaucoma. *Curr Opin Ophthalmol* 2004; **15**:96–101.

Greenfield DS, Weinreb RN. Role of optic nerve imaging in glaucoma clinical practice and clinical trials. *Am J Ophthalmol* 2008; **145**:598–603.

Jonas JB, Budde WM, Panda-Jonas S. Ophthalmoscopic evaluation of the optic nerve head. *Surv Ophthalmol* 1999; **43**:293–320.

Lin SC, Singh K, Jampel HD, et al. American Academy of Ophthalmology; Ophthalmic Technology Assessment Committee Glaucoma Panel. Optic nerve head and retinal nerve fibre layer analysis: a report by the American Academy of Ophthalmology. *Ophthalmology* 2007; **114**:1937–1949.

Sharma P, Sample PA, Zangwill LM, Schuman JS. Diagnostic tools for glaucoma detection and management. *Surv Ophthalmol* 2008; 53 Suppl1:S17–32.

Varma R, Tielsch JM, Quigley HA, et al. Race-, age-, gender-, and refractive error-related differences in the normal optic disc. *Arch Ophthalmol* 1994; **112**:1068–1076.

Chapter 7 The modern multimodal stand-alone ophthalmic imaging center: setup, skills, and operation

Ethan R. Priel

INTRODUCTION

Ever since the invention of the ophthalmoscope by Helmholtz in 1851 (Keeler 2002), the quest to image and record the human fundus in health and disease has brought about far-reaching technological advances. The last several decades have been most momentous, ushering in the transition from large, single-frame, film-based fundus cameras (Chace & Lafayatte 1950) to digital, high-resolution, real-time imaging devices, some of them portable (Deb-Joardar et al. 2007). Along the way, many other ophthalmic imaging systems were developed for corneal topography (Swartz et al. 2007), ultrasound (Lorente-Ramos et al. 2012), and slit-lamp photography, as well as multimodal systems employing different wavelengths (Charbel Issa et al. 2009) and imaging modalities (Halberg 1950, Justice 1978).

Initially, all fundus photography was done by physicians (Martonyi et al. 1994). As far back as 1949 there was a need for 'Organization of a Photographic Department' in Buenos Aires, as reported by Dr Halberg in the BJO (Kempen et al. 2004). Among the considerations undertaken to ensure efficient workflow and use of resources were 'Equipment,' 'Filing and Processing,' and 'Administration'—topics still relevant to this day.

As technology advanced, the expanded imaging options available to the ophthalmic world demanded skill specialization. Ophthalmic photography evolved into a recognized profession, with the Ophthalmic Photographers' Society (OPS) established in the USA in 1969 (Justice 1978), and like-minded professional societies appeared in the UK, Japan, Australia, and more. Within 10 years, certification programs, such as the OPS Certified Retinal Angiographer were put into place (Martonyi CL et al. 1994), to be followed by more task-specific certifications as technology allowed more varied and specialized imaging tasks to be performed.

Hand-in-hand with ophthalmic diagnostic imaging, new treatment modalities appeared and evolved, placing growing demands on hospital-based technical staff. The advent of digital imaging did little to lessen the burden on photographic departments – it simply shifted the pressure to shorten result delivery times.

In addition, the dramatic increase in the number of diabetic patients needing imaging-based eye care, the rising aging population demanding solutions to a variety of degenerative eye diseases, the growing inclusion of images in publications and teaching forums, and finally, the unprecedented number of clinical trials relying on imaging all placed increasing strains on photographic departments. In cases where the department was made up of a lone photographer, things rapidly got out of hand. Lately, with a variety of intravitreal injections becoming the standard-of-care for a growing list of retinal diseases, there has been a dramatic increase in the number of referrals for imaging examinations, often before every scheduled treatment.

Hospitals serve as 'catch basins' and centers of excellence aimed at treating large population masses, either in dense metropolitan settings or at a central location in rural areas. In a world more and more accustomed to instant service and ever-shortening deadlines and where medical negligence lawsuits are a fact of increasing regularity, adding more examinations to the case load described above has increased the pressure on imaging resources. One solution to this problem is to set up a stand-alone center capable of delivering high-quality test results, with shorter waiting times, at an affordable price, keeping pace with technological advances as well as expanding to include new services as required. And, importantly, do so without alienating the surrounding medical community.

Among the services such centers can offer:

- High quality and consistent work due to highly trained staff, state-of-the-art equipment, professionally thought-out work protocols, and quality-assurance procedures
- Rapid access to essential tests thanks to extended clinic hours, patient booking systems and time-slots available for walk-in patients
- Competitive pricing of tests and services thanks to efficient use and short payback time of equipment and facilities
- High patient satisfaction resulting from a professional and orderly facility
- A complete set of results in addition to a written report with interpretation of the test results, for the patient's records, and for use in further medical care

SETUP

When planning an ophthalmic imaging center outside a hospital setting or existing medical center, the following matters need to be considered:

- Location
- Population size to be served
- Size of facility needed and price of rental vs purchase
- Number of hospitals providing same or similar services in the area
- Average waiting time for appointment to imaging services at area hospitals
- Average fees for services/reimbursement in the relevant area
- Availability of professional staff or ability to train applicants
- Establishing good working relations with local medical institutions
- Price of equipment and initial lineup of instruments needed

The location selected for the center should take into account several factors, among them, proximity to major thoroughfares, public transport routes, nearby parking facilities and adjacent office space available for expansion. In considering the appeal of the center, the potential for success is linked to the number of hospitals providing similar services in the area. A fair amount of market research needs to be done concerning the case load of local hospitals, and their position on allowing their resident experts to provide services at alternative centers.

As a rule of thumb, acceptable patient waiting times for ophthalmic diagnostic tests should be kept to 1 week. Unexpected delays often crop up and push the waiting time more towards the 10-day mark. These can be in the form of equipment problems, holidays, or a large influx of patients when one of the area hospitals cannot see patients for a few days, etc. Planning to accommodate the patients, based on a 1-week waiting time, does not mean that this is the only basis for operation. It means that there may be instances where you will be expected to admit patients within an hour—or a day—of their phone call.

Since the concept of a successful stand-alone imaging center is based on it being profitable, a central component of the equation is the price charged for tests. The model presented here is based on a system where patients are covered by some form of insurance that pays for these tests in the public hospitals, and therefore the fees charged at the stand-alone need to be lower than in other institutions where 'public' money covers the tests.

This is actually easier to accomplish than it sounds—since most hospital clinics do not have complete control of their finances, but rather operate under a larger administration which makes it difficult or impossible to set independent policies—such as clinic hours, employment policies, pricing, and purchasing.

If we just take a few of the most significant fixed expenses of any clinic—rent, instrument payback, insurance, and property tax—we can see that by operating a clinic for, say, 12 hours a day, instead of the standard 7 or 8, we can achieve a much higher level of efficiency. This in turn will allow us, among other things, to charge less for services available elsewhere. Note that a separate billing system should be set up in order to accommodate paying ('private') patients.

This mindset forces us, of course, to look at the process of providing medical care (in this case, ophthalmic diagnostic procedures), in a business manner as well. We must constantly be alert in keeping our operation solvent, while remaining committed to the highest professional standards.

When operating in environments where some form of socialized or government backed medical insurance programs are part of the system, best results can achieved by signing agreements with the various insurers approved by the health authorities, since there is great 'power in the numbers' of patients insured by them.

Understanding and accepting new payment agreements with governmental bodies can at times be frustrating, but the number of patients one is able to serve via these agreements often simply demands a different assessment of the economics involved.

For example, such agreements can include a minimum patient load clause, which guarantees the stand-alone imaging center a lump sum based on a minimum number of patients per year, with payment added for patients seen over this amount. In addition, such an agreement allows start-up imaging centers to rent office space, hire personnel and purchase equipment with the security of assured income.

One of the most important components of an imaging center is the constant, evident quality of the work produced by way of hiring and maintaining an excellent technical workforce. In addition, the constant evolution and increasing level of sophistication of ophthalmic diagnostic technology, as well as the ever-growing expectations from the medical community to deliver better and faster results, make the ongoing training—and advanced training—of technical staff of paramount importance.

Proper training can take many forms and levels, and should be an ongoing project. Simply providing the technicians with a basic understanding of the eye, its major components and ailments along with the standard imaging modalities used in the various conditions will not form the basis for a sophisticated and successful imaging center. However, having your staff attend periodic lectures will help to avoid junior technicians misinterpreting and delivering inaccurate results in the absence of more senior technicians.

Some of the more essential staff hiring, training, and education routines are listed below:

- Strong preference to applicants who have completed ophthalmic technician training
- During the employment interview emphasis should be placed on interpersonal skills, meaning that the ability to work with the patients we see every day is as essential a skill as knowing how to operate a camera or visual field machine
- Many technicians need to be introduced to the concept of time management
- The senior technician, or the technical director, should interact routinely with the other technicians in order to ascertain that they are completely conversant in all matters pertaining to their job—from reading and understanding referral letters to knowing how to custom-tailor all imaging modalities according to pathology, patient cooperation and media opacities, if any
- In order to achieve and maintain the highest level of professionalism, periodic in-house lectures and questionnaires should be performed. Occasional guest lectures and attending lectures at conferences are excellent additions to the overall education and esprit-de-corps of the staff
- In such busy centers, it is important to offer technicians the opportunity to learn and grow professionally. Especially for those performing repetitive tasks such as visual field testing, such professional advancement can be very important, insuring their ongoing motivation
- Strongly encourage the technical—as well as secretarial—staff to ask the technical director questions on terminology, diagnosis, and tests. Remaining accessible and insisting that anything out of the ordinary in the daily routine should be investigated and referred upward will greatly reduce the number of mistakes made.

The ongoing operation of such a multifaceted imaging center encompasses many areas that need constant attention:

- Ensuring patient safety
- Maintaining highest-quality results
- Ensuring patient satisfaction from quality of service
- Ensuring referring-physician satisfaction from quality of service
- Keeping abreast of developments in the field of ophthalmic imaging and evaluating new options for inclusion in the list of services offered
- Proper equipment maintenance and data safety
- Keeping the staff motivated, interested in their work, and able to work with requisite professionalism

Several of the tests performed in ophthalmic diagnosis carry risks to the patients—from the wrong eye being dilated to suffering reactions to an intravenous (IV) injection of fluorescent contrast media. The first and best line of defense against mistakes that can cause patient harm is the installation of rock-solid protocols for every single stage of operation. This holds doubly true when patient safety is concerned.

For example, upon checking in a patient at reception, the secretary should make a note—in bold letters—concerning any limitations regarding dilation, such as sensitivity to particular drops. In addition, the patient should be told that when the nurse arrives with the drops, the patient should state again the matter of sensitivity. The nurse, in turn, should be instructed not to take offence at being told this again by the patient, but rather to compliment the patient on raising this concern. The nurse should also sign his/her initials near the notation regarding the sensitivity made by the secretary.

In matters relating to tests that include the IV injection of contrast media, i.e. fluorescein, patients should sign a detailed consent form, after answering pertinent questions, formulated by the medical director of the center. When the patient enters the photography room, appropriate questions should be asked again by the photographer in the room, who is designated as the final defense against mistakes.

A complete emergency medicine kit should be on hand in every facility that performs fluorescein angiography (FA) tests, and immediate emergency medications should be kept within arm's reach for the duration of the work day. In addition, it is useful to have blood pulse oximeters and blood sugar meters available for use in assessing the unwell patient. The physician injecting the dye and other members of the staff should be well versed in the location, purpose, and use of the emergency medical equipment and drugs.

Once or twice a year it is prudent to conduct a refresher session, during which photographers, technicians, and receptionists are asked to assemble an IV setup, hand a particular medicine to the doctor, administer oxygen, etc. These sessions are aimed at making the staff more at ease with emergency situations, as well as familiar with the equipment, thereby freeing the ophthalmologist to devote full attention to the patient.

Maintaining consistently high-quality results is almost a full-time job, which includes both reviewing results from a technical point and ensuring that the tests are performed according to the various diagnoses and referral letters. This is achieved by routinely looking at tests taken by the various technicians, while looking at—among other features—dye arrival times, late-stage images taken for various pathologies, sharp focus of images throughout the study, and the quality of stereo images.

Likewise, for example, optical coherence tomography (OCT) images should be evaluated for scan placement relative to pathology and correct alignment of segmentation lines, slit-lamp photos for even illumination and proper placement of ruler next to lesion, visual field tests for appropriate comments by the technicians as to the reliability of the patient's response, color photos for exposure and stereo quality in relevant photographs.

Patient satisfaction with the level and quality of service is paramount for the success of such a service. It is a tired cliché that the manager of such a service can apologize and explain away an occasional hazy photo or blurry OCT scan, but it is near impossible to account for and apologize for a complaint of rude or unprofessional behavior by one of your staff. This needs to be emphasized to technicians on a regular basis. In such a modern service, there is always more than one customer to satisfy—besides the patient there is the referring physician, whose main concerns are the quality, consistency, and availability of the service being provided. Periodic telephone calls to ascertain satisfaction and occasional letters inserted in the results envelopes help to ensure good working relations with your key customers.

As in all technology-based areas, the field of ophthalmic imaging is changing rapidly, and in order to stay abreast of developments and continue to deliver the most up-to-date test results, one has to both be aware of such developments and be able to afford them. In order to continually be up to date on such matters, the following are some tips that should be practiced regularly:

- Attend meetings and conferences where there are sizable trade shows so that you can review and evaluate the new instruments
- Attend meetings where there are sessions dedicated to imaging, where one is most likely to encounter presentations regarding new and improved, and even experimental, imaging techniques and instruments. Attending lectures on new treatments can yield insight into the various imaging modalities that will be needed in order to evaluate treatment efficacy, etc.
- Establish a good, trusting, working relationship with the leading representatives of the leading imaging equipment suppliers, so that you are assured of first-hand and timely knowledge of developments in the field
- Become a member of the relevant professional associations, subscribe to their publications, and attend their meetings if possible

On the subject of equipment, one should not neglect the all-important areas of proper handling, maintenance, updates, data safety, and, of course, data backups. Anyone using the equipment should be instructed as to the proper use of these delicate instruments, both routine and scheduled care such as cleaning and placing of protective covers at the end of a shift.

Eating and drinking in exam rooms should be strictly forbidden. Complete cleaning of the instruments at the start and end of shifts, with the approved cloth and cleaning fluid, should be carried out, as well as periodic wipe downs during the workday. This will ensure a clean and smooth working instrument for many years, and create a positive impressionfor patients and guests entering the exam rooms.

Special care should be practiced when undertaking the cleaning of lenses that are part of the imaging equipment. Different lenses demand different cleaning routines; it is advisable to print out a small card with the appropriate instructions to be displayed prominently near each instrument. Ideally, one or two competent technicians should be designated for the cleaning of the lenses. This may seem cumbersome to implement during a busy clinic day, therefore not always practical, but it will prove its value in the long run.

Whenever a part seems worn out—even before it breaks down—have it examined by a qualified technician. For example, when a cooling fan of a camera or a computer starts to sound noisy during operation, even though it is still functional—have it replaced as soon as possible. By the same token, software versions need to be updated when applicable. When doing so, make sure that you have first completed a full backup of all relevant data and that the update is carried out by a certified representative of the company supporting the equipment.

The area of data security and safety is hugely important and is best addressed by a competent professional. As with all security matters, soliciting advice is never sufficient; one must adhere to the safety protocols in order for them to be effective.

First, assign each and every user of any computer and imaging device attached to a computer, a unique username and password for accessing the various systems. Once done, have all relevant computer terminals configured so that they enter a 'locked state' after sitting idle for a predetermined period of time. This period should be around 10–15 minutes, but needs to be reasonable for every working environment. This method will greatly reduce the chance of unauthorized access to patient data and other proprietary information.

In addition, reduce the chance that any information relating to patients or your practice will be copied from your system: have all USB ports permanently disabled so that no-one can remove any sensitive patient data. This will of course greatly reduce the chance of your computers becoming contaminated by a virus contained in a USB device—since once the fact that data cannot be downloaded from the computers gets known, almost no attempts to connect such devices to your computers will take place. Of course, you may leave yourself the option of securely downloading data—either by you or a trusted associate, from a designated, limited access computer.

Last, but definitely not least, is the matter of keeping your large staff continuously dedicated, motivated, and committed to the ongoing success of the operation. Sitting in a dark room and repeating the same instructions dozens of times a day to patients may wear out even the most motivated of employees. Therefore, it is in the best interest of all involved, especially those in managerial positions, to take proactive steps to counter such tendencies and work toward creating a supportive and positive work environment, especially as it pertains to those employees performing the diagnostic tests.

Such efforts need to be both innovative and ongoing, starting with supplying comfortable, ergonomic chairs for the technicians, and reupholstering and repadding chairs as needed, and extending to offering periodic access to local and national professional meetings and subscriptions to appropriate publications.

In addition, it is most important to identify those employees who are both motivated and capable, and offer them professional advancement within the organization. This may come in the form of rotating technicians on a daily or weekly basis between different instruments.

Furthermore, holding periodic in-house staff meetings, during which a lecture is delivered on a related subject matter (cataract surgery, glaucoma therapy, cutting-edge imaging, technical tips, etc.), always goes a long way to bolster interest and motivation. During these meetings, one should solicit feedback from the staff on any issue that is important to them and take appropriate action where deemed beneficial.

Another way to preserve interest is to hand out 'home-made' take-home quizzes on matters related to the technical work, which can include photos, charts, abbreviations to decipher, etc., and ask for these to be returned within a week, anonymously. This will achieve many goals—encouraging staff to think and explore on their own without any pressure, as well as providing you with the feedback needed to plan future educational activities. Once in a while, hand out tasks to be completed that are not strictly related to seeing patients—this will give technicians a break from routine while allowing them a larger view of the operation. It may also generate some good ideas as feedback.

There are many more ways in which to keep your technical staff motivated and dedicated—spare no effort in finding them. The future and success of your professional undertaking depends on it, both in the long and short run.

REFERENCES

Chace RR, Lafayatte JH. A modified film carrier for the zeissnordenson fundus camera. *Arch Ophthalmol* 1950; **43**:910–911.

Charbel Issa P, Finger RP, Holz FG, Scholl HP. Multimodal imaging including spectral domain OCT and confocal near infrared reflectance for characterization of outer retinal pathology in pseudoxanthoma elasticum. *Invest Ophthalmol Vis Sci* 2009; **50**:5913–5918.

Deb-Joardar N, Germain N, Thuret G, et al. Systematic screening for diabetic retinopathy with a digital fundus camera following pupillary dilatation in a university diabetes department. *Diabet Med* 2007; **24**:303–307.

Halberg GP. Organization of a photographic department. *Br J Ophthalmol* 1950; **34**:121–125.

Justice J Jr. The Ophthalmic Photographers' Society – a biological sketch. *J Ophthalmic Photogr* 1978; **1**:5.

Keeler CR. The ophthalmoscope in the lifetime of Hermann von Helmholtz. *Arch Ophthalmol* 2002; **120**:194–201.

Kempen JH, O'Colmain BJ, Leske MC, et al. The prevalence of diabetic retinopathy among adults in the United States. *Arch Ophthalmol* 2004; **122**(4):552–563.

Lorente-Ramos RM, Armán JA, Muñoz-Hernández A, et al. US of the eye made easy: a comprehensive how-to review with ophthalmoscopic correlation. *Radiographics* 2012; **32**(5):E175–200.

Martonyi CL, Tomer TL, Wong D. A brief historical review of certification within the ophthalmic photographers' society. *J Ophthalmic Photogr* 1994; **16**:60–64.

Swartz T, Marten L, Wang M. Measuring the cornea: the latest developments in corneal topography. *Curr Opin Ophthalmol* 2007; **18**:325–333.

Thomas RL, Dunstan F, Luzio SD, et al. Incidence of diabetic retinopathy in people with type 2 diabetes mellitus attending the Diabetic Retinopathy Screening Service for Wales: retrospective analysis. BMJ 2012; 344:e874.

Chapter 8 Retinal vascular disorders

Amresh Chopdar

INTRODUCTION

Fluorescein angiography is the most informative procedure for studying retinal vascular disorders in health and disease. It not only demonstrates anatomical details but also explores physiologic competency and pathologic abnormalities. Its spectacular display of architecture and functional signs has broadened our understanding of retinal vascular disease in recent decades.

RETINAL ARTERY OCCLUSION

The main cause of retinal arterial occlusion is a cholesterol plaque or a platelet embolus arising from the carotid system or the heart. Other emboli such as thrombi and vegetations may also arise from the left side of the heart. Microemboli are often visible at a bifurcation of the retinal arterioles. They present with a painless sudden loss of vision affecting the entire visual field or a part of the visual field. Patients may often experience several episodes of transient loss of vision prior to permanent loss. The affected retinal area shows a gray, cloudy swelling. A cherry-red spot in the macular area is a classic sign of central retinal artery occlusion. The blood flow within the occluded vessel appears sluggish and is often broken into segments. This phenomenon is referred to as cattle trucking or railroad wagon rolling (**Figure 8.1**). If a branch of the retinal artery is occluded, the signs remain confined to the affected zone (**Figure 8.2**).

Fluorescein angiography findings

Acute stage

The prearterial phase is difficult to assess due to the masking of the choroidal background fluorescence, which is caused by the cloudy swelling of the retina. The arterial flow remains sluggish and often shows slow progression of the dye front with broken segments barely arriving at the peripheral arterioles. The vessels in the occluded zone may show retrograde venous return from the adjacent nonoccluded zone. Venous return remains delayed and incomplete. The macular area, if affected, remains hypofluorescent throughout the period of angiography (David et al. 1967, 1970, Hayreh & Weingeist 1980).

Resolution

After a few days, the cloudy swelling begins to resolve and the retina may show a mild degree of retinal pigment epithelial changes unmasking the underlying the choroid. The dye begins to flow into the retinal vessels slowly and may show a degree of narrowing and irregularity of caliber. The improvement in circulation is due to either dispersal of the embolus or recanalization of the occluded vessel. Venous return also improves, but the capillary details do not usually recover fully. The optic disc shows some degree of staining during the late phase of the angiogram (**Figure 8.3**).

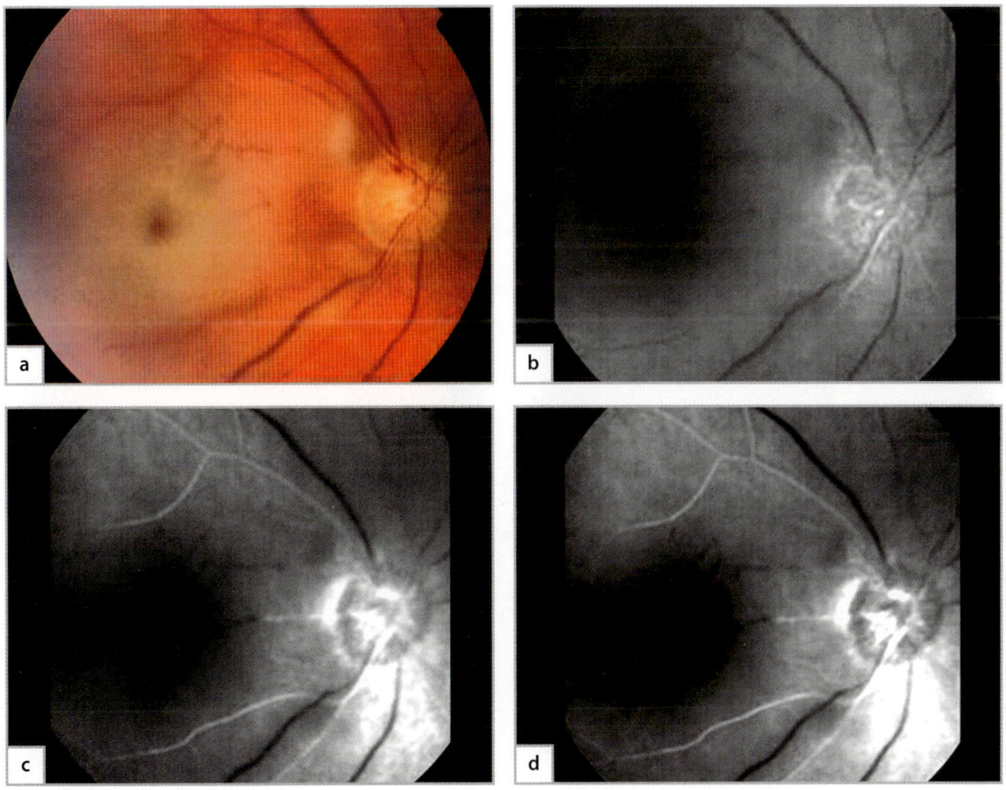

Figure 8.1 Acute stage of central retinal artery occlusion. The right eye shows marked narrowing of the retinal arteriole with cloudy swelling around the macular area and a cherry-red spot. There is also small number of splinter hemorrhages at the upper pole of the optic disc. (b) The arterial phase of the fluorescein angiogram shows deeper choroidal vasculatures on the optic disc with limited dye entry into the central retinal artery. (c) The dye gradually progresses through the branches of the central retinal artery but does not reach its terminal branches. (d) The dye remains limited to the major branches of the retinal arteries without ever reaching the periphery.

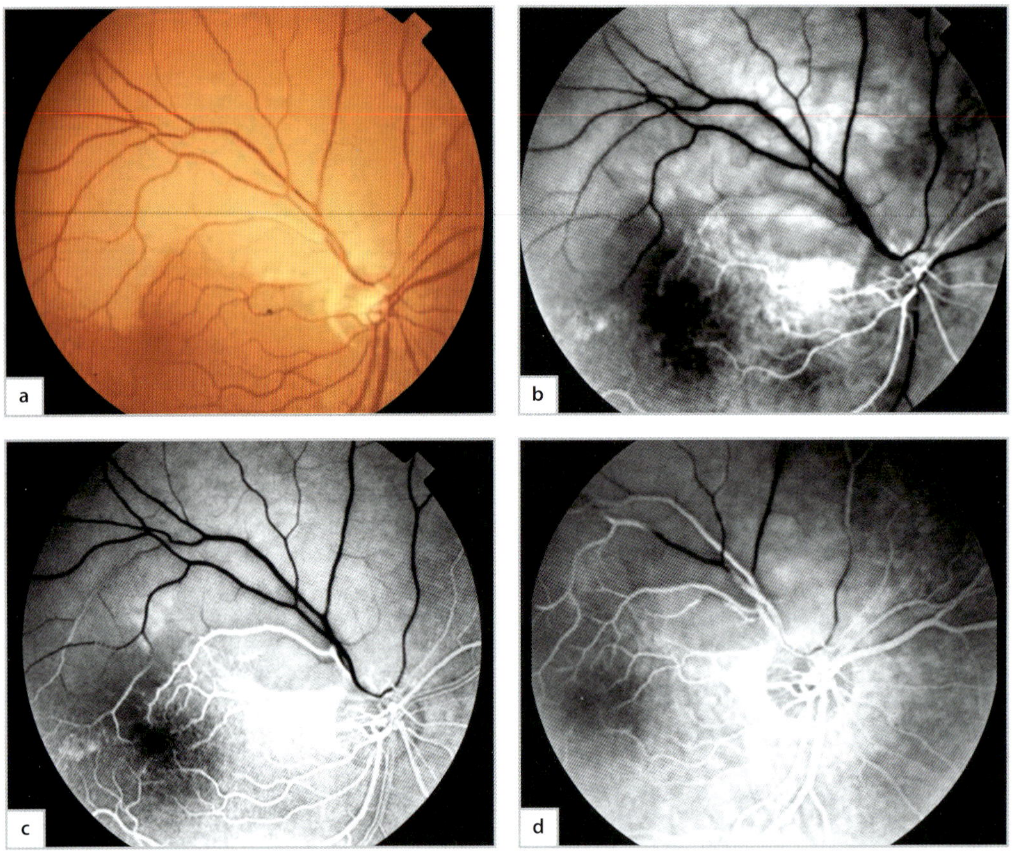

Figure 8.2 Branch retinal artery occlusion. (a) The right eye shows the superior division of the central retinal artery occluded with widespread cloudy swelling of the upper half of the fundus. (b) The arterial phase of the fluorescein angiogram shows patchy choroidal filling but no filling of the superior divisions of the retinal vessels. The inferior branches of the retinal artery fill normally. (c) The arteriovenous phase shows normal choroidal fluorescence. The inferior branches of the retinal arties and parts of the vein fill normally. Retrograde venous return occurs from the temporal regions of the macula toward the upper division of the retinal vein. (d) The late phase shows typical retrograde filling of the veins and branches of the upper part of the fundus. The inferior part of the fundus seems to fill normally.

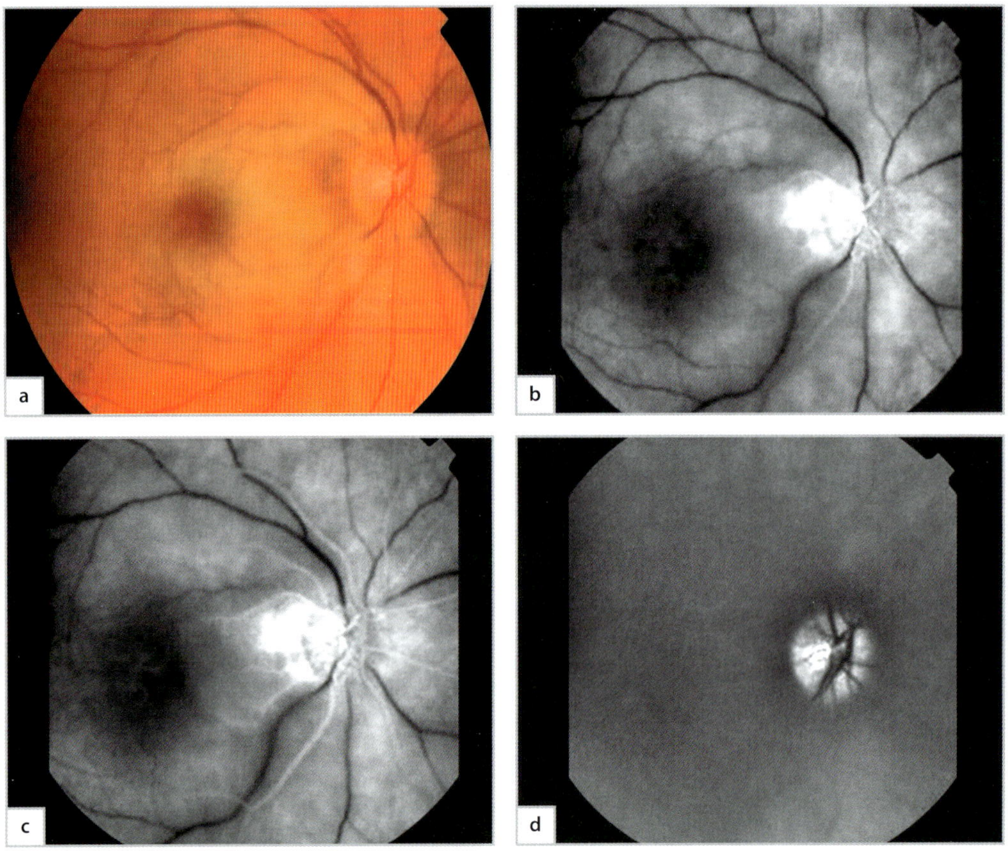

Figure 8.3 Central retinal artery occlusion: resolving stage. (a) The right eye of the same case seen in Figure 8.1 2 weeks after the central retinal artery occlusion shows resolving cloudy swelling of the macular area. (b) Early transit of the fluorescein angiogram shows patchy filling of the choroid, but the dye is slow to enter the narrowed retinal arteries. (c) Further into the transit phase the dye makes its way into the main branches of the retinal arteries. (d) The late phase shows some staining of the optic disc.

Resolved stage

The resolved stage shows a pale atrophic optic disc and marked narrowing of the retinal arterioles. The fluorescein angiogram shows grossly irregular caliber of the retinal vessels and staining of the optic disc toward the late phase (**Figure 8.4**).

CILIORETINAL ARTERY OCCLUSION

Cilioretinal artery occlusion is often associated with the choroidal infarct. The cloudy swelling takes a band-shaped configuration running along the course of the cilioretinal artery from the edge of the optic disc.

Fluorescein angiography findings

During the early phase of the angiography, normal choroidal fluorescence is seen except in the affected area. The occluded area remains hypofluorescent throughout the transit, leading to staining towards the late phase. There is severe restriction of dye flow into the occluded vessel. Venous return is similarly delayed (**Figure 8.5**).

PRECAPILLARY ARTERIOLAR OCCLUSION

Precapillary arteriolar occlusion is a common feature in diseases like hypertension, diabetes, collagen diseases, and autoimmune disorders. The occlusions of the retinal arterioles present as cotton wool spots usually in a vertical orientation due to interruption of the axoplasmic flow along the retinal nerve fibers. The fluorescein angiogram shows initial hypofluorescence due to nonfilling of the local vascular network resulting in retinal edema. The late phase of the fluorescein angiogram shows staining of the area affected (**Figure 8.6**).

RETINAL VEIN OCCLUSION

The clinical picture of retinal vein occlusion is due to a natural block of the vein behind the lamina cribrosa where the superior and inferior divisions meet to form single trunk of the central retinal vein. Alternatively one of its tributaries may be occluded at an arteriovenous crossing in front of the lamina cribrosa in any part of the fundus. The former is called central and the latter branch retinal vein occlusion.

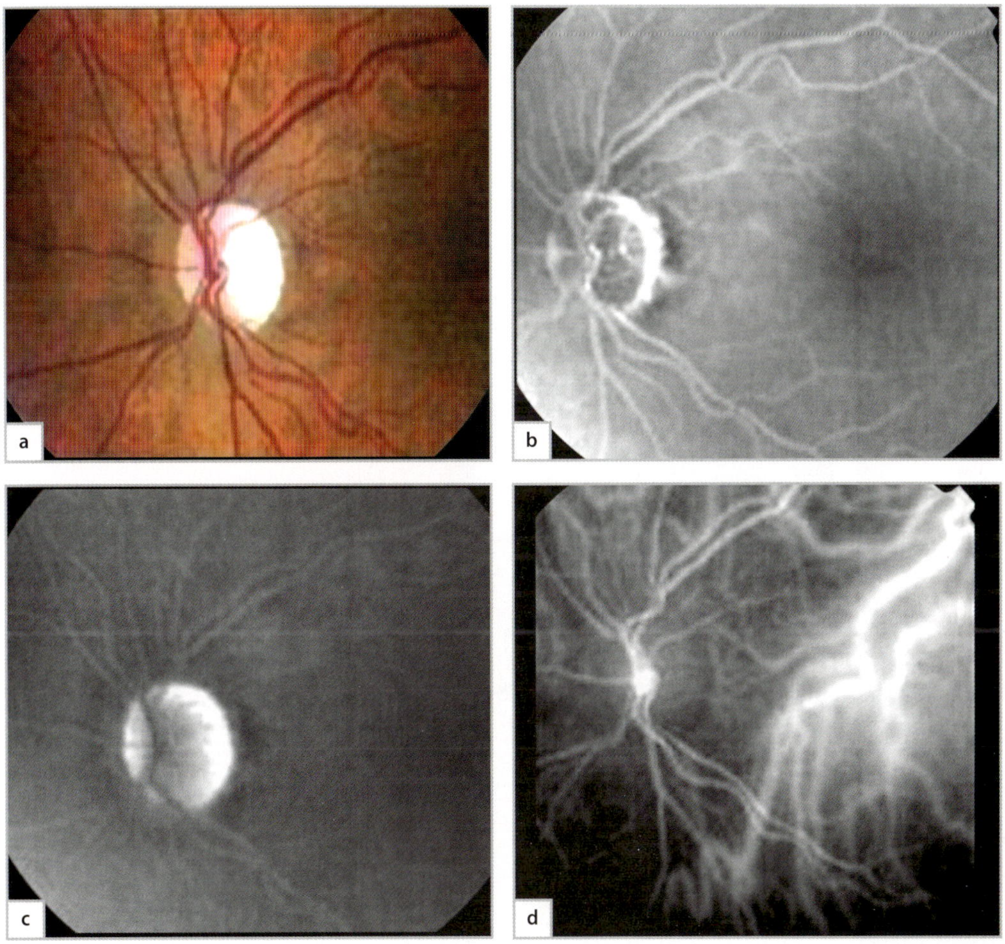

Figure 8.4 Central retinal artery occlusion: resolved stage. (a) The central retinal artery of the right eye in resolved stage shows a pale atrophic optic disc. (b) The arteriovenous phase of the fluorescein angiogram shows almost normal filling of the retinal circulation. (c) The late phase shows moderate degree of staining of the atrophic optic disc.

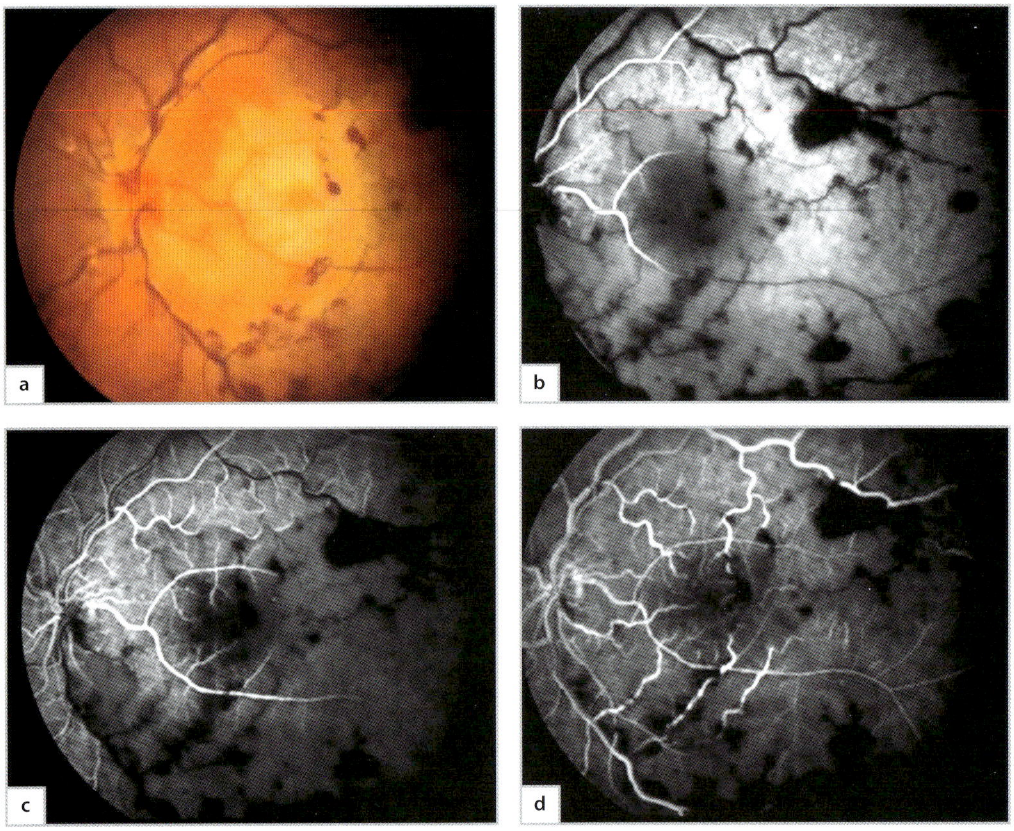

Figure 8.5 Cilioretinal artery occlusion. (a) The left eye shows a blocked cilioretinal artery emerging from the temporal edge of the optic disc supplying the macular area. The occluded zone shows widespread cloudy swelling of the posterior pole including the macula. Superficial retinal hemorrhages are seen in the posterior pole mainly temporal to the macula. (b) The early arterial phase of the fluorescein angiogram shows moderate filling of the background choroid. (c) During the progress of the transit, the dye passes slowly through the cilioretinal artery as well as the inferior branch of the retinal artery. The dye struggles to fill half way into the frame. (d) The late phase shows hardly any further progression of the dye front. The cilioretinal artery never becomes fully filled.

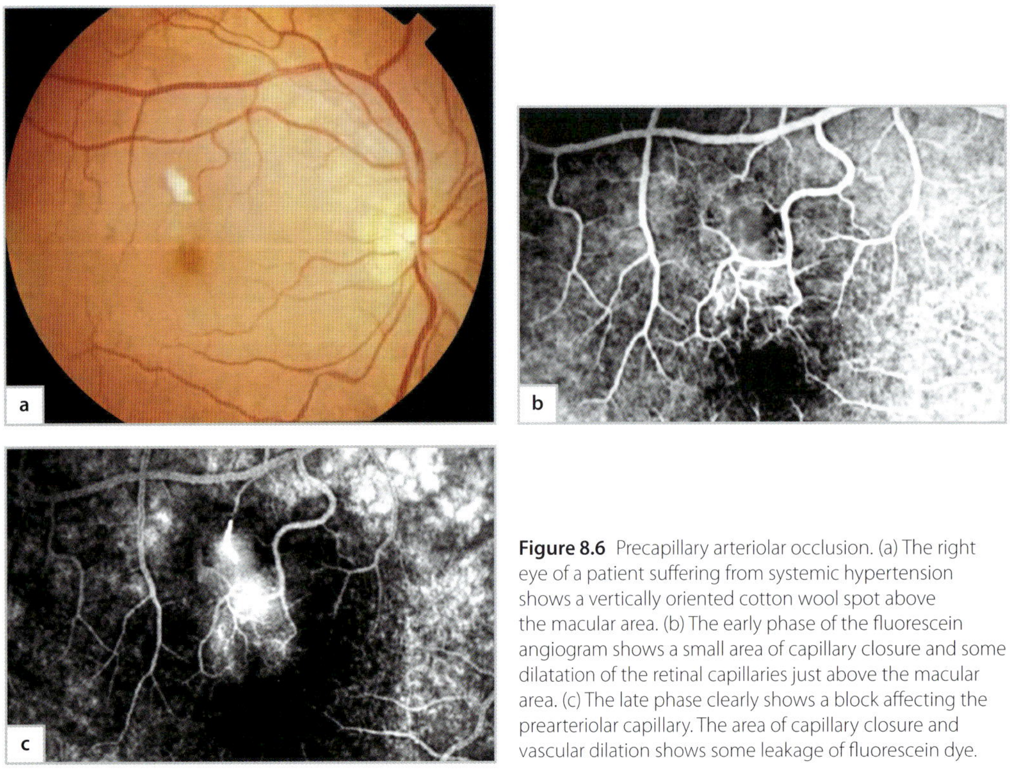

Figure 8.6 Precapillary arteriolar occlusion. (a) The right eye of a patient suffering from systemic hypertension shows a vertically oriented cotton wool spot above the macular area. (b) The early phase of the fluorescein angiogram shows a small area of capillary closure and some dilatation of the retinal capillaries just above the macular area. (c) The late phase clearly shows a block affecting the prearteriolar capillary. The area of capillary closure and vascular dilation shows some leakage of fluorescein dye.

The clinical picture of retinal vein occlusion can be divided into two distinct groups, namely nonischemic and ischemic.

The nonischemic group is associated with slight retinal hypoxia. Patients present with blurred vision, moderate visual loss, and altitudinal field defect. The ophthalmoscopy shows darker congested retinal veins, disc edema associated with variable degree of retinal hemorrhages, and a few or no cotton wool spots. Their vision may worsen due to chronic macular edema. A proportion of cases may show improvement or complete resolution with formation of collaterals anterior to the site of occlusion either at the optic disc or elsewhere. A significant number of patients may convert to ischemic group.

The ischemic group is associated with significant retinal hypoxia due to retinal arteriolar ischemia resulting in profound visual loss. Ophthalmoscopy shows darker, tortuous, engorged retinal veins with a limited amount of confluent hemorrhages. Cotton wool spots are frequently seen surrounding the optic disc and elsewhere in the retina. There may be a variable degree of optic disc edema. This group produces significant neovascularization of the disc and retina (Hayreh 1971, 1976a, 1976b, Laatikainen & Kohner 1976, Hayreh et al. 1978).

Fluorescein angiography findings

In the nonischemic group, the prearterial phase shows patchy choroidal filling associated with some masking. The arterial phase may show sluggish circulation and a degree of irregularity of the retinal arteriolar caliber. All veins and capillaries are markedly engorged and tortuous, and they may show microaneurysamal dilatation. The perifoveal arcade shows marked congestion and dilatation. The late phase shows a considerable amount of staining of the venous wall, leakage of the surrounding retina, and a typical cystoid macular edema. Preservation of the perifoveal arcade is a favorable sign for predicting visual improvement. A few weeks later retinal circulation gradually improves due to collateral formation between the occluded and nonoccluded branches. The retinal hemorrhages take several weeks to months to resolve. Often the visual acuity also improves (**Figures 8.7** and **8.8**).

In the ischemic group, the arterial phase shows masking of the choroidal background fluorescence due to cotton wool spots and retinal edema. The retinal arteriolar filling can be severely delayed or absent due to narrowing caliber and arteriosclerotic changes. There is extensive capillary closure affecting large parts of the retina. Venous return is exceedingly delayed. The veins are highly engorged and tortuous, and they appear discontinued and broken in places hidden from view due to the retinal hemorrhage, cotton wool spots, and edema. It is not unusual to find some veins remaining empty throughout the period of transit. The late phase shows marked leakage of dye from both the disc and the retina, and a strongly stained venous wall (**Figure 8.9**).

However, if the ischemia persists new vessels may form at the optic disc or elsewhere. This neovascularization is the hallmark of severe retinal ischemia. Fluorescein angiography now shows gross retinal arteriolar sclerosis, large areas of capillary closures, and neovascularization. Venous return is also delayed. The new vessels begin to fluoresce early during the transit, and continue throughout to produce marked leakage of dye during the late phase (**Figure 8.10**).

RETINAL VASCULITIS

Retinal vasculitis is seen in younger people affecting mainly veins but arteries may also be affected in certain specific conditions like

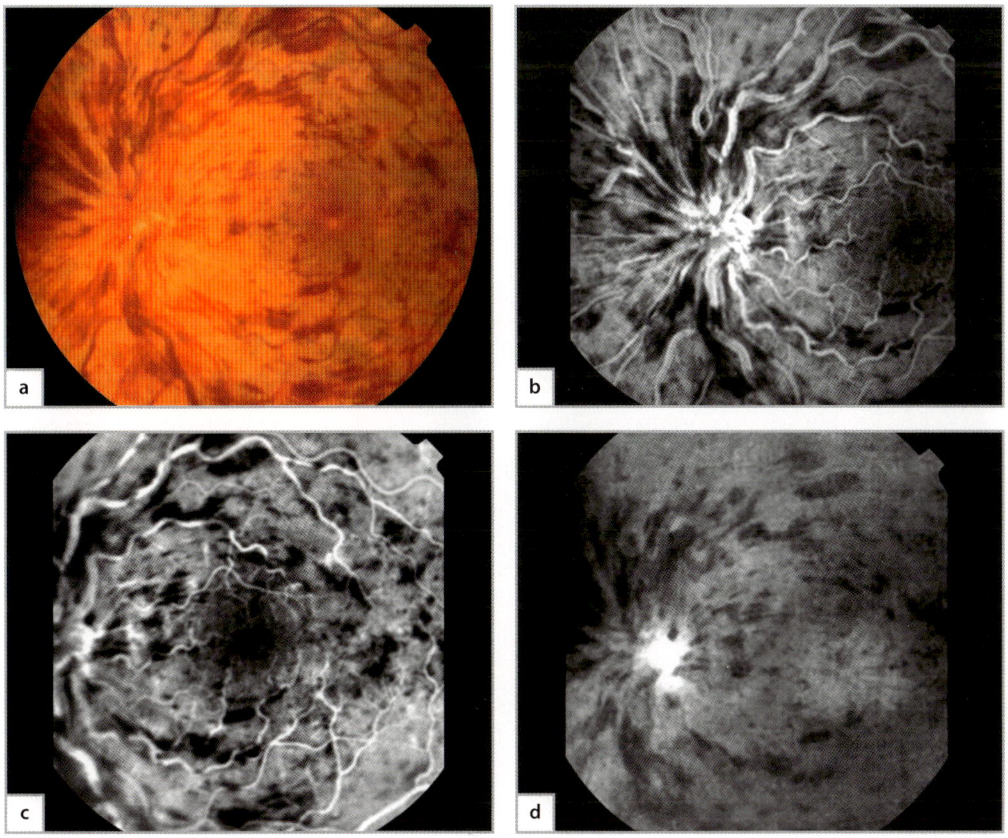

Figure 8.7 Nonischemic central retinal vein occlusion. (a) The left eye shows numerous flame-shaped retinal hemorrhages widely scattered throughout the fundus. The veins are dilated with a moderate degree of optic disc swelling. (b) The early phase of the fluorescein angiogram shows markedly dilated and tortuous retinal veins. The hypofluorescent areas are due to masking by the retinal hemorrhages. (c) The late transit phase continues to show masking from the retinal hemorrhages. There is no evidence of any capillary closure. The capillary detail of the macular area is unclear. (d) The late phase shows no significant evidence of leakage from the fundus as a whole but the macular area is already showing signs of cystoid macular edema.

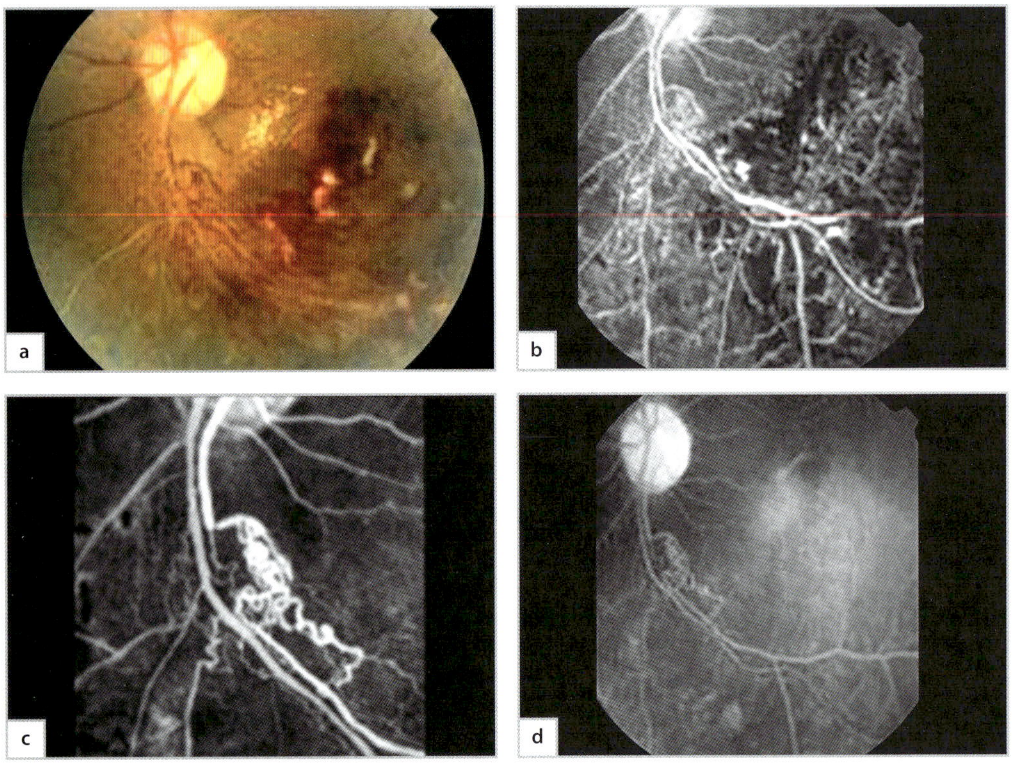

Figure 8.8 Nonischemic branch retinal vein occlusion: resolved stage with collaterals. (a) The right eye shows marked arteriosclerosis, cotton wool spots, and plenty of retinal hemorrhages affecting the entire inferior temporal quadrant of the fundus. (b) The early transit phase of the fluorescein angiogram shows masking due to heavy retinal hemorrhage. There is only a minimal amount of capillary closure. (c) The zoomed frame of the inferior temporal part of the fundus shows collateral formation from the site of the occlusion. (d) The late phase of the same area shows some staining but no evidence of any leak unlike its counterpart in new vessel formation in the ischemic type of vein occlusion.

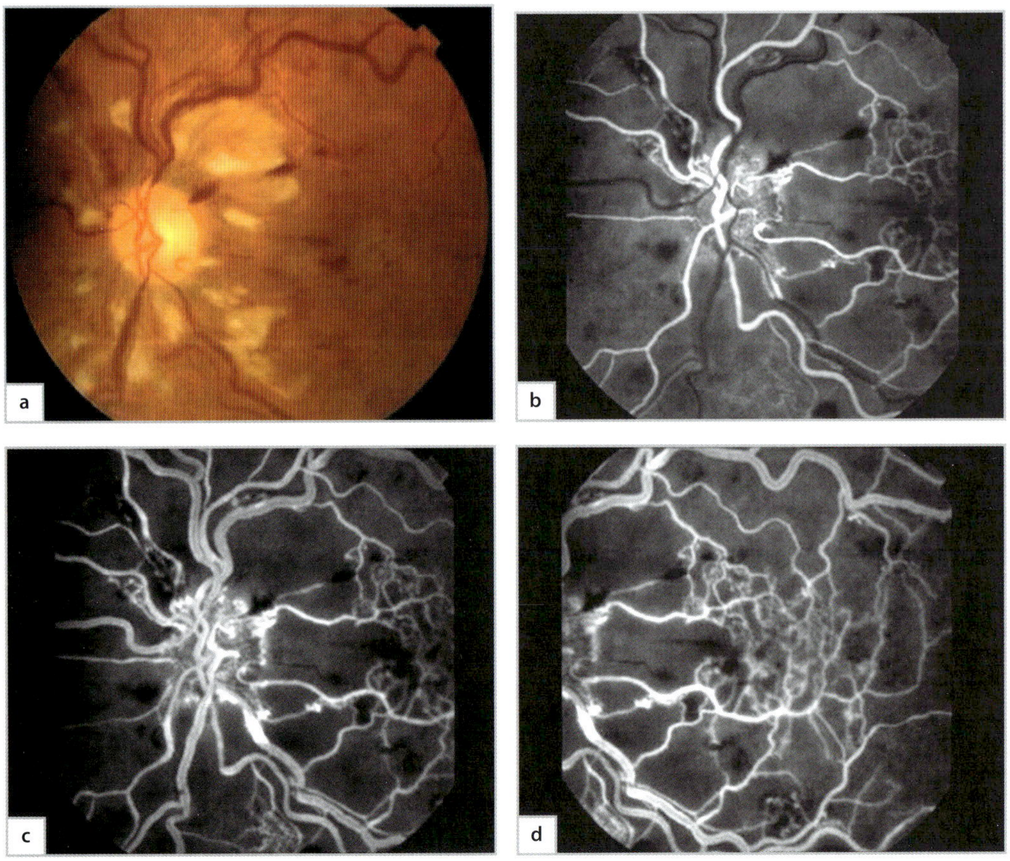

Figure 8.9 Acute ischemic central retinopathy. (a) The left eye shows numerous cotton wool spots around the optic disc and several retinal hemorrhages in the posterior pole. (b) The arterial phase of the fluorescein angiogram shows massive areas of capillary closure involving the entire fundus from the optic disc outward. (c) The late venous phase shows continuing hypofluorescence due to capillary closure. The retinal arteries show a significant degree of arteriosclerosis. The veins are dilated and tortuous. (d) The late phase shows loss of vascular architecture of the macular area, and the retina shows persistent hypofluorescence due to capillary closure.

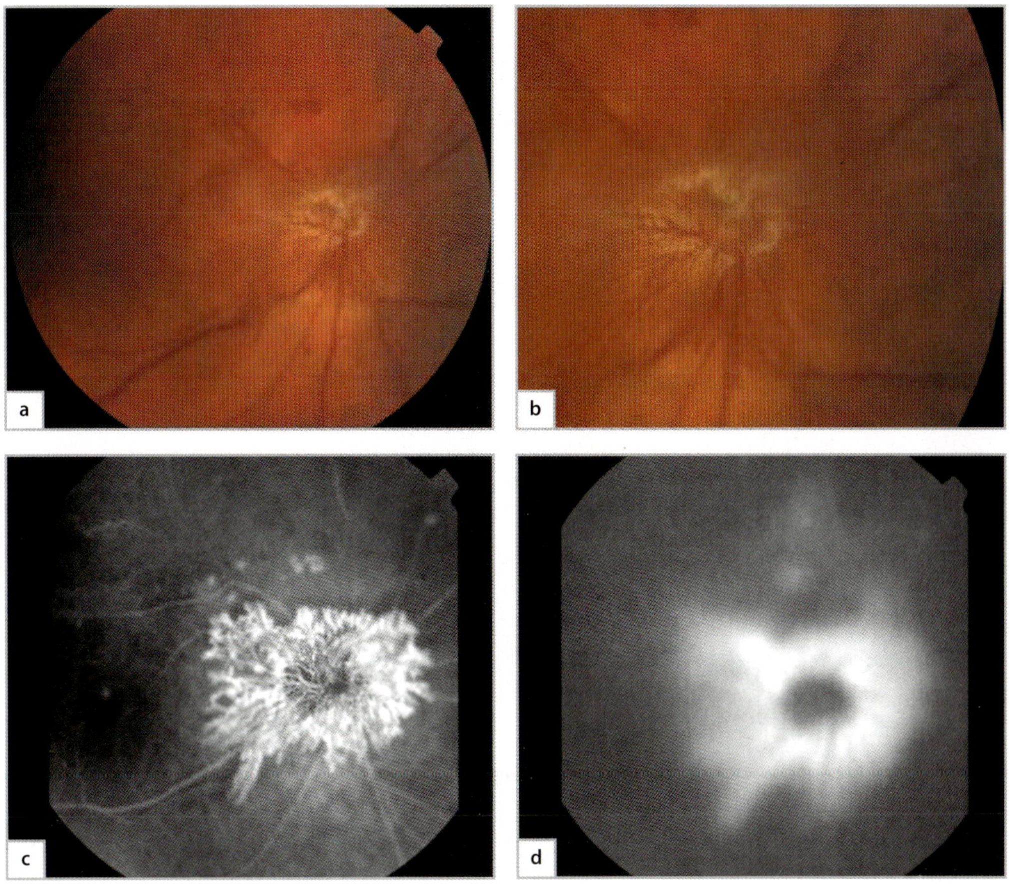

Figure 8.10 Neovascularization from the optic disc following ischemic central retinal vein occlusion. (a) The right eye shows marked arteriosclerosis and neovascularization from the optic disc. (b) The zoomed photograph shows new vessels from the optic disc. (c) The late venous phase of the fluorescein angiogram shows dense hyperfluorescence from the optic disc area. (d) The late phase shows extensive leakage from the optic disc.

polyarteritis and acute retinal necrosis. The clinical picture is often similar to that of retinal vein occlusion with cotton wool spot intraretinal hemorrhages and vascular dilatation. Ophthalmoscopy shows vascular sheathing, anastomosis, and neovascularization involving the peripheral part of the retina (Karel & Divisova 1973, Karel et al. 1974).

Fluorescein angiography findings

The fluorescein angiogram shows the vast areas of vascular dilatation and leakage of dye including staining of the walls of the retinal vein. If new vessels are found, they may lead to leakage of dye (**Figure 8.11**).

ARTERIOVENOUS COMMUNICATION

This is a congenital anomaly often discovered accidentally on routine eye examination. It does not lead to serious complications. Vision is only affected if the macular area is affected by the anastomosis.

Fluorescein angiography findings

The fluorescein angiogram shows an impressive flow of dye through the retinal arterioles and retrograde filling into the veins within the same segment of the fundus. The late phase of the angiogram may show some staining of the walls of the blood vessels but no leakage (**Figure 8.12**).

SICKLE CELL RETINOPATHY

The sickle-shaped red cells resulting from hypoxia fail to pass through the retinal capillary circulation, leading to microvascular occlusion. Occasionally, larger thrombi may form and cause embolization affecting larger branches of the retinal arterioles. The anoxia of the peripheral retina leads to arteriovenous anastomosis and formation of new vessels. This leads to vitreous hemorrhage and retinal detachment. Proliferative sickle cell retinopathy has been divided into five different stages: (1) peripheral arteriolar occlusion, (2) arteriovenous anastomoses, (3) retinal neovascularization, (4) vitreous hemorrhages, and (5) retinal detachment (Condon & Serjeant 1975, Raichand et al. 1977, Goldberg 1971).

Fluorescein angiography findings

The fluorescein angiogram during the early phase shows a total lack of peripheral choroidal and retinal circulation due to arteriolar occlusion. The arterial and early venous phase shows the arteriovenous anastomosis and budding of the new vessels toward the outer periphery of the retina. The late phase shows severe leakage of dye from these new vessels (**Figure 8.13**).

IDIOPATHIC MACULAR TELANGIECTASIA

Idiopathic macular telangiectasia, now called macular telangiectasia, may be unilateral or bilateral, often with lipid exudates and localized

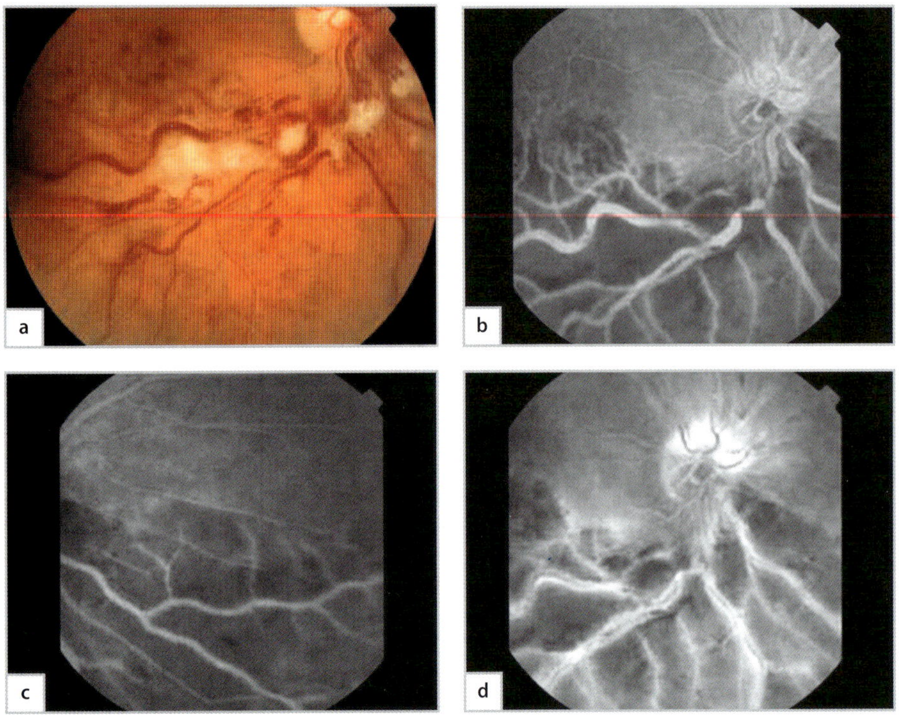

Figure 8.11 Retinal vasculitis. (a) A row of cotton wool spots along the inferior temporal retinal vein commonly described as a candle wax drip. The vein is dilated and tortuous with retinal hemorrhages. (b) The arteriovenous phase of the fluorescein angiogram of the inferior temporal part of the fundus shows a large area of capillary closure and a dilated retinal vein. There is compensatory dilatation of epipapillary capillaries on the upper part of the optic disc. (c) The inferior part of the retina shows marked irregularity of retinal arteriolar capillaries and dilated veins. (d) The late phase shows staining of the lateral walls of the retinal veins with leakage of fluorescein dye from the superior part of the optic disc due to secondary microvascular changes.

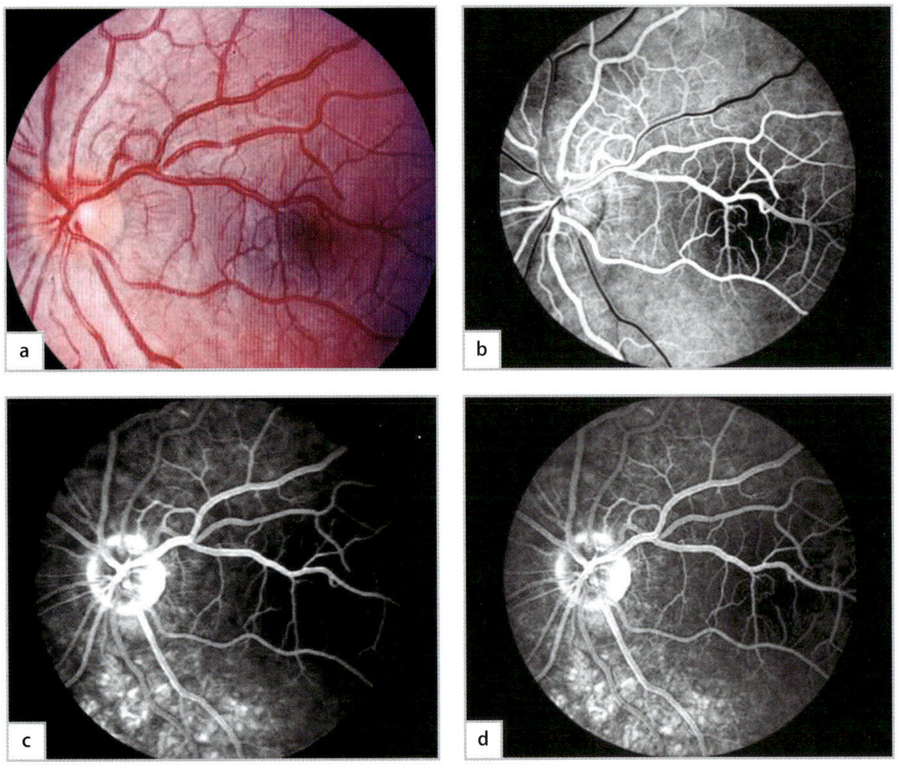

Figure 8.12 Arteriovenous communication. (a) There is an unusual arrangement of vascular tree of the retina. There are numerous arteriovenous communications at the posterior pole. The retinal veins are brighter red than normal. (b) The arterial phase of the fluorescein angiogram shows a branch of the retinal arteriole making a connection with a vein at the temporal part of the macula. (c) The early arteriovenous phase shows the arteriovenous communications as well as retrograde venous return. (d) The late venous phase shows well-filled retinal veins and capillaries. There is no evidence of any leakage of dye.

serous retinal detachment adjacent to the macular area. Full development runs through five different stages. It runs a chronic course and often manifests in the second and third decade of life. Patients complain of episodes of blurring of vision due to fluctuating macular edema (Chopdar 1978, Gass & Blodi 1993).

Fluorescein angiography findings

The fluorescein angiogram shows multiple areas of retinal capillary dilatation, tortuosity, and microaneurysmal dilatation near the macula. The capillaries leak to produce a typical picture of cystoid macular edema (**Figure 8.14**).

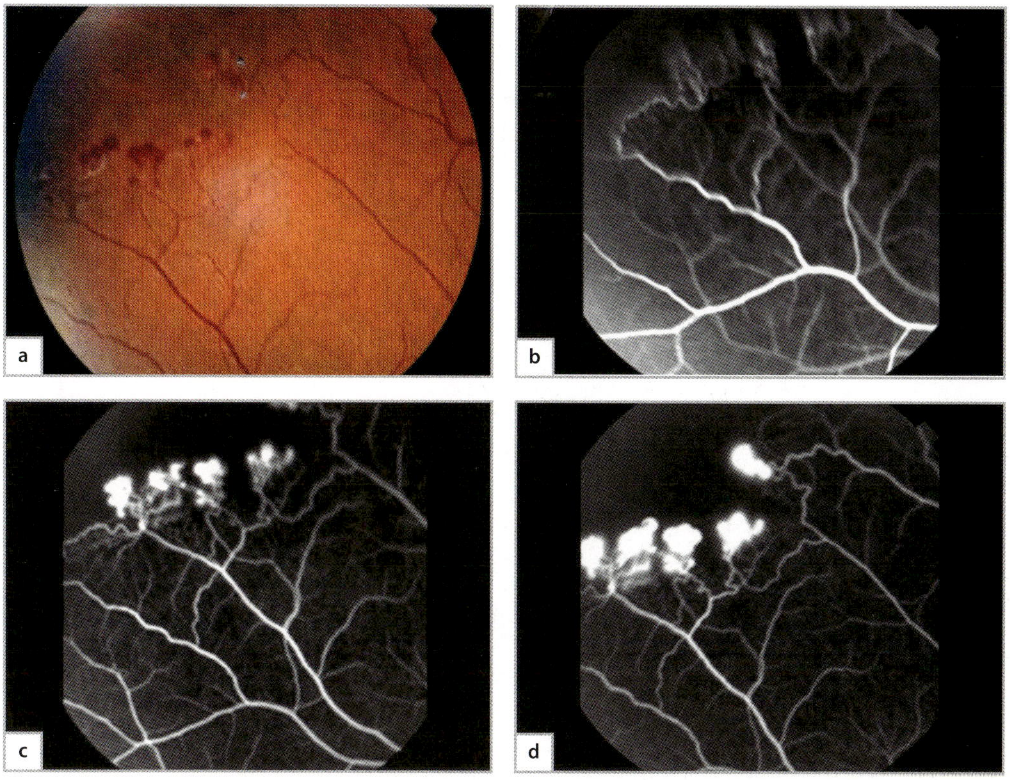

Figure 8.13 Sickle cell retinopathy. (a) The right upper temporal quadrant shows tufts of peripheral neovascularization in a case of sickle cell retinopathy. (b) The early arteriovenous phase of the fluorescein angiogram shows arteriovenous anastomosis of the peripheral vessels. (c) The mid venous phase shows tufts of new vessels growing from the anastomoses toward the peripheral ischemic area of the retina. (d) The later phase shows leakage of fluorescein dye from the new vessels spreading outward.

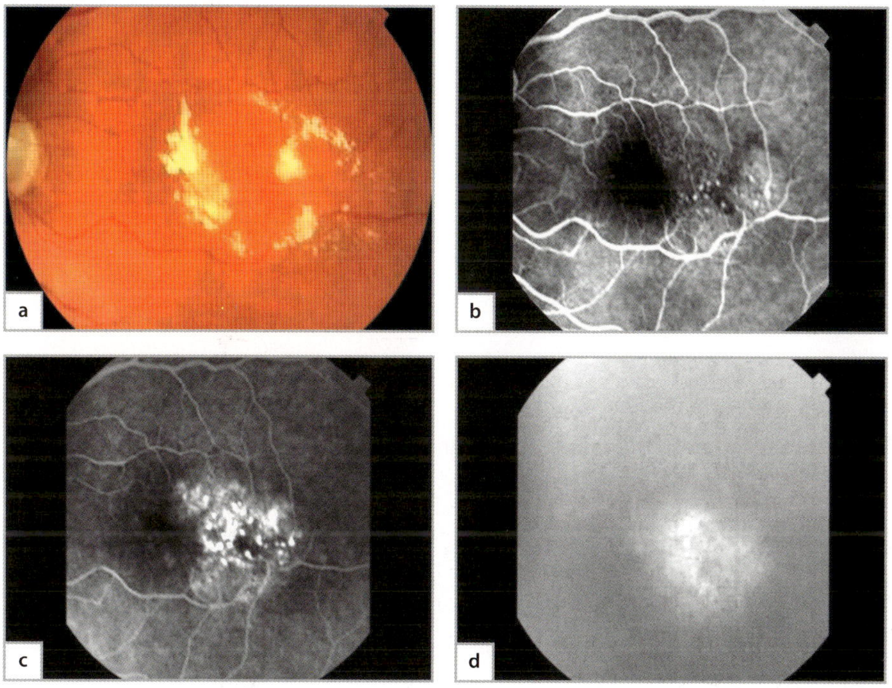

Figure 8.14 Paramacular telangiectasias. (a) The left eye shows a ring of lipid exudate lateral to the macula. Within the ring, several red dots are seen. This area of retina seems to be slightly edematous. (b) The arteriovenous phase of the fluorescein angiogram shows multiple dots of hyperfluorescence similar to microaneurysms associated with retinal capillary dilation and tortuosity. (c) The late venous phase shows many more microaneurysamal changes with increasing hyperfluorescence. (d) The late phase shows minimal degree of leakage from the microvascular changes beginning to create a cystoid change at the temporal aspect of the macula.

MACROANEURYSM

This is one of the most commonly underdiagnosed conditions affecting the fundus. Macroaneurysm is common among elderly patients, particularly those suffering from systemic hypertension and arteriosclerosis. The retinal artery shows a small out-pouching surrounded by a ring of lipid exudate with some retinal edema (Moosavi et al. 2006).

Fluorescein angiography findings

Fluorescein angiography shows marked arteriosclerosis and a slow increase in fluorescence from the aneurysm. The late phase of the angiogram shows some degree of leakage of dye (**Figure 8.15**).

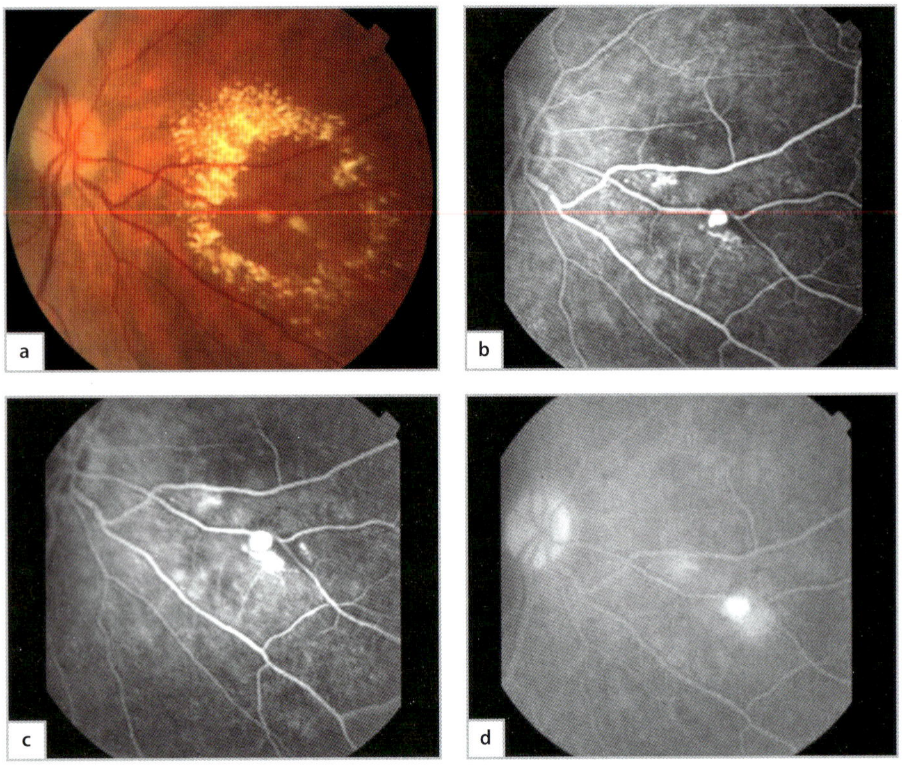

Figure 8.15 Macroaneurysm. (a) The nasal side of the right eye shows a ring of lipid exudate within which there are two gray areas. (b) The same area during the early phase of the fluorescein angiogram shows a saccular dilatation arising from the retinal arteriole within the ring of lipid exudate. Next to this hyperfluorescent spot, there is a small area of capillary closure corresponding to the gray areas seen in the color photograph. (c) The late venous phase shows increase in fluorescence of the spot from the retinal artery. (d) The late phase shows minimal leakage of dye from the macroaneurysm and the staining spreading locally to cover the capillary closure area.

REFERENCES

Chopdar A. Retinal telangiectasis in adults: fluorescein angiographic findings and treatment by argon laser. *Br J Ophthalmol* 1978; **62**:243–250.

Condon PI, Serjeant GR. The progression of sickle cell eye disease in Jamaica. *Doc Ophthalmol* 1975; **31**:203–210.

David NJ, Norton EW, Gass JD, Beauchamp J. Fluorescein angiography in central retinal artery occlusion. *Arch Ophthalmol* 1967; **77**:619–629.

David NJ, Gilbert DS, Gass JD. Fluorescein angiography in retinal arterial branch obstruction. *Am J Ophthalmol* 1970; **69**:43–55.

Gass JD, Blodi BA. Idiopathic juxtafoveolar retinal telangiectasis. Update of classification and follow-up study. *Ophthalmology* 1993; **100**:1536–1546.

Goldberg MF. Natural history of untreated proliferative sickle cell retinopathy. *Arch Ophthalmol* 1971; **85**:428–437.

Hayreh SS. Pathogenesis of occlusion of central retinal vessels. *Am J Ophthalmol* 1971; **72**:998–1011.

Hayreh SS. So-called "central retinal vein occlusion". I. Pathogenesis, terminology, clinical feature. *Ophthalmologica (Basel)* 1976a; **172**:1–13.

Hayreh, SS. So-called "central retinal vein occlusion". II. Venous stasis retinopathy. *Ophthalmologica (Basel)* 1976b; **172**:14–37.

Hayreh SS, van Heuven WA, Hayreh MS. Experimental retinal vascular occlusion-1. Pathogenesis of central retinal vein occlusion. *Arch Ophthalmol* 1978; **96**:311–323.

Hayreh SS, Weingeist TA Experimental occlusion of the central retinal artery. 1. Ophthalmoscopic and fluorescein fundus angiographic studies. *Br J Ophthalmol* 1980; **64**:896–912.

Karel I, Votocková J, Peleska M. Fluorescence angiography in unusual forms of idiopathic retinal vasculitis. *Ophthalmologica* 1974: **168**:446–461.

Karel I, Divisova G. Fluorescence angiography in retinal vasculitis in children's uveitis. *Ophthalmologica* 1973; **166**:251–264.

Laatikainen L, Kohner EM Fluorescein angiography and its prognostic significance in central retinal vein occlusion. *Br J Ophthalmol* 1976; **60**:411–418.

Moosavi RA, Fong KC, Chopdar A. Retinal artery macroaneurysms: clinical and fluorescein angiographic features in 34 patients. *Eye* 2006; **20**:1011–1020.

Raichand M, Goldberg MF, Nagpal K G, et al. Evolution of neovascularisation in sickle cell retinopathy. *Arch Ophthalmol* 1977; **95**:1543–1552.

Chapter 9 Age-related macular degeneration

Raeba Mathew, Sobha Sivaprasad

INTRODUCTION

Age-related macular degeneration (AMD) is the leading cause of central loss of visual acuity in the elderly in the developed countries.

PATHOPHYSIOLOGY

Topographically, the macular area can be subdivided into four distinct zones: the foveola, fovea, parafovea, and perifovea (**Figure 9.1**). In cross-section, the retina has a complex histological structure made up of 10 layers. However, in simpler functional terms, it consists of two main layers: (1) the inner retina and (2) the outer retina consisting of the photoreceptors and the underlying retinal pigment epithelium (RPE). Bruch's membrane is sandwiched between the RPE and the choroid, the main source of blood supply to the outer retina (**Figure 9.2**).

With advancing age, the RPE becomes incompetent, leading to accumulation of waste products, which leads to amorphous deposits called drusen. Gradually the RPE degenerates, creating a geographical atrophic lesion. This is commonly called a non-exudative type of AMD. The exudative or wet form of macular degeneration, develops secondary to a break in Bruch's membrane. The new vessels developing from the choroid insinuate themselves through the breaks and spread under the RPE, leading to the formation of type 1 or occult choroidal neovascularization (CNV). These new blood vessels are fragile, leading to edema, extravasation of blood, and lipid materials. Progressively the new vessels invade the subretinal space, giving rise to a type 2 or classic CNV (**Figure 9.3**).

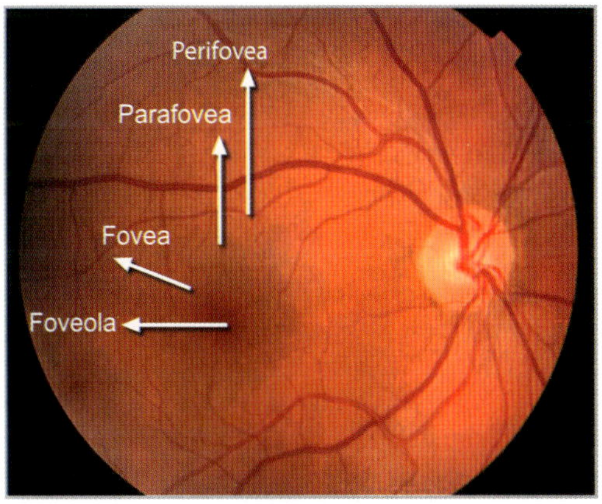

Figure 9.1 Clinical macular area: the four different zones of the macular area.

CLASSIFICATION

In 1995, the international age-related maculopathy (ARM) epidemiological study group (Bird et al. 1995) redefined AMD based on the standard ETDRS (Early Treatment Diabetic Retinopathy Study) grid with three concentric circles diameters of 1, 3, and 6 mm, respectively. ARM was classified into two main groups: early ARM that included drusen and retinal pigment epithelial abnormalities (hyper- or hypopigmentation) and late ARM composed of geographic atrophy (GA), pigment epithelial detachment (PED), CNV, and disciform scarring. The age-related eye disease study (AREDS) group (2000) classified AMD into four levels based on the standard ETDRS grid:

1. Level 1—small drusen <63 μm
2. Level 2—intermediate drusen (63–125 μm) with hypo- or hyper-pigmentation
3. Level 3—large soft drusen (<125 μm) or noncentral GA
4. Level 4—central GA or evidence of neovascular AMD characterized by fibrovascular or serous PED, serous or hemorrhagic sensory retinal detachment, subretinal or subpigment epithelial hemorrhage, and subretinal fibrous tissue (or fibrin)

A recent classification of AMD by the Beckman Initiative for Macular Research Classification Committee (Ferris et al. 2013) reclassified

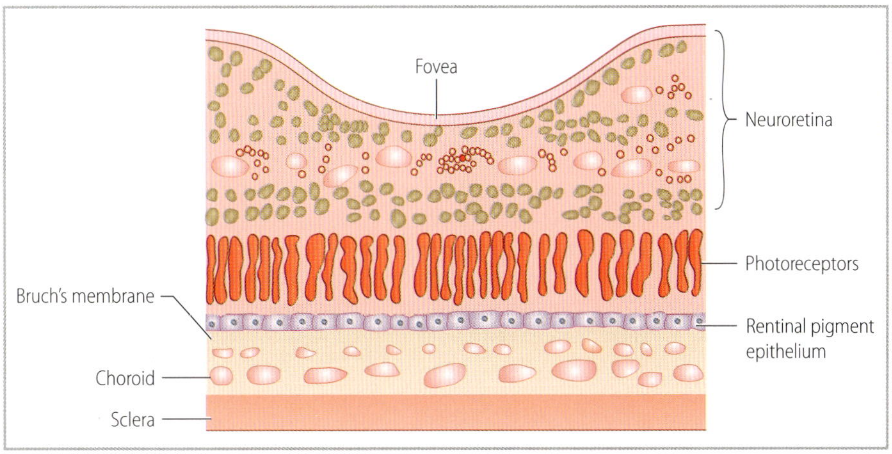

Figure 9.2 Normal macula, showing the two principal layers of the retina and the neuroretina including the photosensitive layers. The retinal pigment epithelium and the Bruch's membrane separate the photoreceptor layer from its vascular supply. The fovea is the thinnest part of the center of the macular area. With permission from Chopdar et al. 2003.

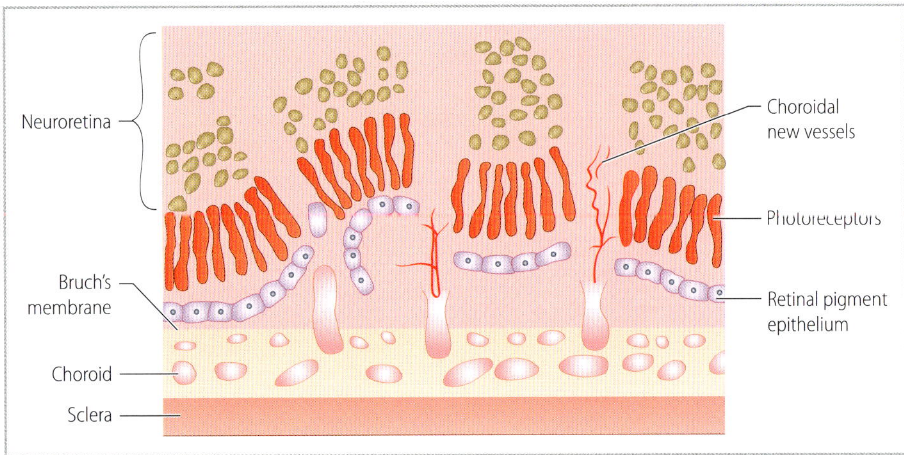

Figure 9.3 Formation of the choroidal neovascular membrane. The choroidal neovascular membrane, grows from the choroid and passes through breaks in Bruch's membrane and eventually through the disrupted retinal pigment epithelium into the subretinal space. With permission from Chopdar et al. 2003.

AMD based on lesions assessed within two disc diameters of fovea in either eye, into five groups:

1. No apparent aging changes—no drusen and no AMD pigmentary abnormalities
2. Normal aging changes—only drupelets (small drusen <63 µm) and no AMD pigmentary abnormalities
3. Early AMD—medium drusen >63–125 µm and no AMD pigmentary abnormalities
4. Intermediate AMD—large drusen >125 µm and/or any AMD pigmentary abnormalities
5. Late AMD—neovascular AMD and/or any GA

DIAGNOSTIC TECHNIQUES

Apart from clinical examination, various objective methods for documentation and quantification of the retinal changes are available at present. Previously, diagnosis and classification of AMD were based mainly on color fundus photographs and fluorescein angiography. Indocyanine green (ICG) angiography was reserved for indeterminate forms of AMD. The recently available optical coherence tomography (OCT) has provided a better understanding of the disease process. The advent of spectral domain OCT (SD-OCT) with better axial resolution, faster acquisition time, real-time tracking of eye movements, and real-time averaging of scanning laser ophthalmoscopic images provide images with a reduced signal to noise ratio. Thus, significant improvement in image quality has allowed precise analyses of the retinal microstructures.

The combination of SD-OCT, enhanced depth imaging that provides information on the choroidal integrity, autofluorescence imaging, and infrared imaging has revolutionized the interpretation, prediction of the prognosis, and follow-up of patients with AMD. Functional analysis using microperimetry helps to evaluate the extent and density of scotoma, assess the fixation patterns in AMD, and pinpoint the area in relation to the scotoma, thus providing additional information for assessment of prognosis. The availability of these new imaging techniques has significantly helped in understanding the functional and morphological correlation in AMD.

DRUSEN

Drusen are small, yellow, round lesions at the level of the RPE within the macula. They may be the first clinical sign of AMD. Initially they may be asymptomatic. They are located posterior to the RPE, lying between the basement membrane of the RPE cells and the inner collagen layer of Bruch's membrane. In due course, they lead to destruction of the overlying RPE and photoreceptors. For practical purposes, drusen may be classified into two categories: hard and soft. Hard drusen do not have the same pathological relevance and are considered to be a sequelae of physiological processes associated with aging. The presence of hard drusen alone is not sufficient to make a diagnosis of AMD. They are usually small in size and have a yellowish appearance with well-defined edges and are considered hydrophobic (**Figure 9.4a–c**).

In contrast, soft drusen are more frequently associated with advanced AMD. They are usually larger than 125 µm, and yellow gray in color with poorly defined edges (**Figure 9.5a–d**). Soft drusen are either highly reflectant or show a neutral appearance on infrared imaging. On histology, they are characterized by poorly defined edges and a tendency to group together. The inner surface of Bruch's membrane appears thickened, and an area of separation from the basement membrane of the RPE may be visible. CNV may potentially develop in this space.

Drusen may evolve over time, leading to advanced stages of AMD. Clusters of drusen in the subfoveal region may alter the RPE photoreceptor layers, leading to areas of atrophy. Soft drusen have a tendency to group together, leading to confluent drusen (<1000 µm in diameter) or drusenoid PED (>1000 µm in diameter) (**Figure 9.6**) (Zayit-Soudry et al. 2007). It has been reported that there is 19% chance of development of geographic atrophy and 23% chance of development of CNV in 5 years if drusen are present.

Fluorescein angiography findings

During the early phase of fluorescein angiography, punctate hyperfluorescence is seen due to window defects resulting from the retinal pigment epithelial atrophy. The fluorescence from the drusen increases in parallel with the concentration of the circulating dye. Towards the late phase of the angiography, most of the smaller hard drusen show a decrease in their fluorescence (**Figure 9.7a** and **b**). However, the larger soft drusen continue to fluoresce and show a moderate amount of staining (**Figure 9.8a–d**).

Reticular pseudodrusen (RPD) or subretinal drusenoid deposits have been recently determined to constitute an independent risk factor for the progression of AMD to advanced stages. They are

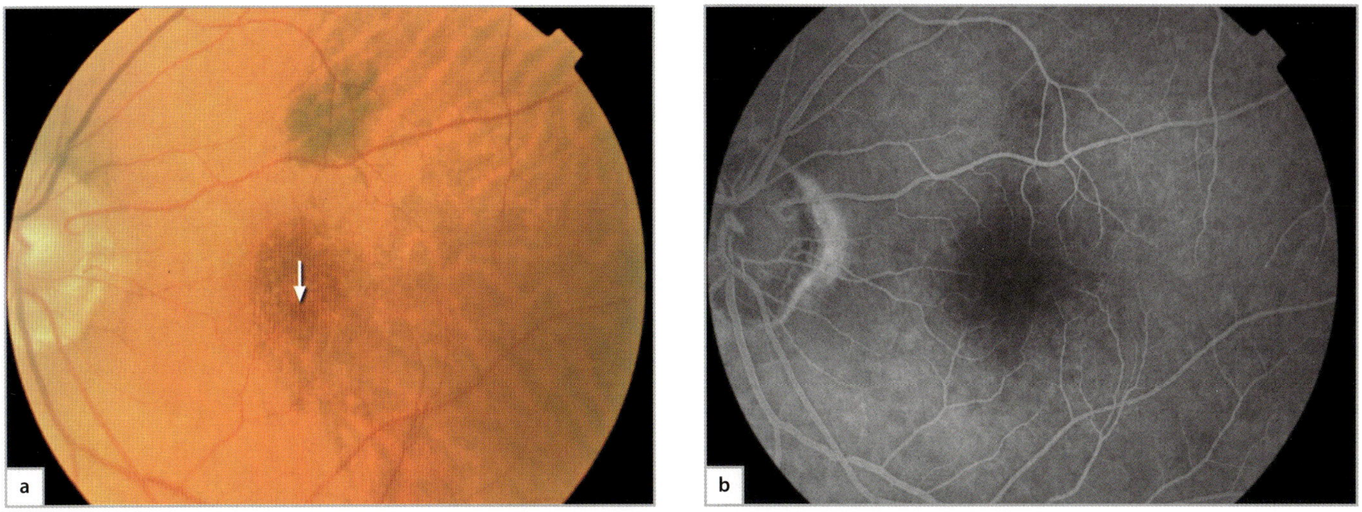

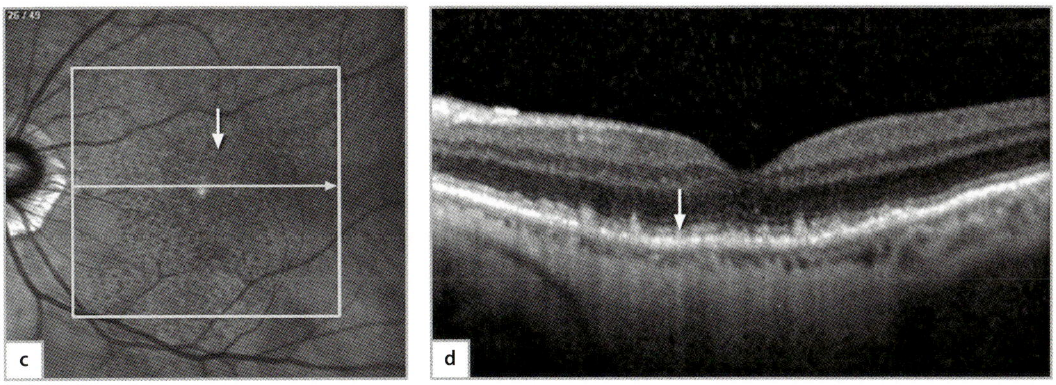

Figure 9.4 Reticular drusen. (a) There are several small drusen in the macular area. There is a mild degree of retinal pigment epithelium defect at the fovea. (b) The mid venous phase of the fluorescein angiogram shows mild hyperfluorescence due to RPE atrophy. (c) The infrared photograph shows the smaller drusen well and the RPE atrophy at the fovea. (d) The spectral domain optical coherence tomography shows the typical reflectance from the drusen in the Bruch's membrane.

sometimes identified on color fundus photographs as indistinct, interlacing, yellowish lesions occurring in the macula, typically along the superior arcades. On autofluorescence, they may be visible as ill-defined, hypofluorescent lesions against a background of mildly elevated autofluorescence. They are best seen on infrared imaging, where they appear as hyporeflectant lesions against a background of mild hyper-reflectance. On fundus fluorescein angiography (FFA), they may appear as defects in choriocapillaris filling in the early-phase images. On indocyanine green angiography (ICGA), a reticular pattern may be identified as a distinctive grouping of hypofluorescent dots present in the mid and late phases of the angiogram. On SD-OCT, they are visualized as granular hyper-reflective material between the RPE and the ellipsoid zone of the photoreceptors in an undulating pattern, unlike the age-related drusen that are located between the RPE and the Bruch's membrane (**Figure 9.9a–c**). They may coexist with soft drusen. They have been described to fade in time and occasionally CNV have been noted to develop in the corresponding areas. RPD have also been reported to lie adjacent to areas of GA or PED.

GEOGRAPHIC ATROPHY

Progressive degeneration of the RPE and the underlying choriocapillaris and overlying photoreceptors leads to GA. The retinal degeneration evolves slowly and the visual loss is gradual. Ophthalmoscopy shows well-demarcated areas of mixture of hypo- and hyperpigmentation of the macular area >175 μm in diameter.

Fluorescein angiography findings

The prearterial phase shows sharply demarcated window defects of the macular area. During transit, an increased amount of patchy hyperfluorescence is seen with a minor degree of staining toward the late phase (**Figure 9.10**).

ICG angiography findings

The early transit shows moderate degree of loss of choriocapillaris. The medium and larger sized choroidal vessels are often preserved. During the progress of the transit, the intensity of fluorescence dies down. The late stage of the angiography shows a mild degree of staining of the sclera underneath.

SD-OCT shows severe disruption or absence of the external limiting membrane and ellipsoid zone, with enhanced visualization of the choroid in these areas. The overlying neurosensory retina shows thinning that may involve the outer nuclear layer, in which case the outer plexiform layer comes directly in contact with Bruch's membrane. On autofluorescence, the area appears as a dense zone of hypofluorescence (**Figure 9.11**).

EXUDATIVE AMD

Exudative macular degeneration is referred to as the wet type of degeneration or neovascular AMD. Patients describe metamorphopsia and rapid deterioration of visual acuity.

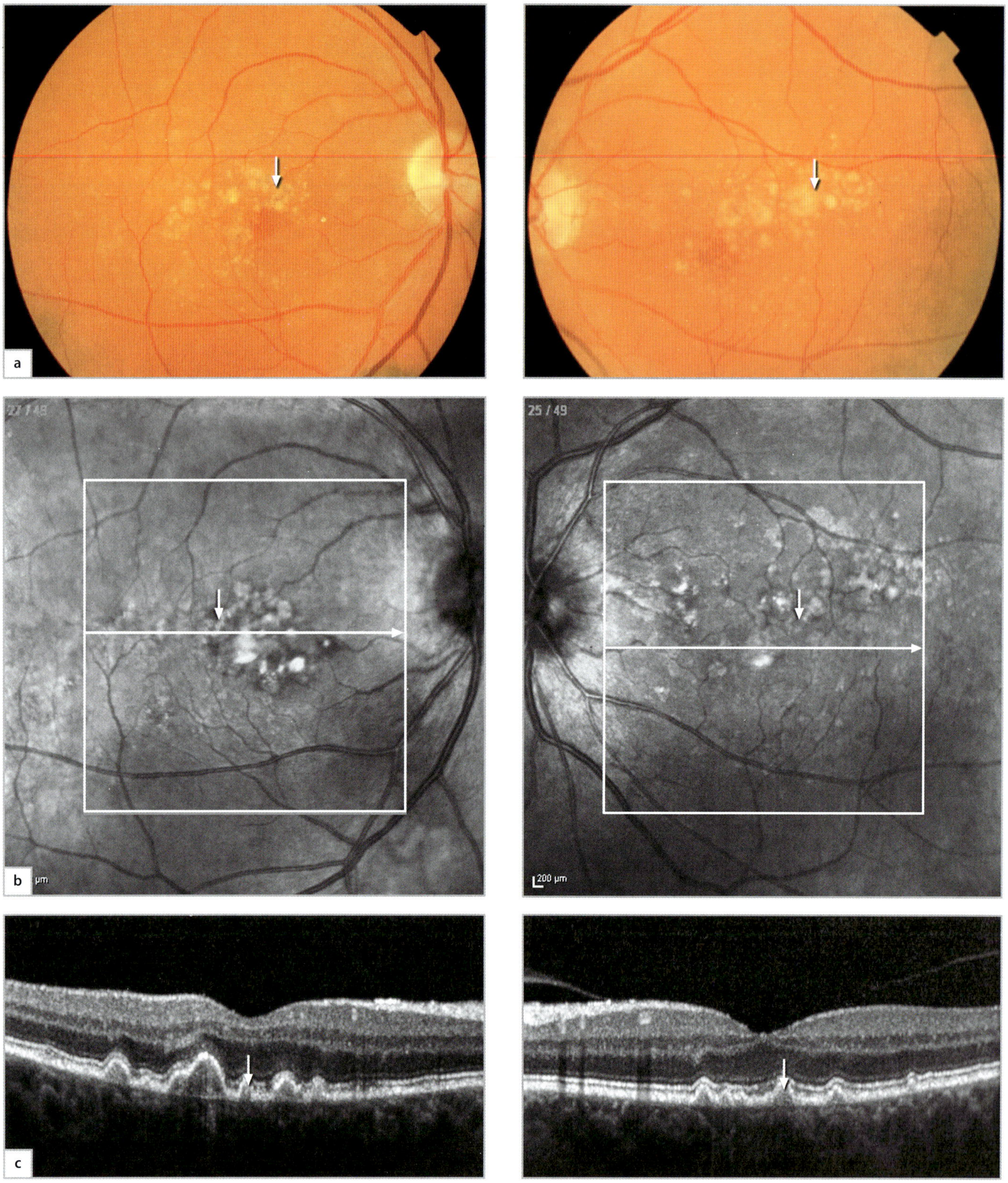

Figure 9.5 Soft drusen. (a) The right and left eye show several soft drusen surrounding the macular area. (b) The infrared images of both eyes clearly show the drusen around the macula. (c) The spectral domain optical coherence tomography (OCT) show raised lesions affecting the Bruch's membrane and retinal pigment epithelium.

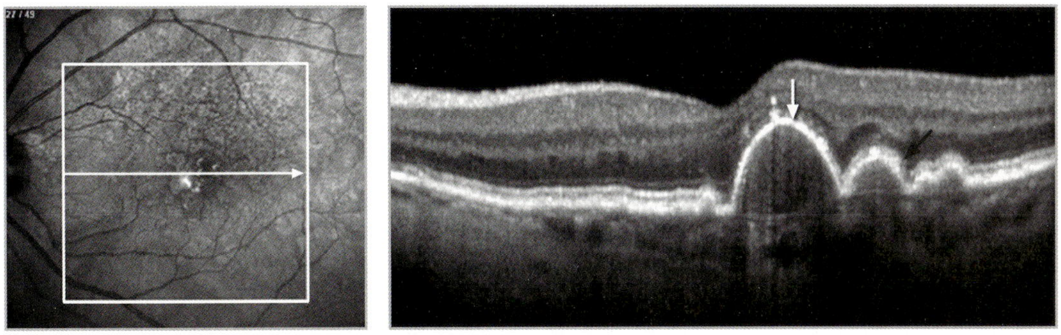

Figure 9.6 Drusenoid pigment epithelial detachment (PED). Spectral domain optical coherence tomography showing large soft drusen (black arrow) and drusenoid PED (white arrow).

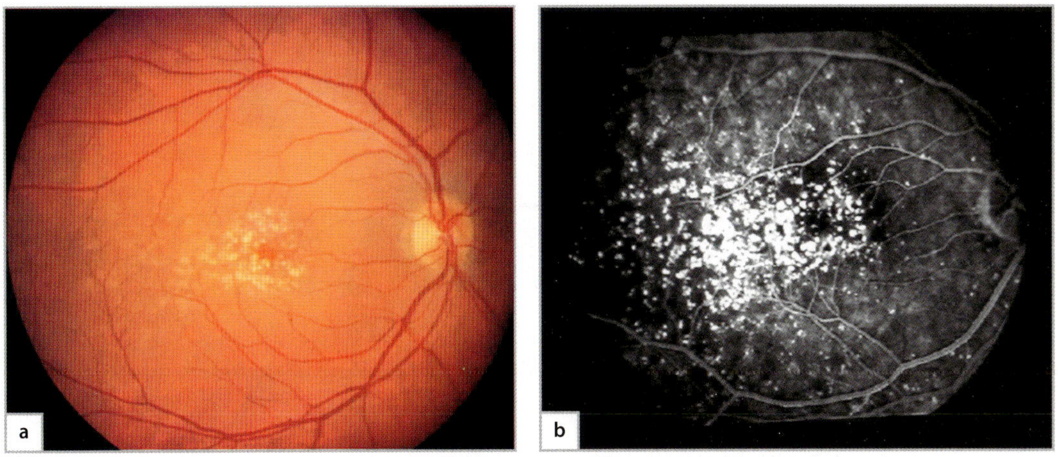

Figure 9.7 Hard drusen. (a) The right eye shows hard drusen mainly around the macular area. (b) The late venous phase of the fluorescein angiogram shows hyperfluorescence of the drusen, which is already showing evidence of diminishing brightness.

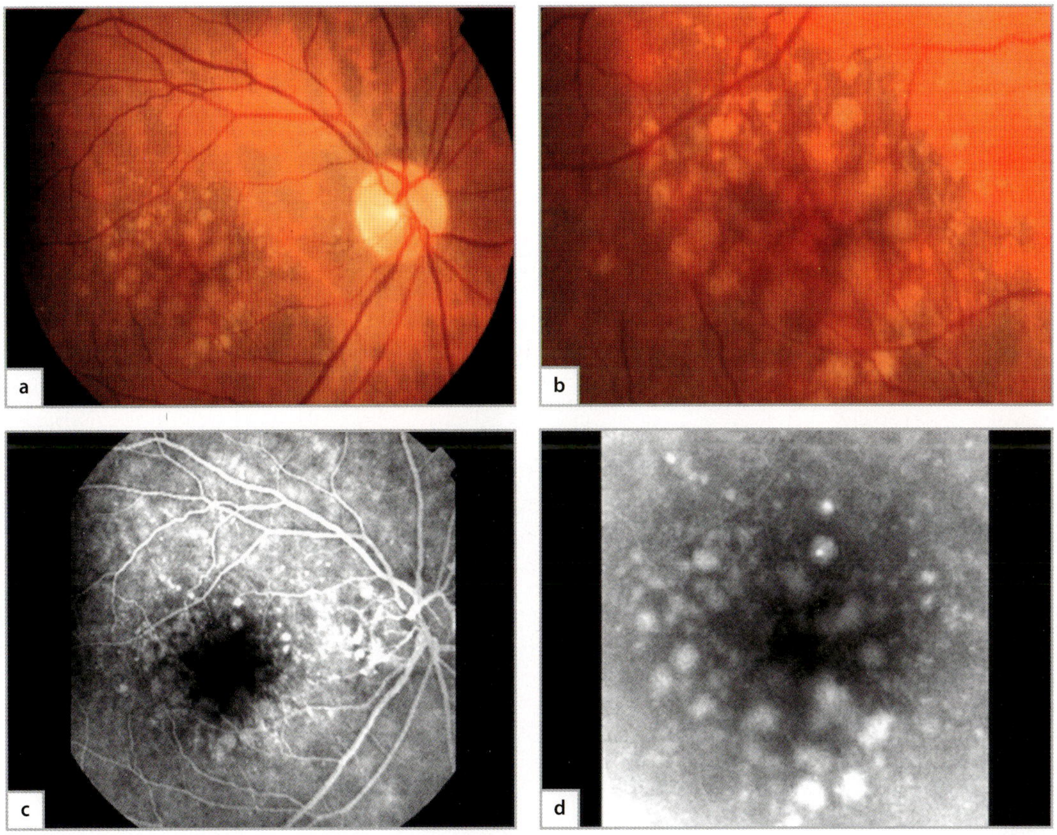

Figure 9.8 Soft drusen. (a) The right eye shows cluster of deep-seated gray white lesions with fuzzy borders at the macular area. (b) The enlarged view of the same area shows all the deep-seated lesions much more clearly. (c) The arteriovenous phase of the fluorescein angiogram shows faint hyperfluorescence of some of the larger lesions. (d) The enlarged view of the macular area during the late phase shows increase in hyperfluorescence of all those gray white lesions.

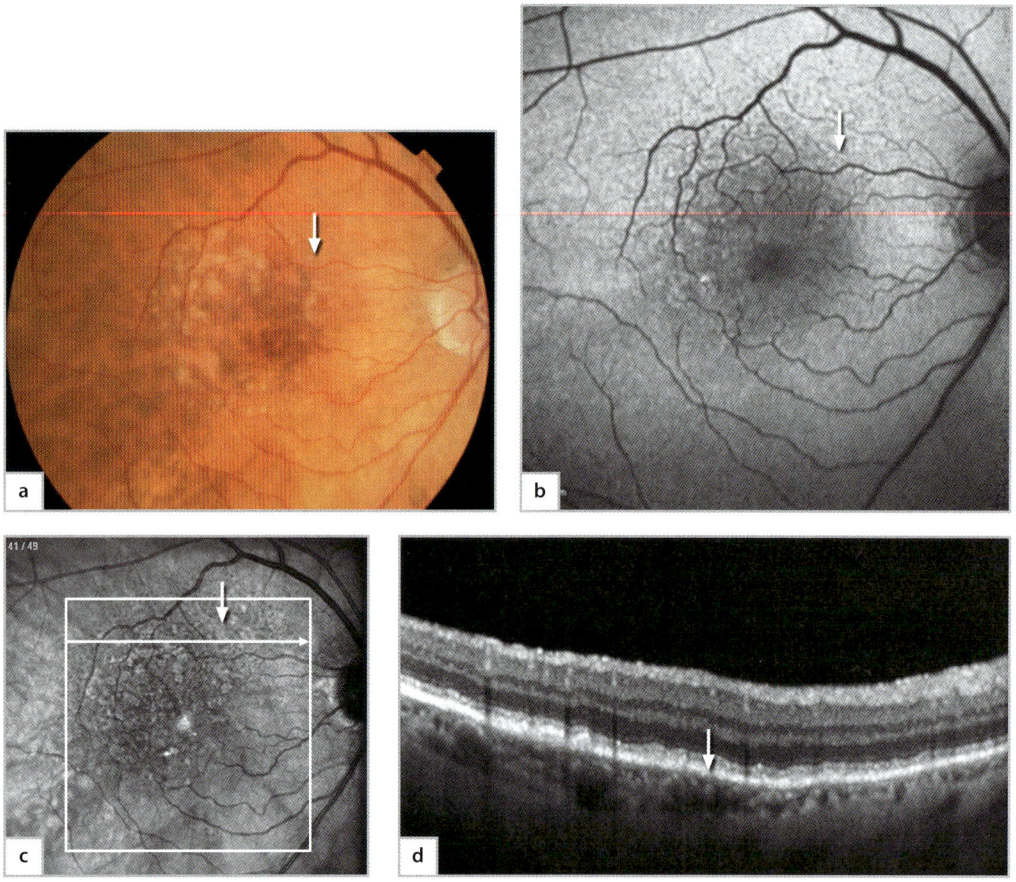

Figure 9.9 Reticular pseudodrusen. (a) The right eye shows poorly defined pseudo reticulad drusen in the superior part of macula. (b) The infrared autofluorescence image shows the drusen much more clearly. (c) The area of cut for part (d). (d) Spectral domain optical coherence tomography shows the drusen lay between the retinal pigment epithelium and neurosensory retina.

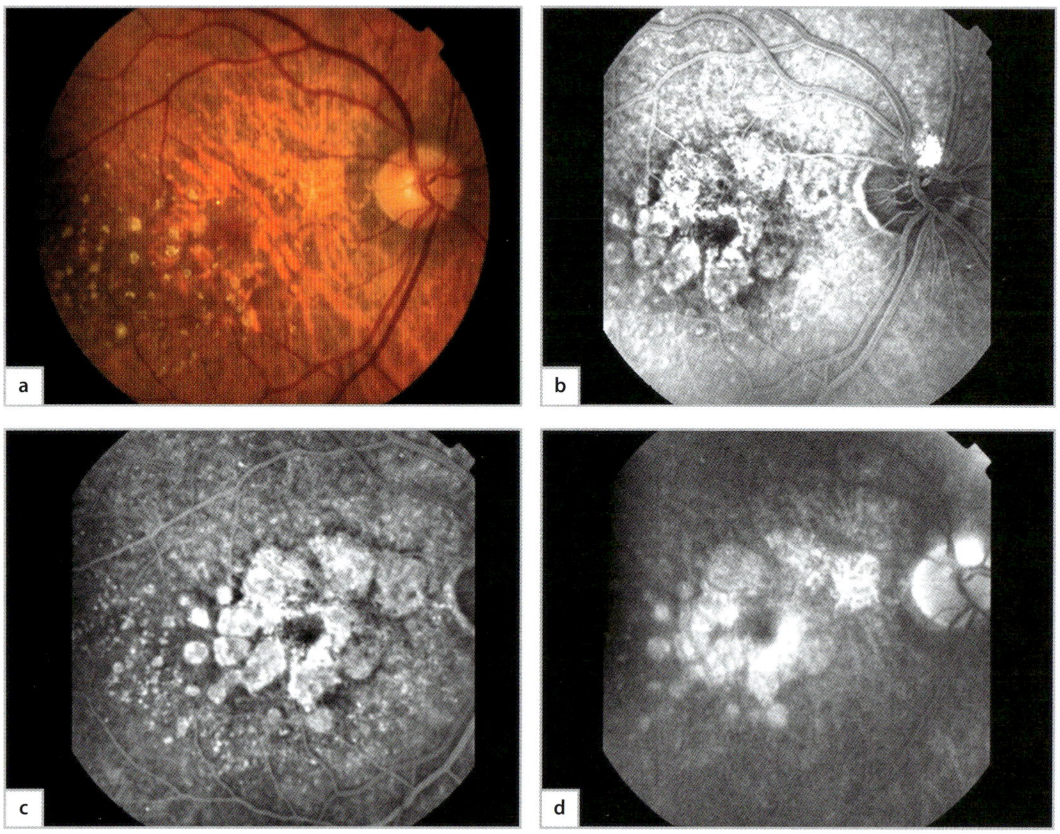

Figure 9.10 Dry age-related macular degeneration. (a) The right eye shows retinal pigment epithelial degeneration associated with many colloid bodies. (b) The red-free photograph shows the retinal pigment epithelium around the macular area. (c) The arteriovenous phase of the fluorescein angiogram shows hyperfluorescence from the retinal pigment epithelium (RPE) atrophic areas. The intensity of hyperfluorescence is very similar to that of the background. (d) The late phase shows staining of the underlying sclera through the atrophic RPE. There is no evidence of any leakage of dye.

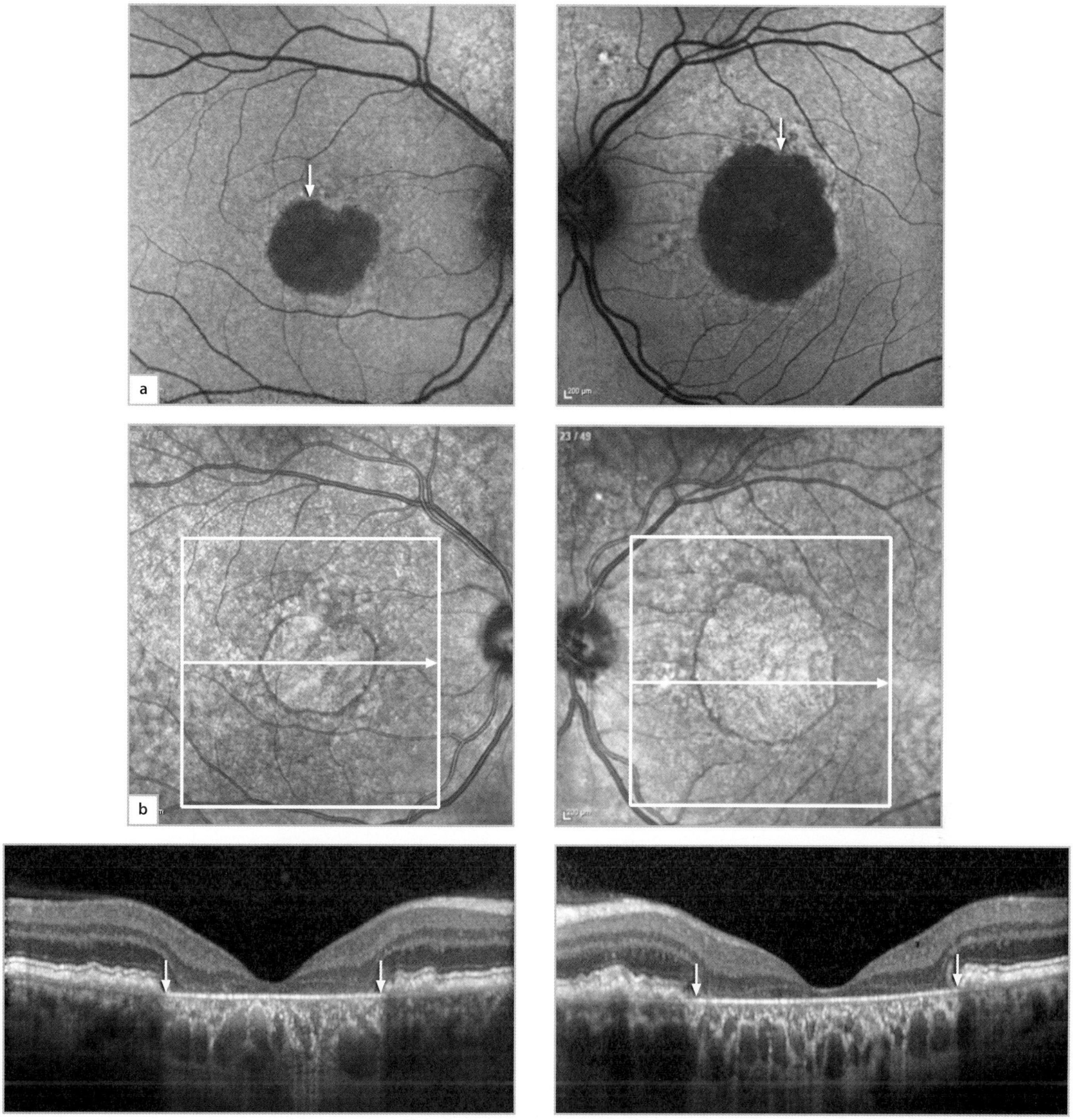

Figure 9.11 Geographic atrophy. (a) The autofluorescence images of both eyes show areas of well-demarcated hypofluorescence. (b) The spectral domain show areas of loss of retinal pigment epithelium and photoreceptor layers with thinning of the overlying retina and enhanced visualization of the choroid (Cukras et al. 2010). The bottom row corresponds to the areas of cut, as seen in part (b). All OCT illustrations are shown: first the site of the cut section in the topography followed by the real OCT.

RETINAL PIGMENT EPITHELIUM DETACHMENT

The detachment of the RPE from the basement membrane is the first stage of the disease process. This occurs due to a break in Bruch's membrane that initially elevates the entire retina along with the pigment epithelium, without disrupting the neurosensory layers. The subpigment epithelial space usually fills with serous fluid derived from the choriocapillaris. The detached area appears as a grayish yellow looking raised lesion, with a sharply outlined margin. Later the tight junctions between the epithelial cells slowly break down, allowing the serous fluid to gain access to the subretinal space. As this is a natural cleavage line, the serous fluid soon separates the neurosensory layer of the retina from the pigment epithelium, resulting in a widespread neurosensory retinal detachment, thus masking the sharp outline seen from the underlying PED.

Fluorescein angiography findings

When the detachment is confined under the RPE, the prearterial phase shows a small area of masking of choroidal background fluorescence, followed by a small hyperfluorescent spot at the center. During the progress of the transit, a steady increase in fluorescence occurs, covering a larger area of leakage toward the late phase. The margin remains sharp and well defined throughout the different phases of angiography. When the serous detachment extends to the subretinal space, the dye leaks into this space and spreads widely, and the sharp margin seen previously is lost (**Figure 9.12**).

ICG angiography findings

During the early phase of ICG angiography, a faintly hypofluorescent well-demarcated lesion is seen corresponding to the PED. The intensity remains unchanged throughout the transit; however, there is a mild-to-moderate degree of hyperfluorescence toward the late phase due to leakage of dye into the PED (**Figure 9.13**). SD-OCT shows dome-shaped elevation of the RPE that appears optically empty with visualization of the thin line of Bruch's membrane and a choroidal shadow (**Figure 9.14**).

OCCULT CHOROIDAL NEOVASCULARIZATION

In adverse circumstances, new vessels budding from the choriocapillaris gradually insinuate themselves through the breaks in Bruch's membrane. These new vessels invade the subpigment epithelial space and spread under the PED and may be referred to as vascularized PED. This type of CNV is also described as type 1 neovascularization or occult CNV. These choroidal new vessels lack tight junctions and are prone to leakage. The choroidal new vessels continue to grow under the subpigment epithelial space and radial branches are sent out to cover the base. The PED eventually surrounds the CNV and grows around it. The PED may eventually regress and become fibrotic. This leads to radial tractions lines under the RPE, giving a typical cartwheel appearance.

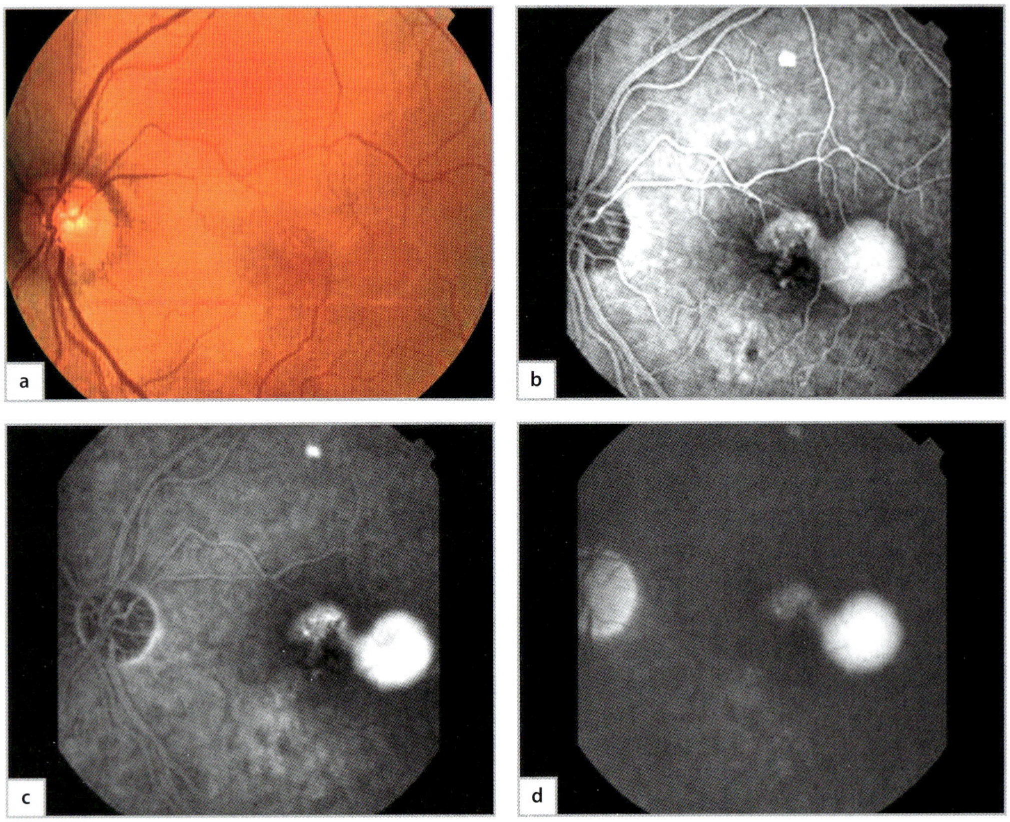

Figure 9.12 Fundus fluorescein angiography of pigment epithelial detachment (PED). (a) The left eye shows a well-circumscribed lesion on the temporal border of the macula. There is mild degree of retinal pigment epithelium (RPE) changes seen just above the macula. (b) The arteriovenous phase of the fluorescein angiogram shows a round well-demarcated hyperfluorescent round lesion temporal to the macula. There is also some hyperfluorescence seen just above the macular area due to RPE atrophy. (c) The late transit phase shows increase in fluorescence of the round lesion, whereas the hyperfluorescence of the lesion just above the macula has slightly reduced. (d) The late phase shows considerable hyperfluorescence of the round lesion lateral to the macular area. The fluorescence of the lesion just above the macular areas has reduced. The consistent increase in fluorescence from the round lesion is due to accumulation of fluorescein dye into the pocket of PED.

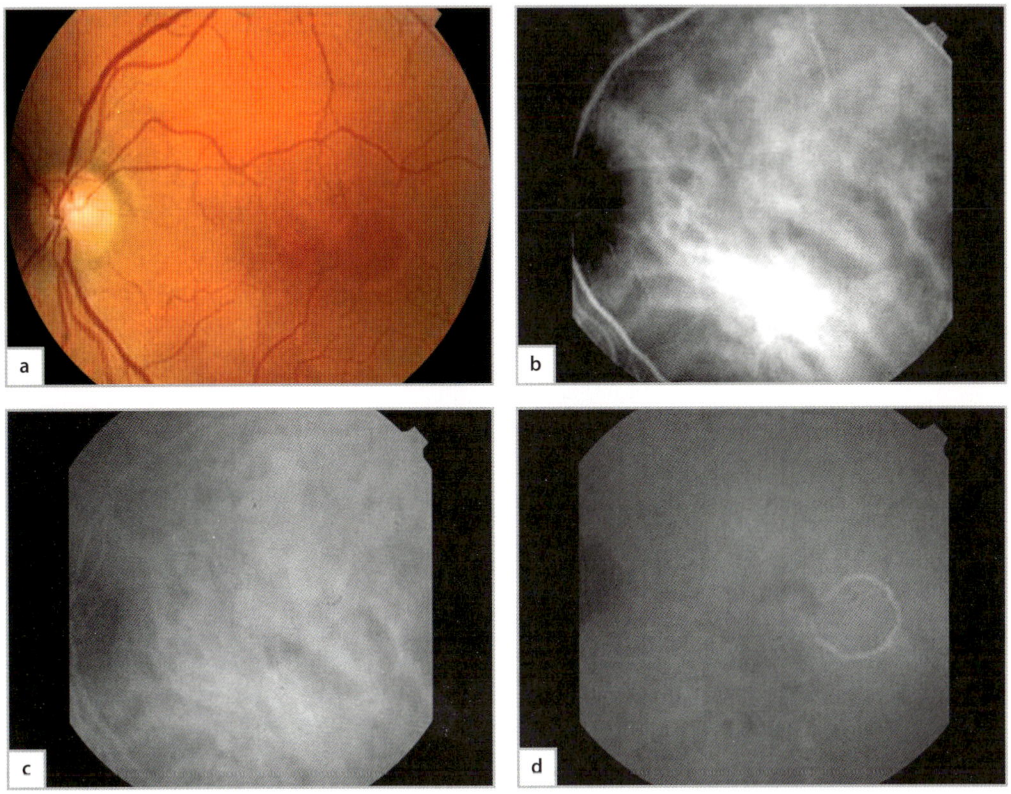

Figure 9.13 Indocyanine green (ICG) angiogram of pigment epithelial detachment (PED). (a) The left eye shows a well-circumscribed round lesion lateral to the macular area. (b) The early arteriovenous phase of ICG angiography shows normal choriocapillaris. Just lateral to the macula, the margin of the round lesion is seen. (c) The late transit phase shows the round lesion has remained unchanged. (d) The late phase of the ICG angiogram shows the outline of PED with minimal staining.

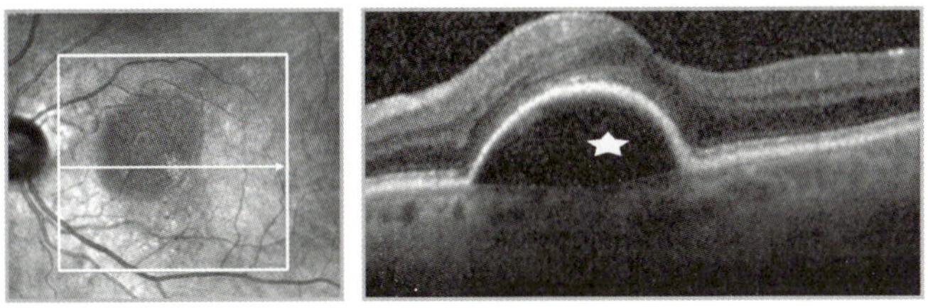

Figure 9.14 Pigment epithelial detachment (PED). Spectral domain optical coherence tomography of the left eye shows a serous PED. A thin line of Bruch's membrane is visible posterior to the PED, indicating deposition of serous fluid underneath.

Fluorescein angiography findings

Fluorescein angiography usually shows an irregular area of RPE elevation consisting of speckled fluorescence in the mid phase, leading to moderate leakage toward the late phase. The leakage may be widespread or localized to one small area where a discrete notch is demonstrated, rather like the eye of a kidney bean. The second form of occult CNV is described as late leakage from an indeterminate source, which is characterized by leakage in the late phase with no discernable leakage in the early and mid phases.

Once the CNV grows in a radial pattern and the PED and CNV complex becomes fibrotic, the radiating lines simulating a cartwheel are easily visible during the early phase leading to moderate leakage and staining towards the late phase (**Figure 9.15a–e**)

ICGA angiography findings

Occult CNV associated with vascularized PED usually shows several different forms of leakage in ICG angiography.

1. Hot spot: this is an area of hyperfluorescence in the mid and late phase of angiography measuring <1 disc diameter. Hot spots are usually seen at the margin of the PED but may also be located elsewhere
2. Plaque: plaques are described as an area of hyperfluorescence appearing during the mid and late phase of angiography, of >1 disc diameter and usually affecting a wider area involving the PED (**Figure 9.16**)
3. Occult CNV: the transit phase ICG angiogram shows some evidence of dilated choroidal vessels but no clear demonstration of CNV. The late phase ICG angiogram shows diffuse leakage of dye into the macular area (**Figure 9.17**)

SD-OCT may show the dome-shaped PED with hyper-reflectivity visible posterior to the PED which is considered to represent the CNV being adherent to the basal surface of the RPE along the PED (**Figure 9.18**). The overlying retina shows signs of activity that appears as intraretinal fluid and subretinal fluid.

CLASSIC CHOROIDAL NEOVASCULARIZATION

Once the CNV spreads along the subpigment epithelial space, the integrity of the RPE is lost and this allows the CNV to gain access into the subretinal space. CNV spreads in the subretinal space as classic CNV

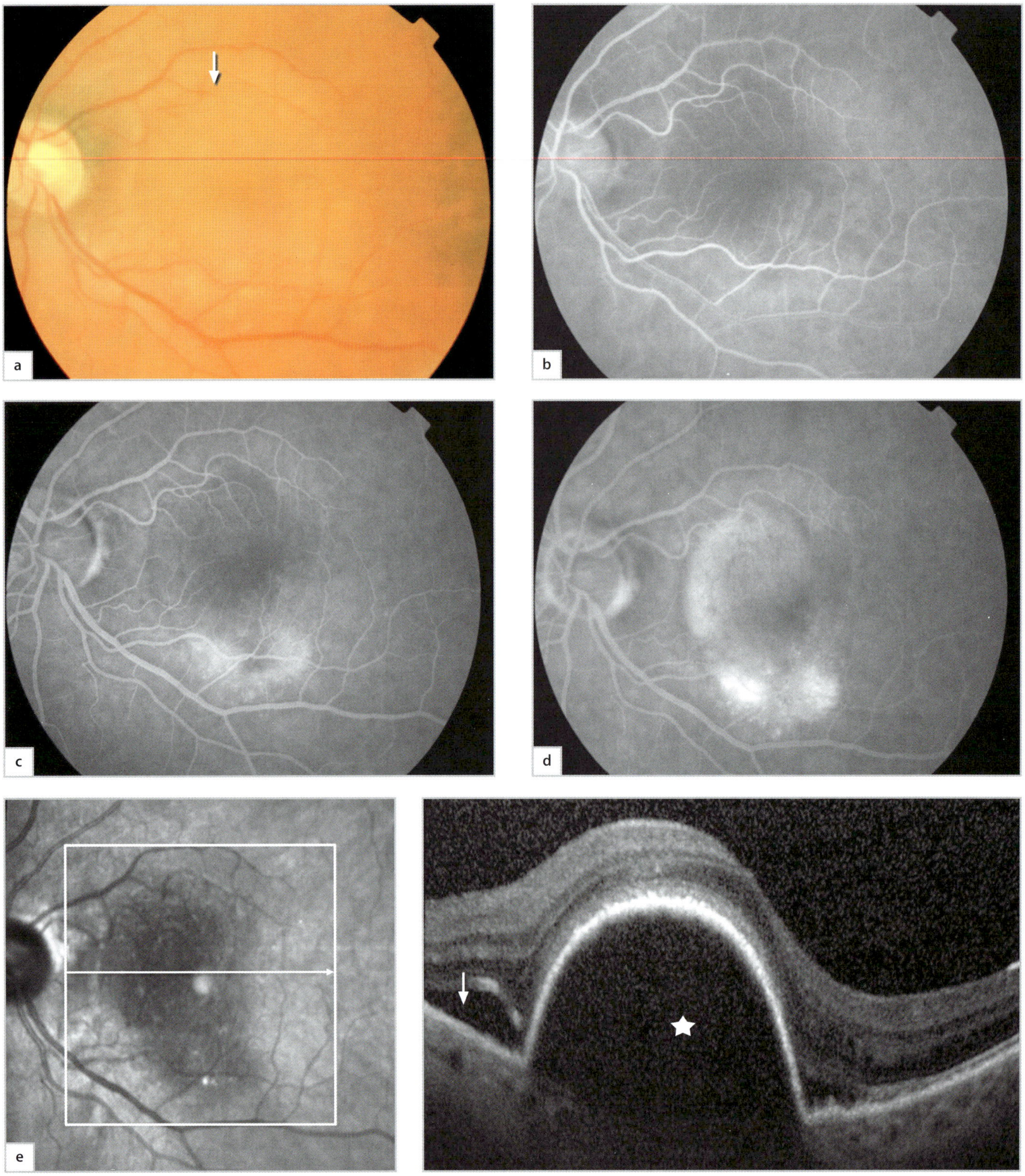

Figure 9.15 Occult choroidal neovascular membrane (CNV). (a) The left eye shows faint demarcation outline of the pigment epithelial detachment (PED). (b) The arteriovenous phase of the fluorescein angiogram shows mild hypofluorescence of the macular area. (c) The late venous phase shows horseshoe-shaped hyperfluorescence in the lower border of macula. The outline of the PED is now beginning to show its demarcation. (d) The late phase shows moderate leakage into the lesion. Note that the lower border shows relatively brighter appearance due to excessive leakage due to an underlying occult CNV. (e) Spectral domain optical coherence tomography from a different case with the scan line through the foveal area shows PED with a shallow subretinal fluid.

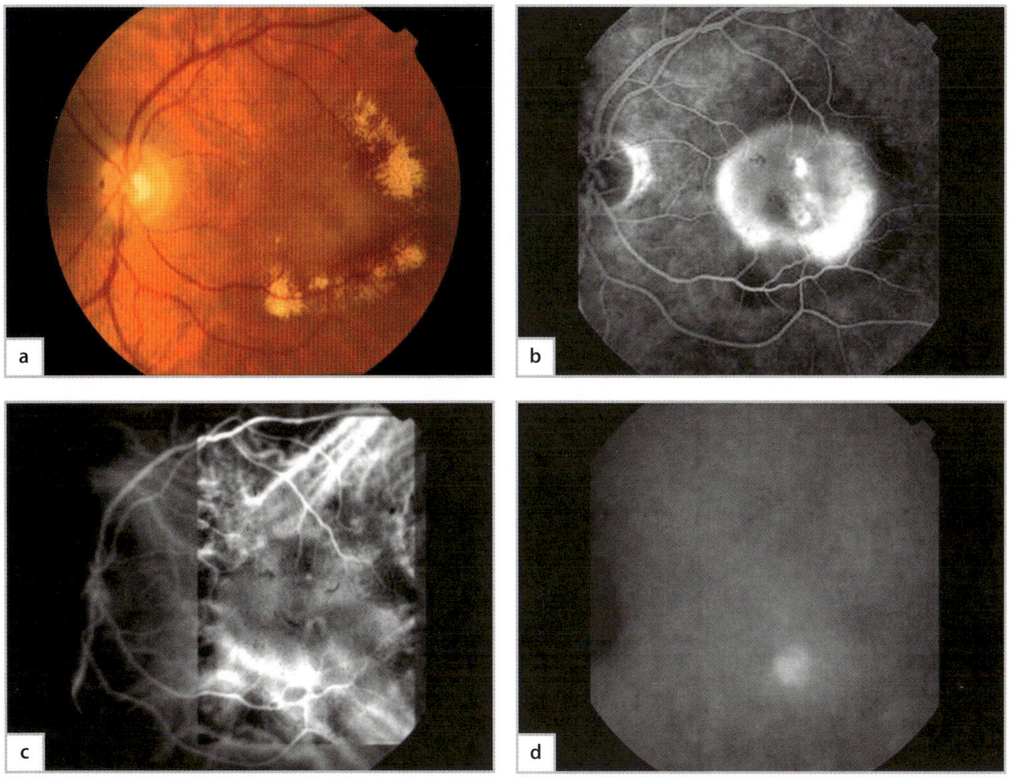

Figure 9.16 Vascularized pigment epithelial detachment (PED) plaque. (a) The left eye shows a PED lateral to the macular area. It is surrounded by a ring of lipid exudate. (b) The mid transit phase of the fluorescein angiogram shows the PED and underneath there is hyperfluorescent spot at about 12 o'clock position. (c) The mid transit phase of the indocyanine green (ICG) angiogram shows hyperfluorescent area beneath the PED. (d) The late phase of the ICG angiogram shows a lager area of hyperfluorescence underneath the PED plaque of hyperfluorescence.

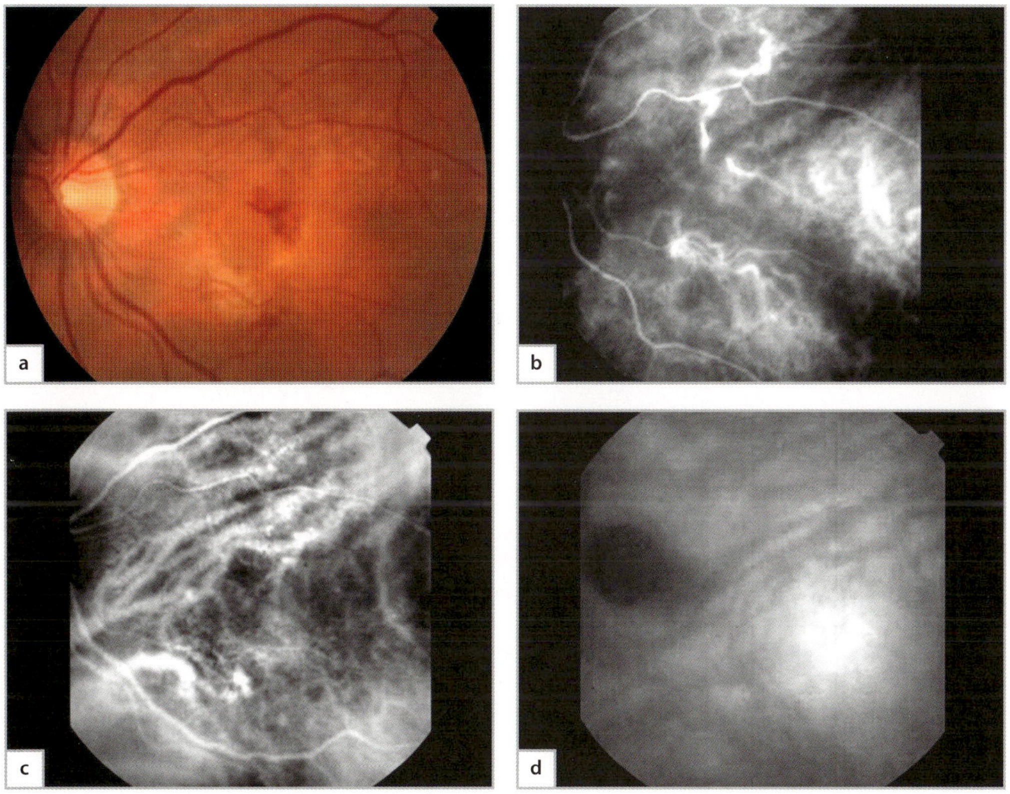

Figure 9.17 Indocyanine green (ICG) angiogram of occult choroidal neovascularization (CNV): same case as Figure 9.9. (a) The left eye shows intraretinal hemorrhage and diffuse macular edema with subretinal fibrosis. (b) The early phase of the ICG angiogram shows some dilatation of choroidal vessels but no defined view of CNV. (c) The late transit phase shows dilated choroidal vessels under the macular area but no clear demonstration of CNV. (d) The late phase shows a diffuse area of leakage at the macula.

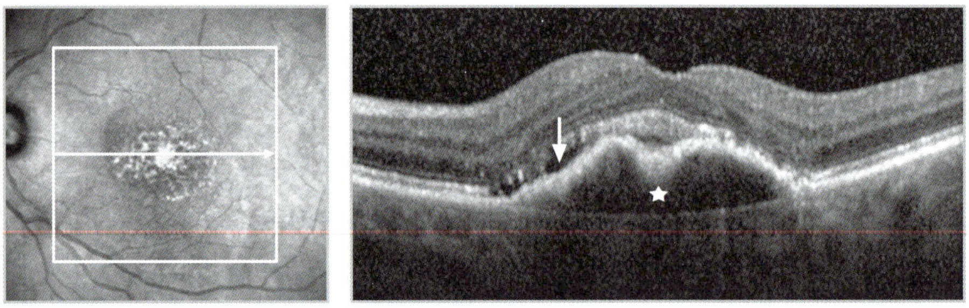

Figure 9.18 Occult choroidal neovascular membrane. Spectral domain optical coherence tomography of the left eye shows pigment epithelial detachment with hyper-reflectivity posterior to the retinal pigment epithelium and presence of subretinal fluid.

or type II CNV. The angiogram of such CNV shows a very distinctive pattern. Clinically, the patient's vision is substantially compromised with metamorphopsia and central scotoma. Ophthalmoscopy shows an exudative detachment with associated deep-seated gray area with small amount of intraretinal hemorrhage.

Fluorescein angiography

During the very early phase, there may be a transient period of hypofluorescence due to masking from the exudation. The CNV develops a typical lacy pattern of early hyperfluorescence that increases in fluorescence throughout the transit phase. Towards the late phase, the leakage may be so profuse that the lacy pattern of the CNV may be 'drowned' within the leakage. The outer edges of the CNV show a rim of hypofluorescence due to mild hemorrhages arising from the newly laid fragile capillaries. Long-standing cases may show cystoid macular edema.

ICG angiography

ICG angiography is not always required to confirm the diagnosis. It shows the CNV complex during the early phase but in less detail.

SD-OCT

On SD-OCT, type 2 membranes are noted anterior to the RPE band and posterior to the photoreceptor layer. Disorganization of the overlying photoreceptor layer has been seen to be associated with intraretinal fluid, rather than subretinal fluid (**Figure 9.19a–e**).

RETINAL ANGIOMATOUS PROLIFERANS

Sometimes this has been referred to as type 3 CNV. The characteristics of retinal angiomatous proliferans (RAP) are described in three stages. They are believed to arise from the neuroretina and extend downward to the choroid. Stage one is characterized by the formation of minute intraretinal vascularization, leading to neurosensory separation. In stage two, intraretinal vasculature invades the subretinal space and in stage three it develops a chorioretinal communication. Clinically, these may present with a small area of intraretinal hemorrhages, exudates, and cystoid macular edema. Fluorescein angiography shows bright hyperfluorescence associated with the tip of a retinal vessel during the early phase, increasing in the mid phase and with leakage in the late phase, leading to cystoid macular edema. The ICG angiogram shows classic vascular abnormalities and chorioretinal communication during the mid to late phase, with moderate leakage. For these reasons, diagnosis of RAP is often made with confidence during the stage three of the disease.

The SD-OCT is very characteristic in stage three, when the retinochoroidal anastomosis can be visualized clearly, associated with signs of activity indicated by intraretinal or subretinal fluid (**Figure 9.20a–e**).

Polypoidal choroidal vasculopathy appears as branches of the choroidal vessels with terminal aneurysmal dilations that resemble polyps. They vary in size and shape and are often associated with PED and neurosensory detachment of the overlying retina. Although the vasculopathy predominantly affects the peripapillary region, it may also involve the macular region and any other areas of the fundus. Fluorescein angiography does not reveal the nature of the dilation but shows an area of nonspecific leakage. However, early phase ICG angiogram shows the branching and the polypoidal nature of the abnormalities clearly, leading to very localized area of leakage toward the late phase. Some of the polyps may be seen to pulsate in video ICG angiography, especially when performed on Spectralis HRA + OCT. The area covered by ICG leakage is usually much smaller than the area of leakage seen on fluorescein angiography.

On SD-OCT, the polyps may be visualized as characteristic spikes that arise from areas deep to the RPE, with visualization of hyperreflective material within, which may represent the polypoidal structures (**Figure 9.21a–d**).

DISCIFORM DEGENERATION

Over time, the CNV undergoes the reparative process by increased fibrosis. A dense fibrous scar is formed that is circular in appearance, resembling a disc. The name disciform macular degeneration is derived from its shape.

Fluorescein angiography findings

The early phase shows variable amount of hyperfluorescence from the CNV, with a moderate degree of staining of the whole area in the late frames. Chorioretinal shunts may be seen within the scar.

ICG angiography findings

It is unnecessary to perform ICG angiography. It may show hypofluorescence during the early phase and mild staining toward the late phase. SD-OCT shows areas of dense subfoveal hyper-reflectivity that may be associated with loss of the ellipsoid zone and external limiting membrane (**Figure 9.22a–c**).

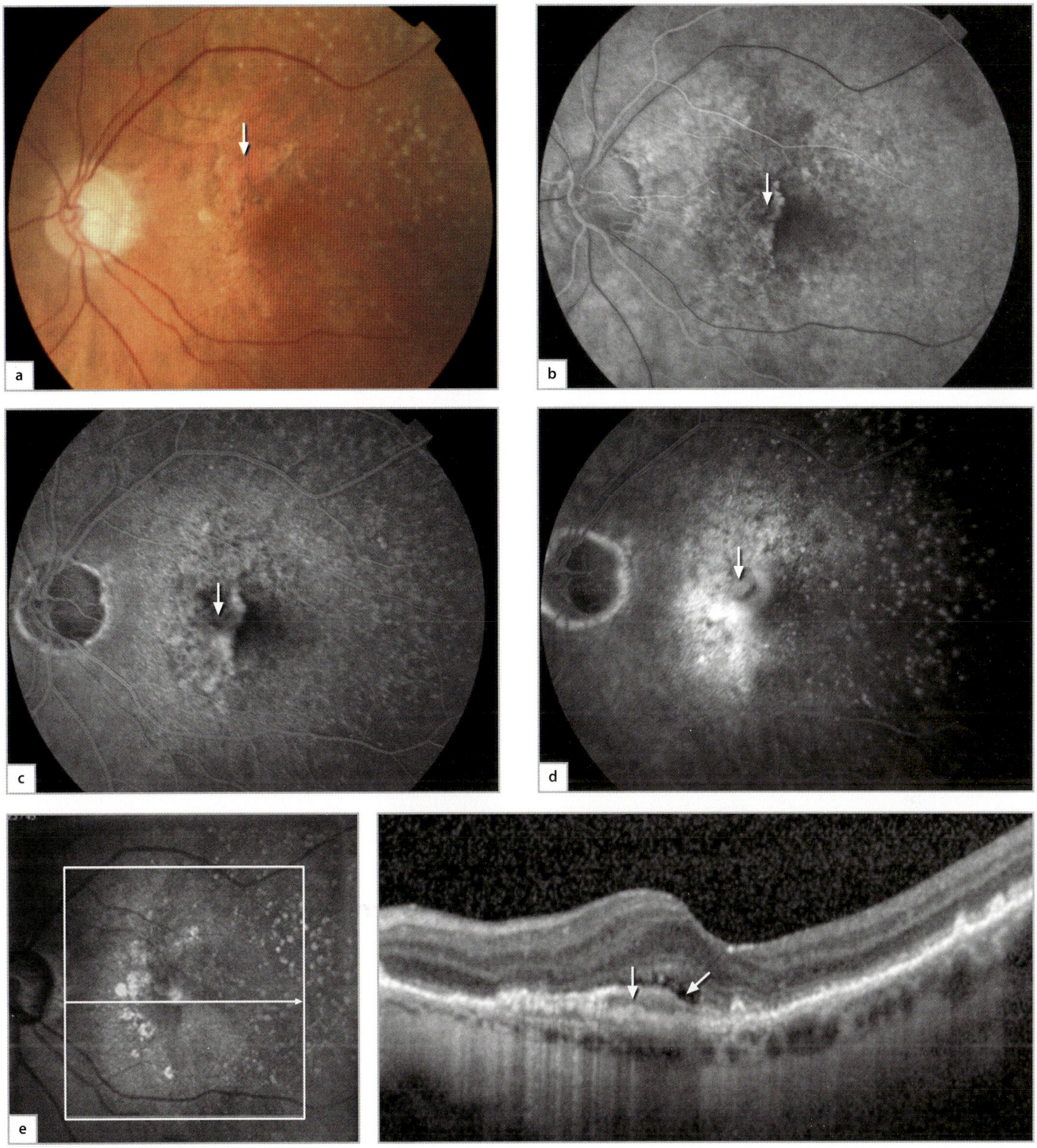

Figure 9.19 Classic choroidal neovascular membrane (CNV). (a) The left eye shows a grayish area nasal to the macular area. (b) The arterial phase of the fluorescein angiogram shows atypical lacy pattern of hyperfluorescence area developing nasal to the macula. (c) The late venous phase shows increase in fluorescence due to progressive leakage from the CNV. (d) The late phase shows profuse leakage drowning the lacy pattern seen earlier. (e) The spectral domain optical coherence tomography shows an area of hyper-reflectivity lying anterior to the retinal pigment epithelium with overlying subretinal fluid.

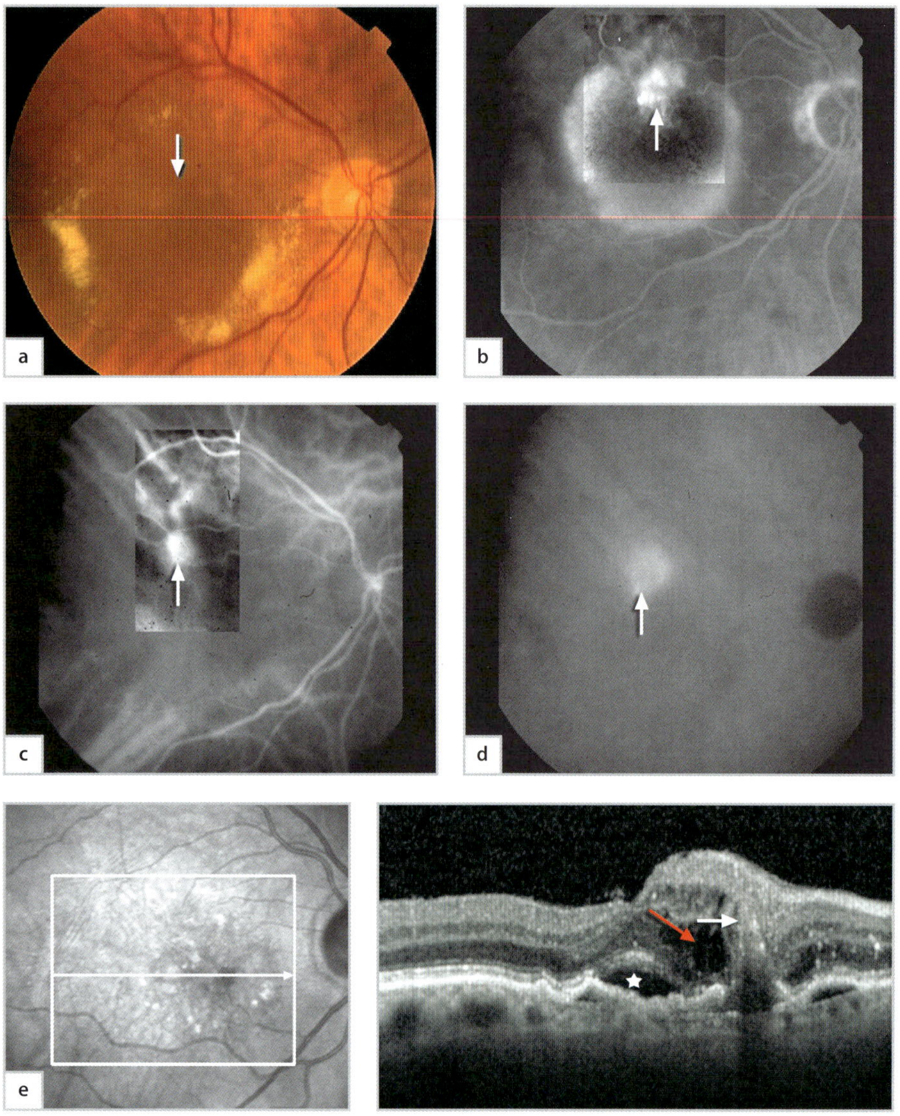

Figure 9.20 Retinal angiomatous proliferation. (a) The right eye shows an area of macular edema with circinate lipid exudate. (b) The arteriovenous phase of the fluorescein angiogram shows several dots of hyperfluorescence at the 12 o'clock position. The outline of the lesion is also seen as a ring of hyperfluorescence. (c) The arteriovenous phase of the indocyanine green (ICG) angiogram shows a distinct retinochoroidal vascular anastomosis at the 12 o'clock position with increase in hyperfluorescence. (d) The late phase of the ICG angiogram shows leakage confined to the microvascular changes seen superiorly. (e) Spectral domain optical coherence tomography from a different case shows the retinochoroidal anastomosis (denoted by the white arrow) with intraretinal fluid (red arrow) and subretinal fluid (star).

FUNCTIONAL CHANGES IN AMD

Microperimetry

The classification of fixation pattern is based on the location and stability using MP-1 software as recommended by Fuji et al. (2003). The site of fixation marks out the center of the foveal avascular zone (FAZ), and the stability of fixation is the ability to maintain a steady fixation at the preferred retinal site.

Classification of different types of fixation

1. Predominantly central fixation is when > 50% of the preferred fixation points are located within 2° of the FAZ
2. Poor central fixation is when < 50% but > 25% of the preferred fixation points are within 2° of the FAZ
3. Predominantly eccentric fixation is when < 25% of the preferred fixation points are located within the 2° of the FAZ

Stability of fixation

The stability of fixation is based on the steady adjustment of the preferred retinal site.

1. Stable fixation is when > 75% of the fixation points located within 2° of the FAZ
2. Relatively unstable fixation is when < 75% of the fixation points are located within 2° of the FAZ, but > 75% of the fixation points are located within 4° of the FAZ
3. Unstable fixation is when < 75% of the fixation points are located within 4° of the FAZ (**Figure 9.23**)

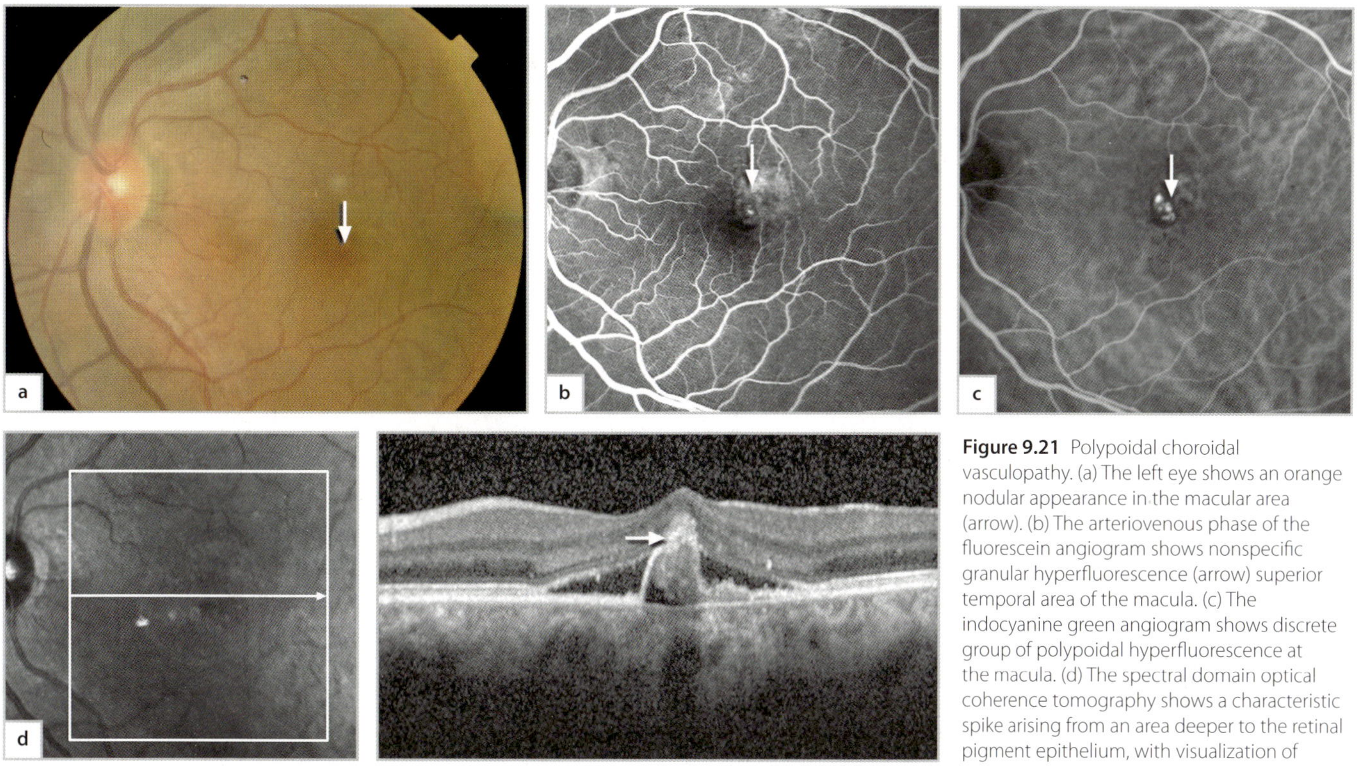

Figure 9.21 Polypoidal choroidal vasculopathy. (a) The left eye shows an orange nodular appearance in the macular area (arrow). (b) The arteriovenous phase of the fluorescein angiogram shows nonspecific granular hyperfluorescence (arrow) superior temporal area of the macula. (c) The indocyanine green angiogram shows discrete group of polypoidal hyperfluorescence at the macula. (d) The spectral domain optical coherence tomography shows a characteristic spike arising from an area deeper to the retinal pigment epithelium, with visualization of hyper-reflective material within (arrow).

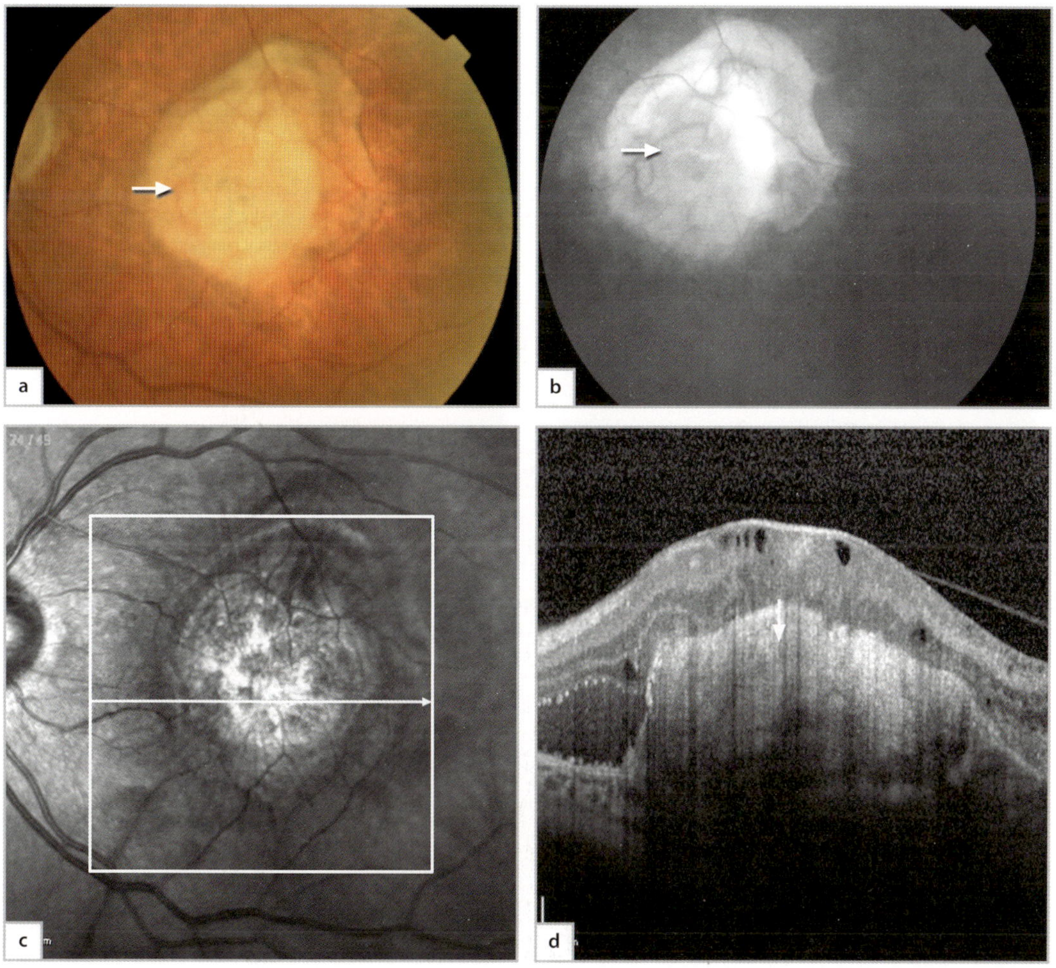

Figure 9.22 Disciform degeneration. (a) The left eye shows a disc-shaped fibrovascular scar at the macular area. (b) The late phase of the fluorescein angiogram shows marked staining. Through the stained area, deep-seated choroidal vasculatures are also seen. (c) The spectral domain optical coherence tomogram shows an area of dense subfoveal hyper-reflectivity.

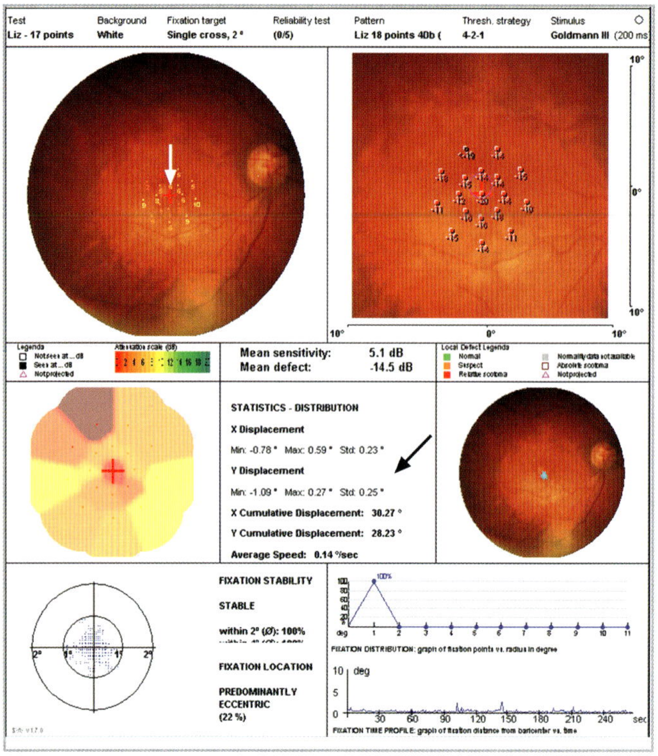

Figure 9.23 Microperimetry of the right eye of a patient with neovascular age-related macular degeneration shows areas of reduced sensitivity shown in orange and red areas (white arrow). Fixation is eccentric but stable (denoted by the black arrow).

REFERENCES

Age-Related Eye Disease Study Research Group. Risk factors associated with age-related macular degeneration. A case-control study in the age-related eye disease study: age-related eye disease study report number 3. *Ophthalmology* 2000; **107**:2224–2232.

Bird AC, Bressler NM, Bressler SB, et al. An international classification and grading system for age-related maculopathy and age-related macular degeneration. The International ARM Epidemiological Study Group. *Surv Ophthalmol* 1995; **39**:367–374.

Chopdar A, Chakravarthy U, Verma D. Age related macular degeneration. *BMJ* 2003;**326**:485–488.

Cukras C, Agrón E, Klein ML, et al. Age-Related Eye Disease Study Research Group. Natural history of drusenoid pigment epithelial detachment in age-related macular degeneration: age-related eye disease study report no. 28. *Ophthalmology* 2010; **117**:489–499.

Ferris FL, 3rd, Wilkinson CP, Bird A, et al. Clinical classification of age-related macular degeneration. *Ophthalmology* 2013; **15**:036.

Fujii GY, De Juan E Jr, Humayun MS, et al. Characteristics of visual loss by scanning laser ophthalmoscope microperimetry in eyes with subfoveal choroidal neovascularization secondary to age-related macular degeneration. *Am J Ophthalmol* 2003; **136**:1067–1078.

Zayit-Soudry S, Moroz I, Loewenstein A. Retinal pigment epithelial detachment. *Surv Ophthalmol* 2007; **52**:227–243.

Chapter 10 Macular dystrophies

Amresh Chopdar

INTRODUCTION

Macular dystrophies are inherited genetic disorders affecting the young. Nearly always both eyes are affected and visual symptoms begin early in childhood progressing steadily into adulthood. Visual loss, color vision defects, and photophobia are the most predominant features. An early and accurate diagnosis is required to plan schooling and career.

STARGARDT'S DISEASE

In 1909, Stargardt described a form of macular dystrophy of autosomal recessive inheritances, affecting children between the age of 8 and 15 years. The degeneration progresses rapidly and leads to severe visual loss. Ophthalmoscopy shows a granular appearance of the fovea associated with a variable amount of retinal pigment epithelial atrophy, often surrounding the fovea. The lesions are bilaterally symmetrical and in 50% of cases yellow-white flake-like deposits in the retinal pigment epithelium (RPE), similar to those seen in fundus flavimaculatus, may be observed (Noble & Carr 1979). Stargardt's disease may also be transmitted in an autosomal dominant fashion. Histology shows a complete loss of photoreceptors and RPE.

Fluorescein angiography findings

The retina shows a generalized masking of the choroidal fluorescence during the early phase of the fluorescein angiogram. Such an appearance is common in many other types of macular dystrophies and is referred to as a dark fundus. During the progress of the transit, punctate hyperfluorescence appears surrounding a hypofluorescent fovea. Often alternating concentric rings of hypo- and hyperfluorescence are seen to surround the fovea, resembling a target disc, hence the popular name of bull's eye maculopathy. Maximum hyperfluorescence is seen during the venous phase. Thereafter, the intensity reduces with the concentration of dye in circulation. There is no evidence of leakage of dye. In advanced cases, a large area of retinal pigment epithelial defect is seen (**Figure 10.1**).

FUNDUS FLAVIMACULATUS

Many of Stargardt's patients also had yellow-white flaky lesions in the posterior pole of the retina. Franceschetti (1965 a and b) was the first to describe the appearance of multiple yellow-white, irregularly shaped, flaky deposits at the level of RPE, widely distributed in the posterior pole in patients with a specific type of macular dystrophy. The retina in between the flakes was normal. He also recognized the autosomal recessive inheritance pattern and named it fundus flavimaculatus. In advanced cases of disease, the macular area may show areas of retinal pigment epithelial atrophy. Klein and Krill in 1967 histochemically proved the deposits were mucopolysaccharides in the inner half of the retinal pigment. Hadden and Gass in 1976 studied a large series of patients and confirmed the strong association between these two conditions.

Fluorescein angiography findings

The phenomenon of a dark fundus is very evident in fundus flavimaculatus. The changes seen outside the macula depend on the amount of flaking present. This can vary from minimal to widespread involvement. The arterial phase shows increasing hyperfluorescence of the yellow-white flakes progressing throughout the transit, which fade away toward the late phase. The contrast of hyperfluorescence against the dark fundus can be very striking. Some of these flakes may also show hypofluorescence, particularly during the early stage of their development, before resulting in retinal pigment epithelial degeneration. There is no evidence of leakage of dye during the late phase. The areas in between the flakes show hypofluorescence during the prearterial phase due to temporary choroidal masking. However, toward the venous phase the distinction is less clear. The retina in between the hyperfluorescence is normal (Ernest and Krill 1966) (**Figure 10.2**). The

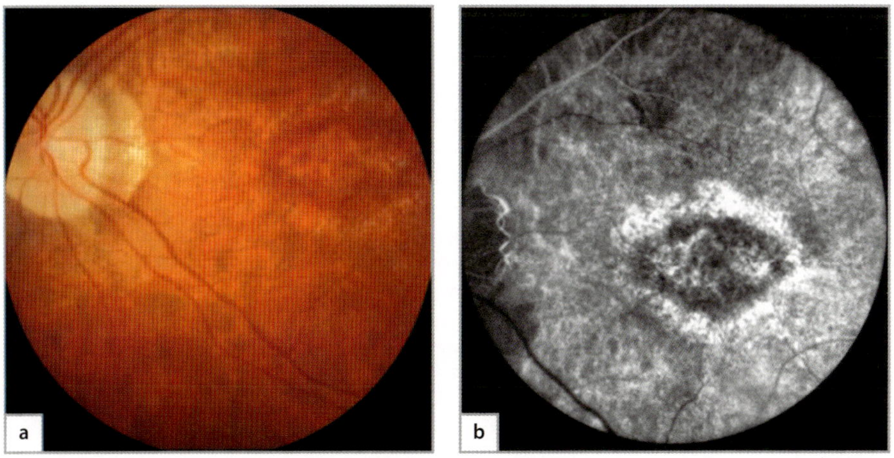

Figure 10.1 Stargardt's disease. (a) The left eye shows alternating dark and light rings surrounding the macula resembling a target. (b) The mid transit phase of the fluorescein angiogram of the left eye shows central speckled hyperfluorescence surrounded by a ring of hypofluorescence, which is in turn surrounded by a hyperfluorescence ring reflecting the changes seen in (a).

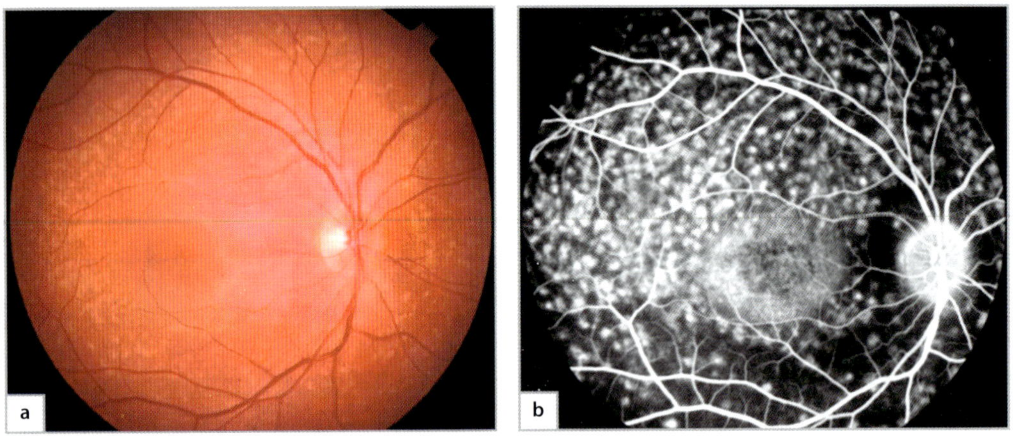

Figure 10.2 Fundus flavimaculatus. (a) The right eye shows subtle flakey deposits in the deeper layer of the retina. The macula displays a dull reflex. (b) The arteriovenous phase of the fluorescein angiogram shows many hyperfluorescent spots scattered all over the fundus. In between the hypofluorescent areas, the retina is normal. The macular area shows atypical target appearance as seen in Stargardt's disease. The background looks considerably dark for a Caucasian fundus. This phenomenon is known as dark fundus, which is seen in many cases of macular dystrophies.

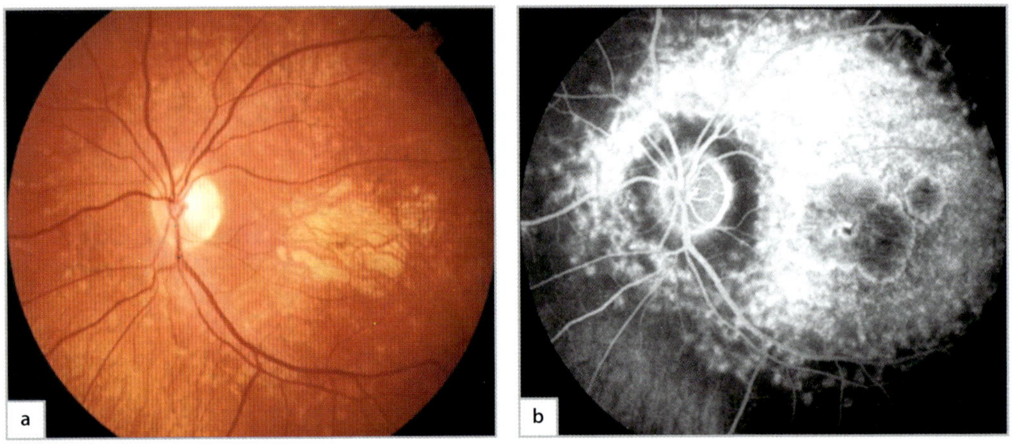

Figure 10.3 Advanced stage of fundus flavimaculatus and Stargardt's disease. (a) The left eye shows typical flakey deposits in the deeper layer of the retina and also a large area of marked retinal pigment epithelial atrophy in the macular area. (b) The late phase of the fluorescein angiogram shows many hyperfluorescent spots scattered widely in the posterior pole. The macular area shows an area of window defect at the center with minimal staining.

advanced stage of the disease atrophic of RPE shows intense staining but no evidence of leakage (**Figure 10.3**).

BULL'S EYE MACULOPATHY

Bull's eye maculopathy is a descriptive name given to the macular changes seen; they resemble a target practicing board with concentric rings. The ophthalmoscopic appearance of mild retinal pigment epithelial degeneration and a slightly darker looking fovea is less conspicuous than the angiographic picture. A typical bull's eye macula lesion is seen in a variety of macular dystrophies such as progressive cone-rod dystrophy, various forms of toxic maculopathy due to chloroquine, tamoxifen, and other dominant foveomacular dystrophies.

Fluorescein angiography findings

The fovea remains hypofluorescent, while the surrounding fluorescence increases steadily during the progress of the transit and may produce a mild leakage or staining toward the late phase of the angiography. This surrounding fluorescence may show alternating concentric hypo- and hyperfluorescence, depending on the degree of pigment epithelial degeneration (**Figure 10.4**).

VITELLIFORM MACULAR DYSTROPHY (BEST'S DISEASE)

Sometimes referred to as Best's vitelliform dystrophy of the fovea, this is an autosomal dominant dystrophy (Best 1905 Blodi and Stone 1990). During the previtelliform stage, the fovea appears normal, but the electro-oculogram (EOG) shows defined abnormalities. A typical vitelliform lesion (egg yolk) appears during the first decade of life, leading to an amorphous scrambled egg-like appearance in the next few decades of life, finally ending with an atrophic chorioretinal scar. A subretinal neovascular membrane may form, leading to a disciform macular degeneration-like lesion in young patients. The EOG often reveals marked abnormalities, but the electroretinogram may remain normal. There is an adult variety of vitelliform dystrophy that looks similar clinically to a normal EOG.

Fluorescein angiography findings

During the early stage of the disease, there is generalized masking of the choroidal background fluorescence due to its characteristic dark fundus phenomenon. In the previtelliform stage, the natural hypofluorescent area of the fovea shows considerable widening without other abnormalities (**Figure 10.5**). In its early vitelliform (egg yolk) stage, the

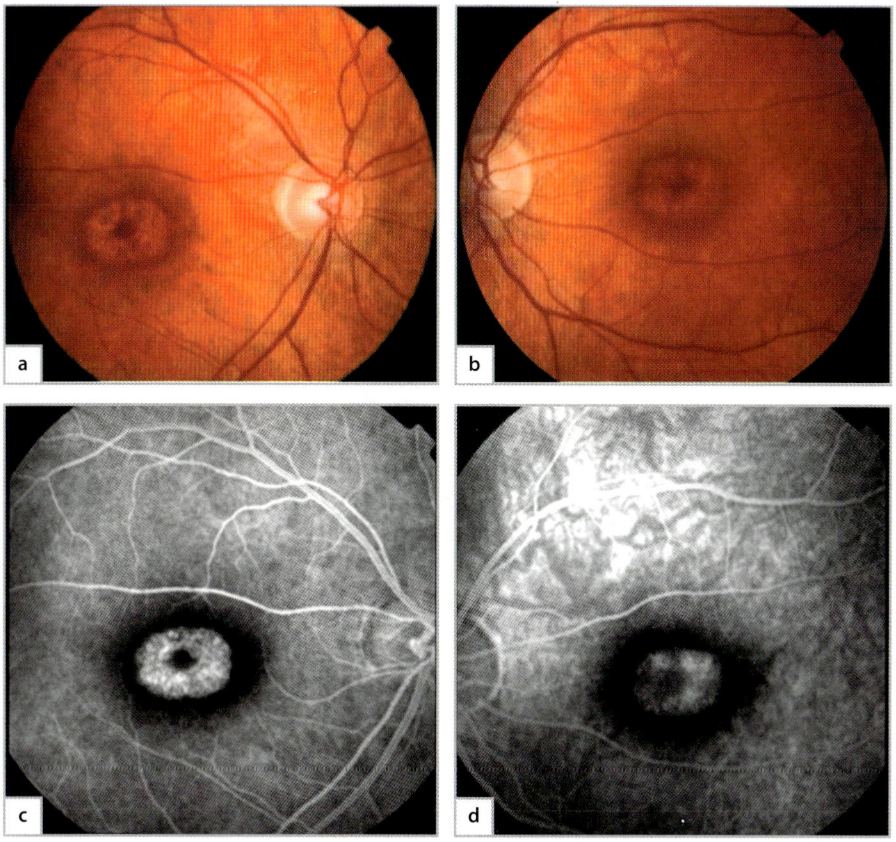

Figure 10.4 Bull's eye maculopathy. The right and left eye show a typical target appearance of the macular area in each eye. The bottom row shows the same two eyes during the later phases of the fluorescein angiogram, which show a dark fundus in each eye. The target appearance of the macular area is well demonstrated with a hypofluorescent center surrounded by a hyperfluorescent ring.

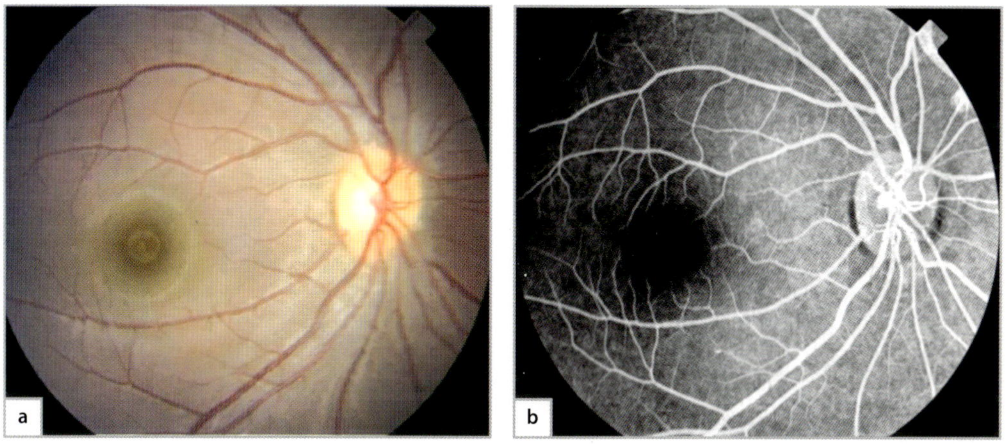

Figure 10.5 Best's disease previtelliform stage. (a) The left eye of a young child shows a circular lesion at the macula. (b) The arteriovenous phase of the fluorescein angiogram shows a wider area of capillary-free zone at the macula with loss of capillary detail.

wider hypofluorescent fovea changes to show several hyperfluorescent spots at its margin during the venous phase. During the late phase, the dye leaks into the cyst and stains with fluorescein (**Figure 10.6**).

Once the scrambled egg stage has developed, the macular area shows a mixture of hypo- and hyperfluorescence due to granular fragmentation of the amorphous materials and retinal pigment epithelial degeneration. The contrast of fluorescence increases throughout the transit and finally produces a minimal degree of staining (**Figure 10.7**). The final stage is when pigment epithelial changes progress to marked retinal pigment epithelial atrophy. The transit of the fundus fluorescein angiography (FFA) shows a large area of hyperfluorescence during the early phase and staining during the late phase.

PSEUDOVITELLIFORM (ADULT) CYST

Unlike Best's disease, this adult type is not hereditary in nature. They may be binocular or uniocular. The EOGs are also normal. Visual deterioration is often mild and most cases are discovered during routine eye testing. The yellow material filling the fovea may liquefy to produce a typical fluid level as in a hypopyon, thus clinically referred to as pseudohypopyon. In long-standing cases, RPE atrophy takes place and a round yellow-gray lesion is seen at the macular area (Fishman et al. 1977).

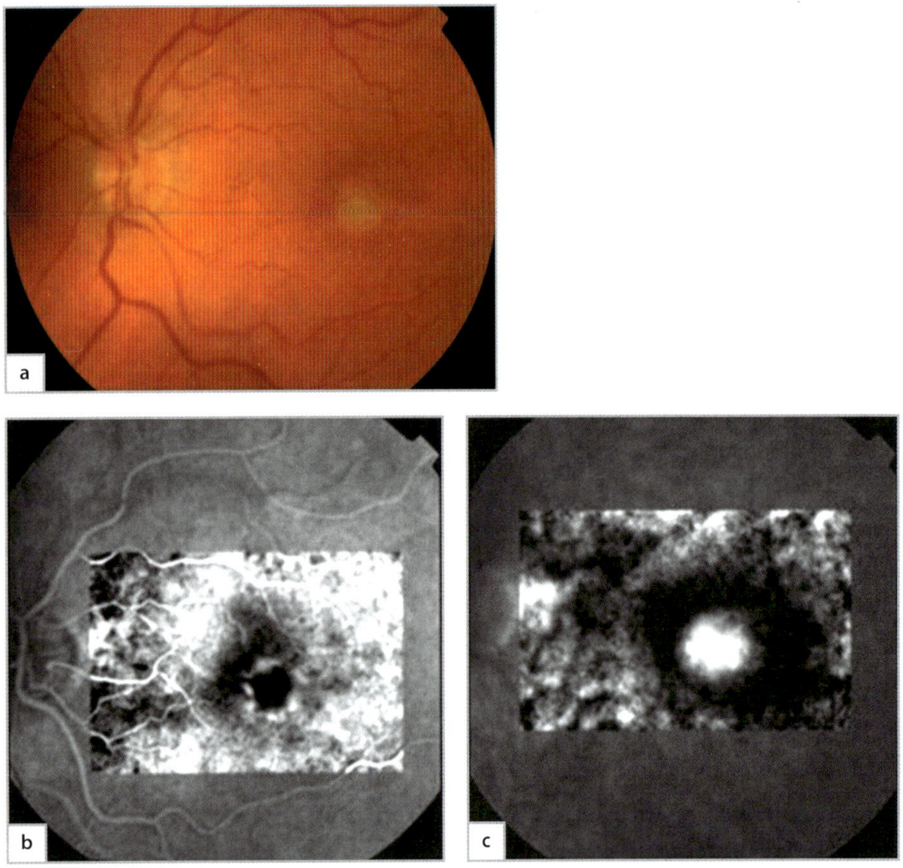

Figure 10.6 Best's disease vitelliform stage. (a) The left eye of a young adult shows a small yellow bleb at the macular area. (b) The early phase of the fluorescein angiogram shows punctate hyperfluorescence from the edge of the perifoveal arcade. The center of the fovea remains hypofluorescent due to the concentration of yellow pigment. (c) The late phase shows moderate degree of leakage into the vitelliform cyst.

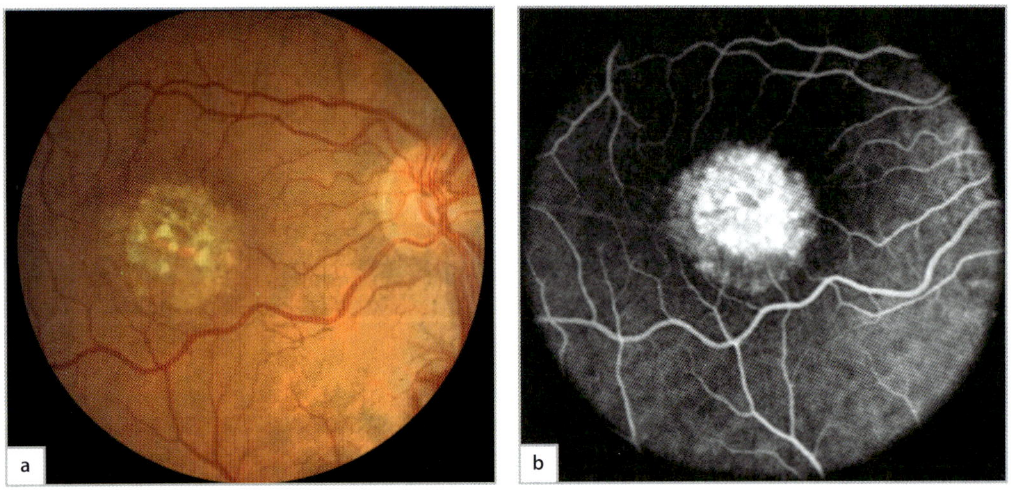

Figure 10.7 Best's scrambled egg stage. (a) The right eye shows the granular fragmentation of the amorphous materials within the vitelliform cyst. (b) The arteriovenous phase of the fluorescein angiogram shows punctate hyperfluorescence within the cyst.

Fluorescein angiography findings

The fluorescein angiogram is very similar to those seen in the vitelliform stage of the hereditary type. Hyperfluorescence starts from the outer margin of the lesion, which increases in fluorescence during the transit and fades away toward the late phase. The central area containing the yellow material remains hypofluorescent. In chronic cases where the yellow pigment has undergone resolution, the perifoveal area shows hypofluorescence due to scattered pigment, and the RPE atrophy at the fovea shows a mild degree of hyperfluorescence toward the late phase (**Figure 10.8**).

RETICULAR DYSTROPHY OF THE RETINA

There is a large variety of pattern dystrophies of the macula. They are named according to the perceived appearance of the lesion.

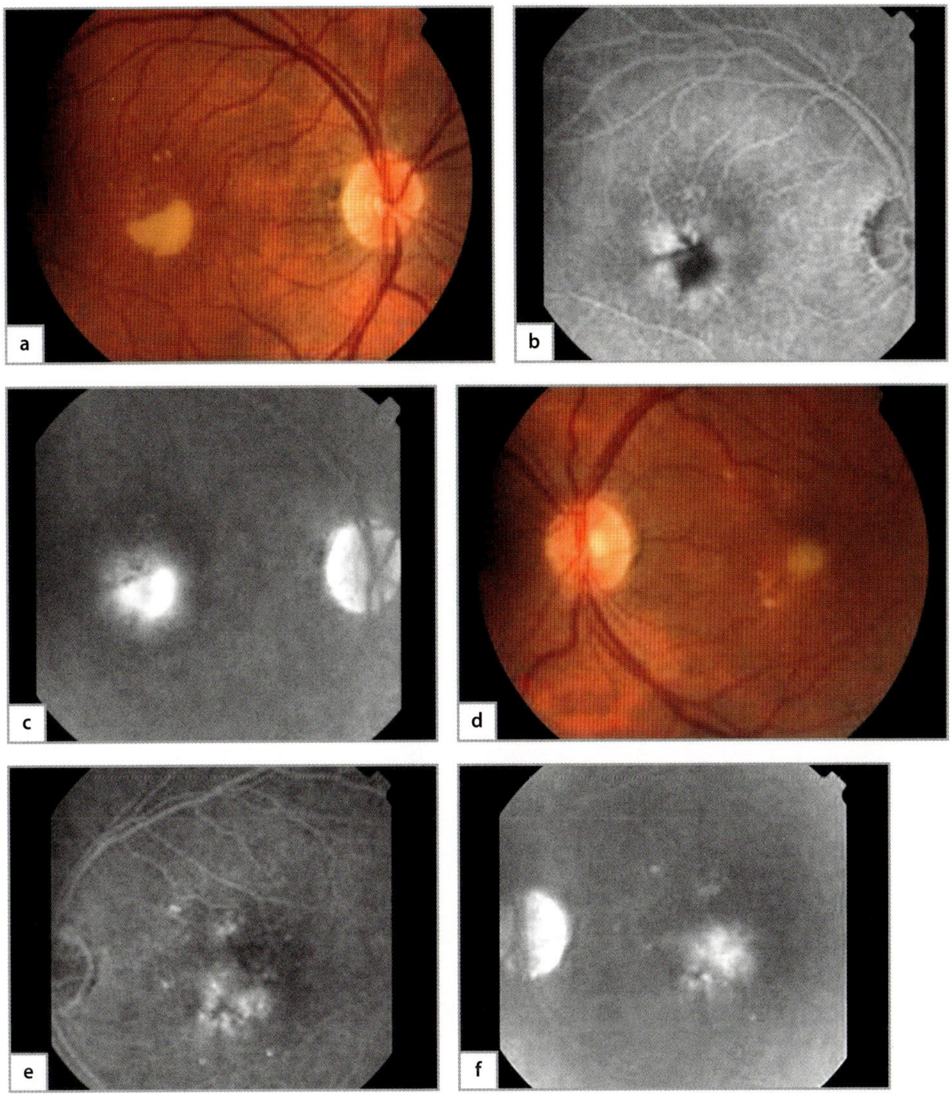

Figure 10.8 Adult pseudovitelliform macular degeneration. (a) The right eye shows a pseudohypopyon vitelliform cyst at the macular area. (b) The late transit phase of the fluorescein angiogram shows hyperfluorescence around the margin of the original cyst. (c) The late phase shows staining of the cyst area. (d) The left eye from the same case shows a typical vitelliform cyst at the macular area. The area just below the cyst shows moderate degree of retinal pigment epithelial atrophy. (e) The late transit of the left eye shows hypofluorescence at the macular area occupied by the vitelliform cyst. The area below the cyst shows hyperfluorescence due to retinal pigment epithelial degeneration. (f) The late phase shows moderate degree of staining of the macula and adjacent area.

Reticular dystrophy is one such dystrophy. This is a rare and unusual form of hereditary retinal pigment epithelial dystrophy first described by Sjogren in 1950 (Chopdar 1976a). It shows a network of polygonal pigmented lesion all over the retina, including the macula.

Fluorescein angiography findings

The early phase of the angiography shows persistent masking of choroidal background fluorescence along the black lines throughout the transit to demonstrate the networking. The retinal circulation over the pigment is unaffected. There is no evidence of leakage (**Figure 10.9**).

CONE-ROD DYSTROPHY

Cone-rod dystrophy is a homogenous group of macular dystrophies characterized by progressive visual loss, loss of color vision, and photophobia. Scotopic vision is less affected. It can be inherited by both autosomal dominant and recessive trait. The recessive type often manifests during the early teens with a typical bull's eye pattern of macular changes. Some patients may show pigment clumpings and RPE changes at the macular area (Krill and Duetman 1972).

Fluorescein angiography findings

The fluorescein angiogram shows a typical dark fundus due to persistent hypofluorescence of the choroid. The pigment clumps at the center of the macula and usually masks fluorescence, at the same time a typical window defect is seen surrounding the macular area due to RPE changes. The foveal center remains hypofluorescent throughout the angiography period. Thus, there is a typical target disc appearance (**Figure 10.10**).

MACULAR COLOBOMA

Whether macular coloboma is a true developmental anomaly remains unresolved. The macular area shows an oval, white lesion with some pigmentation on the edges with very little sign of true inflammation. This is a true hiatus of the retina at the macular area exposing the underlying sclera. Unlike congenital toxoplasmosis, which is often

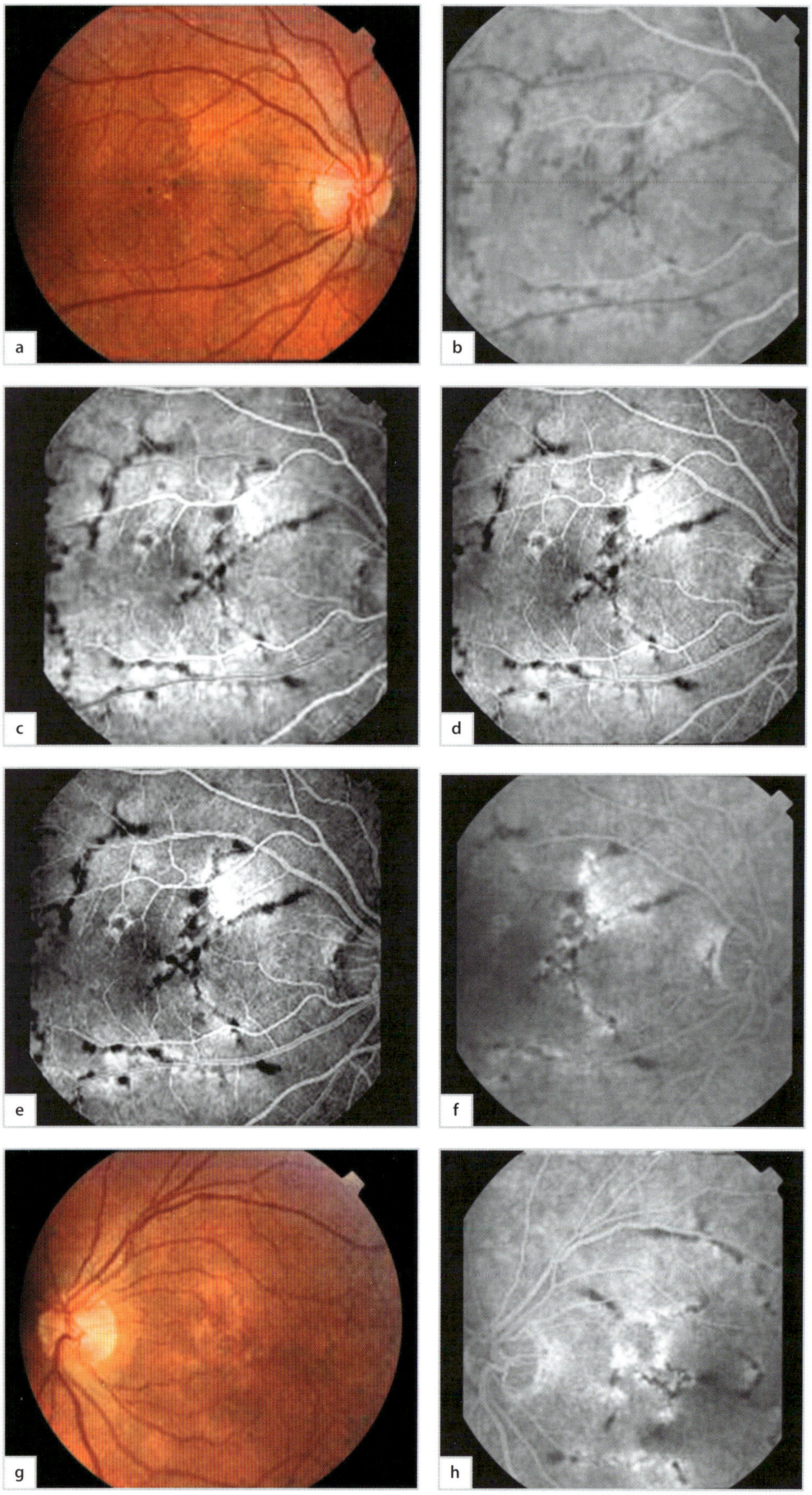

Figure 10.9 Reticular dystrophy. *For caption, see opposite.*

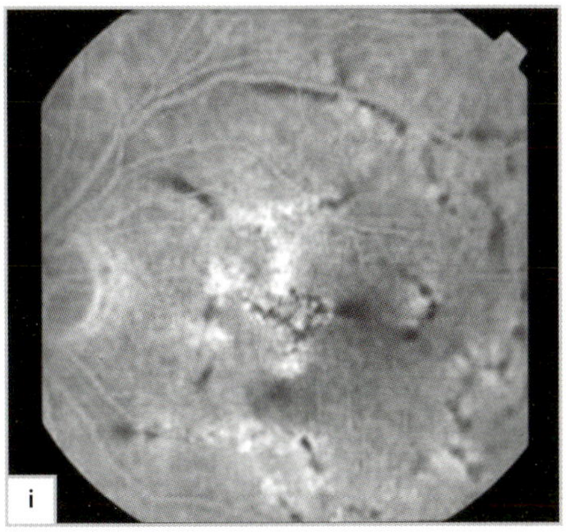

Figure 10.9 Reticular dystrophy. (a) The right eye shows some amount of pigmentation in the deeper layer of the retina. (b) The left eye shows changes similar to the right eye. (c) The arteriovenous phase of fluorescein angiogram of the right eye shows the networking of polygonal pigmentation affecting a very wide area of the fundus including the macula. (d) The arteriovenous phase of the left eye shows a typical fishnet pattern of pigmentation of the posterior polar region and consistent hypofluorescence from the pigment.

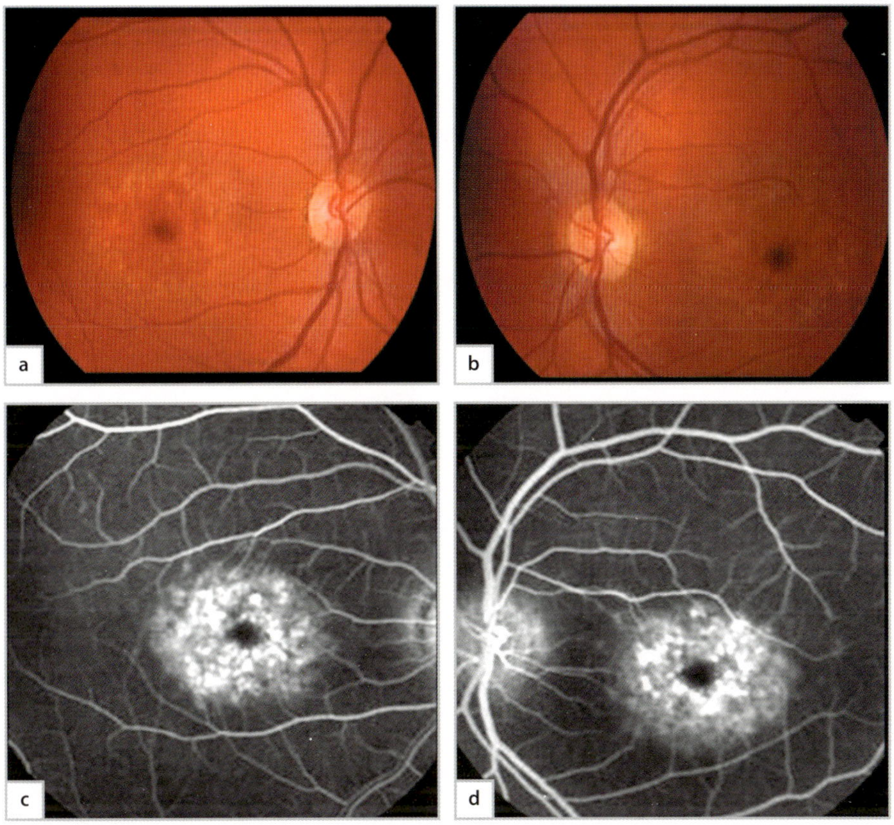

Figure 10.10 Cone-rod dystrophy. (a) The right eye shows some pigment clumping at the center of the fovea surrounded by a mixture of speckled pigment distribution limited to the macular area. (b) The left eye shows almost a similar picture to that of the right eye. (c) The fluorescein angiogram of the right eye during the venous phase shows a darker looking background due to masking of choroidal fluorescence. The hypofluorescence at the center is due to masking of the pigment clumps seen in (a). The central hypofluorescence is in turn surrounded by granular hypo- and hyperfluorescence, resulting in a target appearance. (d) The left eye shows very similar picture to that of the right eye.

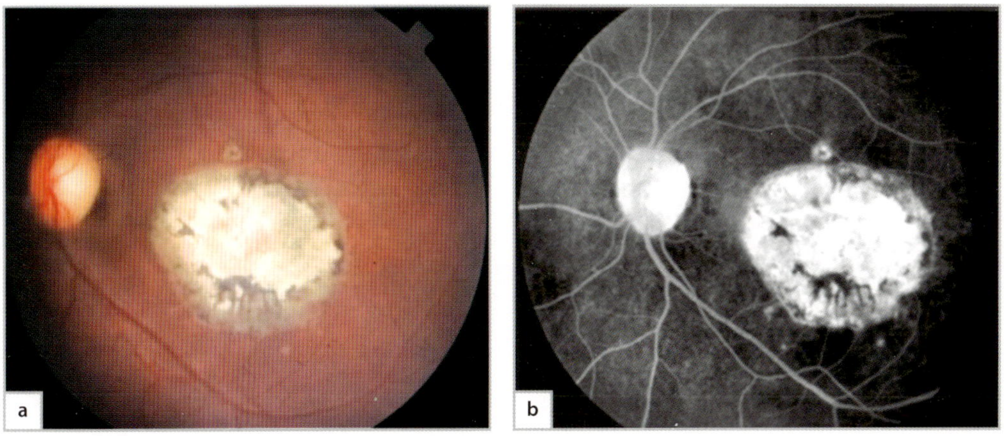

Figure 10.11 Coloboma of the macula. (a) A large area of retinal hiatus exposing the underlying sclera. There is a small amount of dispersion of light brown uveal pigment. (b) The late venous phase of the fluorescein angiogram shows staining of the underlying sclera and masking of the pigment.

confused with coloboma, the pigmentation is light brown and there is no clumping.

Fluorescein angiography findings

The early phase of the angiogram shows the remainder of the larger sized choroidal blood vessels through a central defect that increases in fluorescence during the transit. The rest of the retina shows no abnormality. The entire area produces an intense staining toward the late phase. The pigment continues to mask the underlying fluorescence throughout the period of angiography (**Figure 10.11**).

REFERENCES

Best F. Uber eine hereditare Maculaaffektion, Beitrage ur Verebungslehre. *Ztschr f Augenh* 1905; **13**:199.
Blodi CF, Stone EM Best's vitelliform dystrophy. *Ophthalmic paediatrics and genetics* 1990; **11**:49–59.
Chopdar A Reticular dystrophy of retina. *Br J Ophthalmol* 1976a; **60**:342–344.
Ernest JT, Krill AE. Fluorescein studies in fundus flavimaculatus and drusen. *Am J Ophthalmol* 1966; **62**:1–6.
Fishman GA, Trimble S, Rabb MF, Fishman M. Pseudovitelliform macular degeneration. *Arch Ophthalmol* 1977; **95**:73–76.
Franceschetti A, Francois J. Fundus flavimaculatus. *Arch d'Ophthalmol (Paris)* 1965a; **25**:505–530.
Franceschetti A. A special form of tapetoretinal degeneration: Fundus flavimaculatus. *Trans Am Acad Ophthalmol Otolaryngol* 1965b; **69**:1048–1053.
Hadden OB, Gass JDM. Fundus flavimaculatus and Stargardt's disease. *Am J Ophthalmol* 1976; **82**:527–539.
Klein BA, Krill AE. Fundus flavimaculatus: clinical, functional, and histologic observations. *Am J Ophthalmol* 1967; **64**:3–23.
Kobrin JL, Apple DJ, Hart WB. Vitelliform dystrophy. *Int Ophthalmol Clin* 1981; **21**:167–184.
Krill AE, Duetman AF. Dominant macular degeneration. The cone dystrophies. *Am J Ophthalmol* 1972; **73**:352.
Noble KG, Carr RE. Stargardt's disease and fundus flavimaculatus. *Arch Ophthalmol* 1979; **97**:1281–1285.
Sjogren H. Dystrophia reticularis laminae pigmentosa retinae. *Acta Ophthalmol* 1950; **28**:279–295.
Stargardt K. Ueber familiaere, progressive degeneration in der Makulagegund des Auges. Albrechte von Greafes's Arch. *Kln Exp Ophthalmol* 1909; **71**:534–550.

Chapter 11 Choroidal disorders

Amresh Chopdar

IDIOPATHIC CENTRAL SEROUS CHOROIDOPATHY

Central serous retinopathy or idiopathic central serous choroidopathy is a disease affecting the choriocapillaris and the retinal pigment epithelium (RPE) in young adults between the ages of 20 and 45 years old. The exact nature of the pathology is uncertain, but it is believed to be due to the dysfunction of the choriocapillaris leading to development of a small retinal pigment epithelial detachment. Occasionally, this may lead to a wider neurosensory detachment of the retina. Pigment epithelial detachment varies widely in numbers, sizes, and locations. Resolution often takes place spontaneously within a few weeks. Recurrences may occur in certain individuals. People predisposed to anxious personality and those prone to allergy and atopy are more likely to suffer from central serous choroidopathy. The patients present with a sudden onset of visual symptoms of metamorphopsia, micropsia, and central scotoma. The visual acuity is only reduced modestly and can be improved by a small hypermetropic correction. Ophthalmoscopy shows a round neurosensory separation affecting the macular area. Careful inspection of this detached area may show a small gray-yellow spot within it, which may represent the retinal pigment epithelial detachment and mark the site of leakage of fluorescein dye during angiography. In some cases, precipitates may deposit in the inner surface of the retina (Gemenetzi et al. 2010).

Fluorescein angiography findings

The prearterial phase of the fluorescein angiogram shows patchy choroidal filling but no persistent filling defect. There may be a transient masking of choroidal background fluorescence corresponding to the serous detachment of the retina. Later frames show a variety of patterns of leakage (Yoshioka & Sugita 1970).

Inkblot (spot) leakage

This is the commonest form of leakage. A tiny spot appears with a well-defined margin and increases in size throughout the transites, producing a moderate degree of leakage during the later phases. During the late phase of the angiography, the dye extends into the subretinal space and may mask the sharp outline of the initial spot (**Figure 11.1**).

Smokestack (mushroom shaped) leakage

This type of leakage is usually associated with widespread neurosensory detachment of the retina. The underlying leakage begins as a small spot but soon the dye makes an upward expansion as it enters

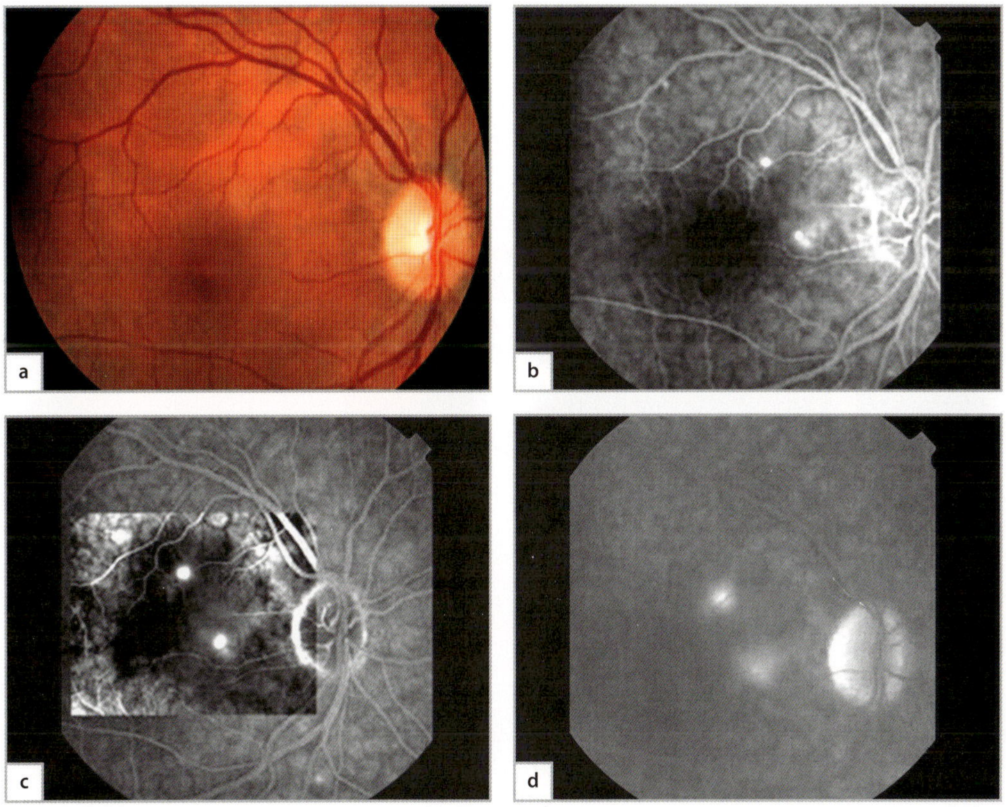

Figure 11.1 Idiopathic central serous choroidopathy: spot leakage. (a) The right eye shows a very ill-defined shallow serous retinal detachment superior temporal to the optic disc. (b) The prearterial phase of the fluorescein angiogram shows two pinhead-sized hyperfluorescent spots , one superior and the other one nasal to the macular area. (c) An enhanced frame of the late venous phase shows the spots increasing in hyperfluorescence due to continuing leakage. (d) The late phase shows increased leakage with fuzzy borders.

the subretinal space. After it has reached a certain height, the top flattens and whole thing collapses downwards. The late phase of the angiogram shows leakage of dye slowly saturating the subretinal fluid and hiding the smokestack, due to heavy drench of fluorescein dye in the subretinal fluid (**Figure 11.2**).

Punctate staining

Retinal pigment epithelial degeneration following resolution shows punctate hyperfluorescence during the early part of the transit as window defects. The hyperfluorescence increases slowly during the transit, but fades away toward the late phase (**Figure 11.3**).

CHOROIDAL FOLDS

A space-occupying lesion in the orbit may push the choroid inward, taking with it the RPE and the overlying neuroretina, resulting in visible striations in the posterior pole commonly known as choroidal folds. Sometimes these may occur a result of lower intraocular pressure or even without any cause. The choroid gathers around the optic disc in a concentric manner (Cangemi et al. 1978, Cohen & Gass 1994–1995).

Fluorescein angiography findings

During the early retinal arterial phase, hyperfluorescent striae are seen to run across the retina; they correspond to the crests of the folds. The troughs remain relatively hypofluorescent; thus, alternative hyper- and hypofluorescent bands run across the retina. The intensity of fluorescence increases with the concentration of circulating dye during the transit and fades away toward the late phase (**Figure 11.4**).

CHOROIDITIS

During the acute phase, the lesion is seen as a gray-white irregular patch in the fundus, affecting both the choroid and the retina. At first it is gray, but when healed it produces a moderate degree of pigment clumping and chorioretinal atrophy. The commonest identifiable causes are toxoplasmosis and histoplasmosis.

TOXOPLASMOSIS

Toxoplasmic chorioretinitis is a protozoal infection caused by *Toxoplasma gondii.* Infection can be either congenital or acquired. The congenital form commonly affects the macula area in the eye or is associated with other systemic diseases. The acute chorioretinitis shows as a gray-white lesion affecting the choroid and the overlying retina with ill-defined edges. Once the lesion has healed, it leaves a patch of atrophic scar at the macula with pigment clumping. In extreme cases, it may resemble a macular coloboma (Perkins 1973).

Fluorescein angiography findings

Acute chorioretinitis

Initially the retinal edema masks the background choroidal fluorescence during the early phase of the angiography, but there is a moderate degree of staining toward the late phase.

Healed lesion

The prearterial phase shows a few remaining larger sized choroidal vessels seen through the atrophic RPE. The pigment clump masks the choroidal background fluorescence throughout the transit and late phase. The late phase shows some staining of the underlying sclera as a large window defect, but no evidence of any leakage (**Figure 11.5**).

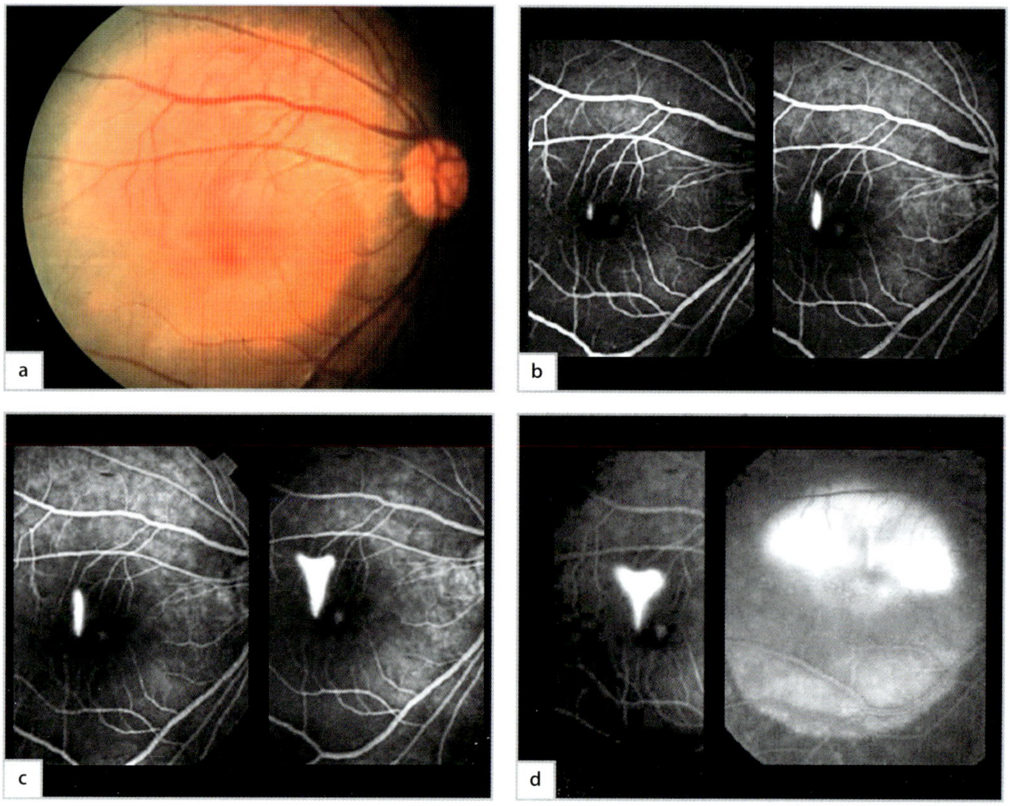

Figure 11.2 Idiopathic central serous choroidopathy: smoke stack leakage. (a) The right eye shows a bullous retinal detachment of the macula. (b) The arteriovenous phase of the fluorescein angiogram shows a small leakage that commences medial to the fovea and gradually extends upward. (c) The later phases show leakage continuing to spread in an upward direction. (d) The late phase shows the gradual collapse of the shape of the leakage to fill the serous exudate.

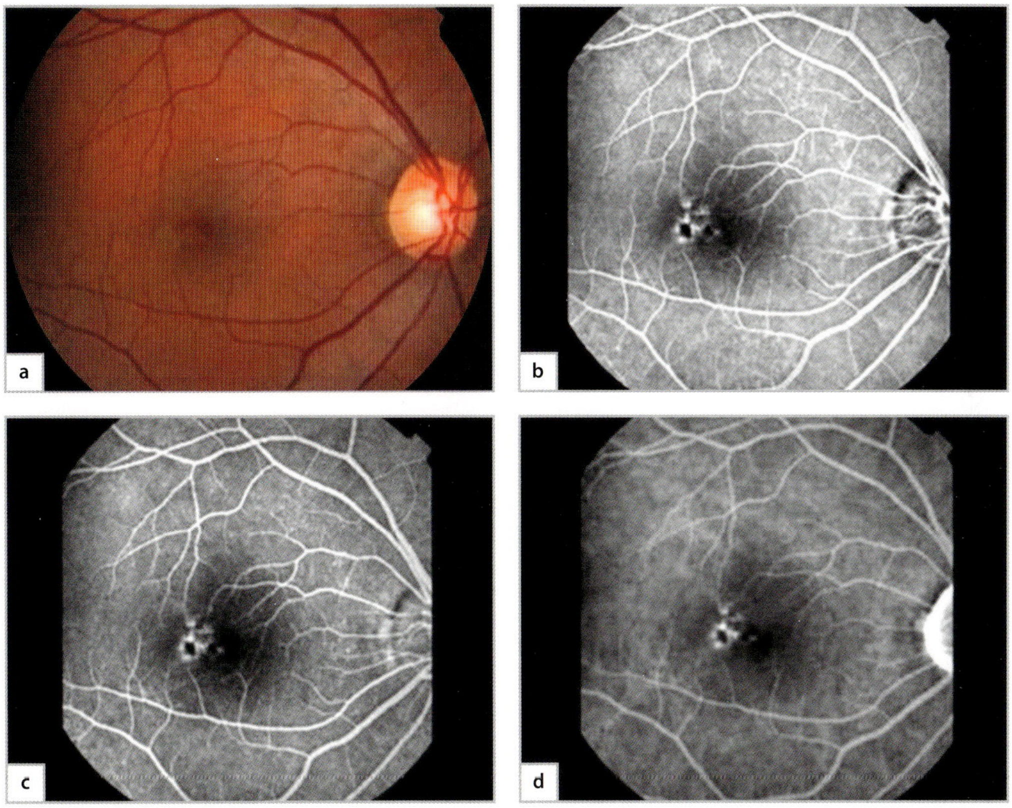

Figure 11.3 Resolved idiopathic central serous choroidopathy. (a) A minor degree of retinal pigment epithelial changes following full resolution. (b) The arteriovenous phase of the fluorescein angiogram shows mixture of hypo- and hyperfluorescence lateral to the macula. (c) A later phase shows diminishing degree of fluorescence. (d) The late phase shows minimal staining of the underlying sclera.

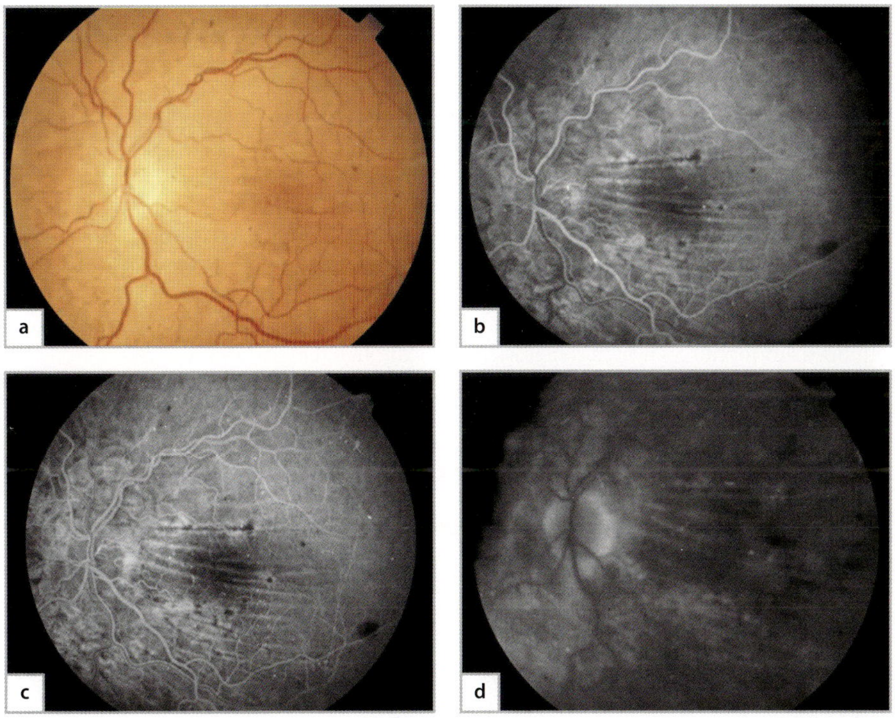

Figure 11.4 Choroidal folds. (a) The left eye shows parallel radiating folds across the macular area. A few hemorrhages are seen in the posterior pole. (b) The arterial phase of the fluorescein angiogram shows alternating hypo- and hyperfluorescence in radiating lines across the macular area. There are several blots in hypofluorescent areas due to masking of choroidal background fluorescence, which is most likely due to the retinal hemorrhages seen on the photograph. (c) The arteriovenous phase shows increasing hypo- and hyperfluorescence across the macular area. There are similar alternating concentric rings around the optic disc. The troughs of the folds remain hypofluorescent whereas the apexes of the folds show hyperfluorescence. (d) The late phase shows staining of a few remaining folds.

PRESUMED OCULAR HISTOPLASMOSIS

This is commonly seen in the eastern part of the USA, but has been reported from many other parts of the world. *Histoplasma capsulatum* is the causative organism; it is found in the soil. Often the ocular involvement is due to silent past systemic infection. The patient is a normal healthy individual showing past lesions in the lungs, and occasionally calcification in the liver and spleen. The histoplasmin test is positive in a majority of cases. The diagnosis is often based on ocular findings. The macula shows a green-yellow raised lesion surrounded by retinal hemorrhage and proliferation of pigment. The peripheral part of the retina shows multiple punched-out atrophic lesions, some of them full thickness.

Fluorescein angiography findings

The fluorescein angiogram shows a central choroidal neovascular membrane with leakage toward the late phase. The intraretinal hemorrhages mask the background fluorescence. The peripheral lesions show hyperfluorescence due to scleral staining. Many punched-out hyperfluorescent spots are seen scattered within the fundus (**Figure 11.6**).

CENTRAL AREOLAR CHOROIDAL DYSTROPHY

This is an autosomal dominant macular dystrophy. During the early stage of the disease, the fundus shows milder degree of granular pigmentary changes at the macular area. As the degenerative progresses, the RPE shows increasing amount of atrophic changes associated with moderate loss of choriocapillaris. In advanced stages, a circular dense chorioretinal scar is seen with almost total loss of RPE and the underlying choroid. The visual loss progresses with the advancing disease, leading to profound loss during the advanced stage of the disease (Noble 1977, Noble et al. 1977, Chopdar 1993).

Fluorescein angiography findings

The angiogram during the early stage of the disease shows confluent punctate hyperfluorescence with a darker hypofluorescent fovea. This gives a typical bull's eye pattern similar to other macular dystrophies. In the advanced stage, fluorescein angiography shows a distinct demarcation between the affected and nonaffected areas. The affected area shows marked loss of RPE and chorioretinal atrophy. The late phase of the angiography shows staining of the lesion (**Figure 11.7**).

ANGIOID STREAKS

Angioid streaks are breaks in Bruch's membrane; associated changes in the RPE show multiple red lines radiating from the optic disc toward the peripheral parts of the retina. They are commonly seen in pseudoxanthoma elasticum, Paget's disease, Ehlers–Danlos syndrome, sickle cell disease, and other diseases affecting Bruch's membrane. Angioid streaks often lead to disciform degeneration (Smith et al. 1964, Federman et al. 1975, Clarkson 1982).

Fluorescein angiography findings

Fluorescein angiography during the early phase shows patchy filling of the choroid and the beginning of linear hyperfluorescence radiating from the optic disc towards the peripheral part of retina. The later phase of angiography shows increasing hyperfluorescence and staining of these radiating hyperfluorescence tracks (**Figure 11.8**).

CHOROIDAL RUPTURE

Choroidal rupture commonly occurs following blunt impact to the eye. Ruptures are often concentric around the optic disc. Initially hemorrhage may be seen in the fundus, but once this has cleared the breaks are easily seen as a white concentric ring around the optic disc. Formation of a subretinal neovascular membrane is the most common complication and threatens vision (Luxenberg 1986).

Fluorescein angiography findings

The prearterial phase shows a concentric hypofluorescence semicircle. The concave border faces towards the optic disc. At times it is possible to see one or two larger sized choroidal vessels through the rupture. Throughout the transit, it is easy to see the retinal vessels bridging the gap. The two edges of the rupture begin to fluoresce toward the late venous phase and continue to produce a moderate degree of staining, which can be seen easily through the gap (**Figure 11.9**).

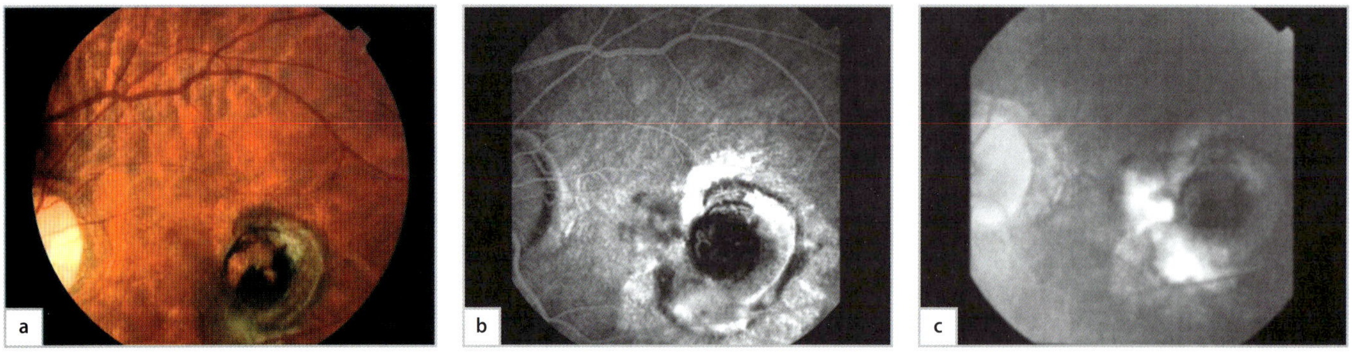

Figure 11.5 Toxoplasmic choroiditis. (a) The left eye shows a large circular punched-out heavily pigmented lesion surrounded by a moderate degree of retinal pigment epithelial atrophy at the macula. (b) The arteriovenous phase of the fluorescein angiogram shows a combination of hypo- and hyperfluorescence at the macula due to retinal pigment epithelial atrophy and heavy pigmentation. (c) The late phase shows staining from the atrophic areas and continuing masking from the pigment.

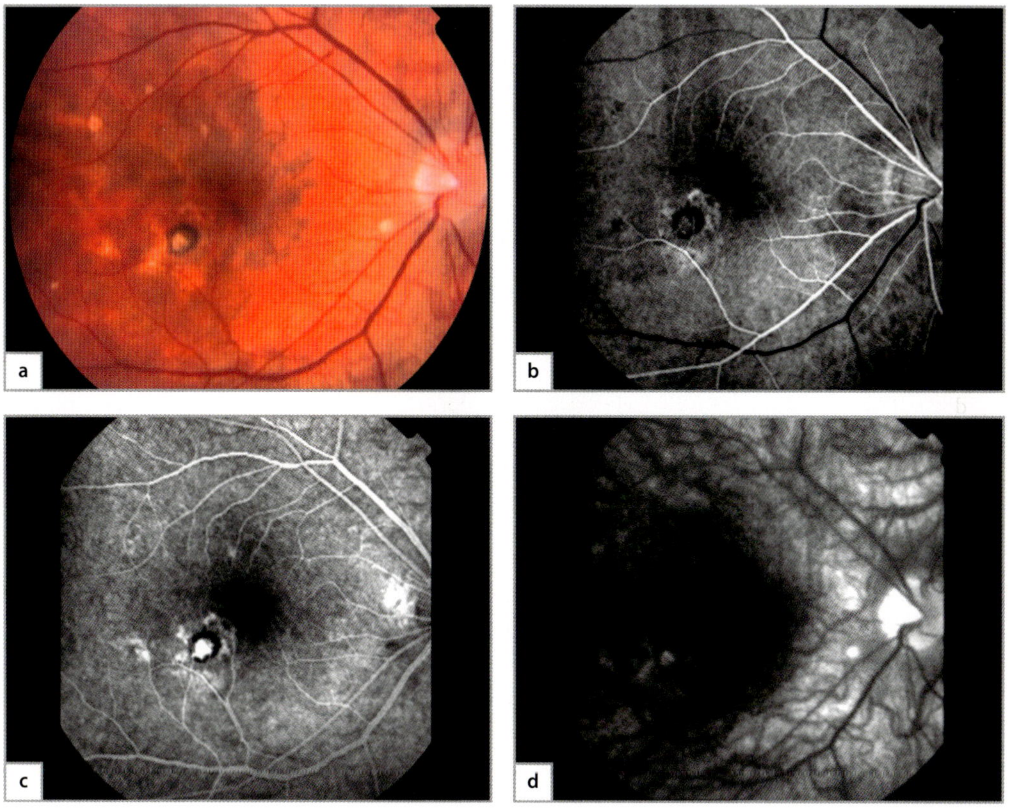

Figure 11.6 Presumed ocular histoplasmosis. (a) The right eye shows a dark pigmented lesion close to the inferior part of the macula. There are several punched-out atrophic lesions scattered in the posterior pole. (b) The arterial phase of the fluorescein angiogram shows a dark hypofluorescent ring corresponding to the pigment deposit, surrounded by a hyperfluorescent zone both outside and inside the hypofluorescent ring. (c) The arteriovenous phase shows intense staining of the central area but some fading of the outer circle. There are several faint hyperfluorescent spots in the posterior pole. (d) The late phase shows generalized fading of fluorescence from the fundus.

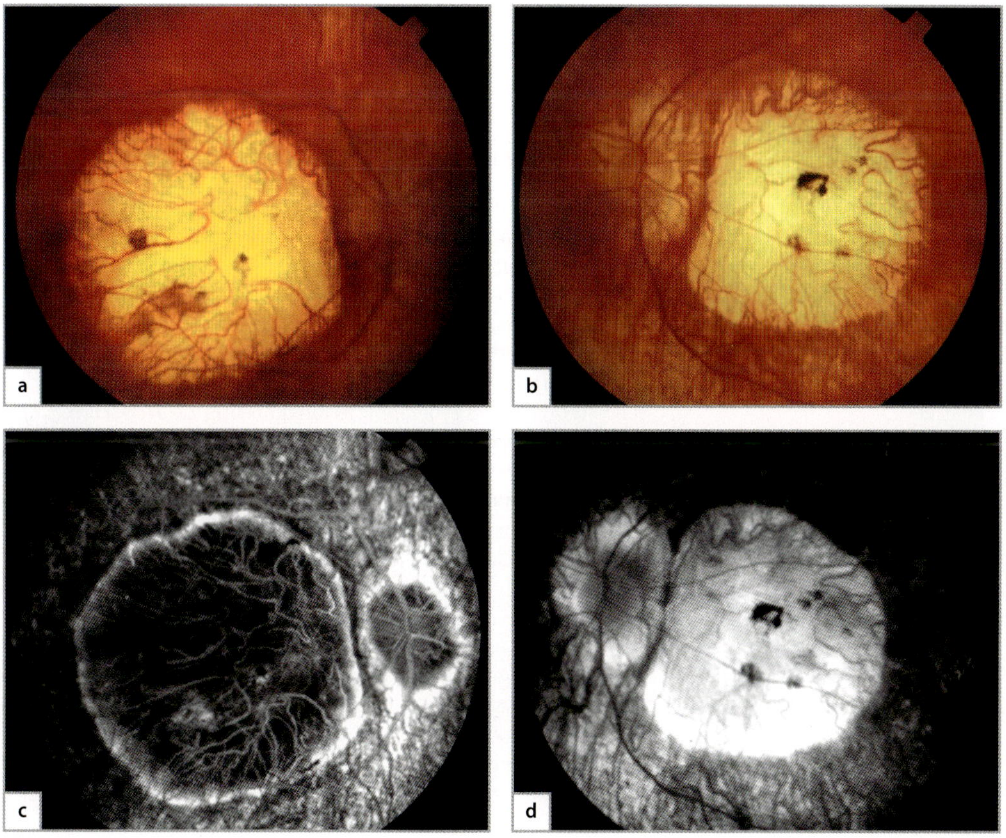

Figure 11.7 Central areolar choroidal dystrophy. (a) The right eye shows a large area of chorioretinal atrophy at the macula exposing the sclera and a few remaining larger sized choroidal vessels. (b) The left eye shows a similar large area of chorioretinal atrophy at the macula exposing the sclera and a few remaining larger sized choroidal vessels. (c) The late venous phase of the fluorescein angiogram of the right eye shows a large hyperfluorescent ring outlining the area of chorioretinal atrophy within the macula. There is also a generalized retinal pigment epithelial degeneration. (d) The late phase shows marked staining of the underlying sclera, outlining the large chorioretinal atrophy of the macular area.

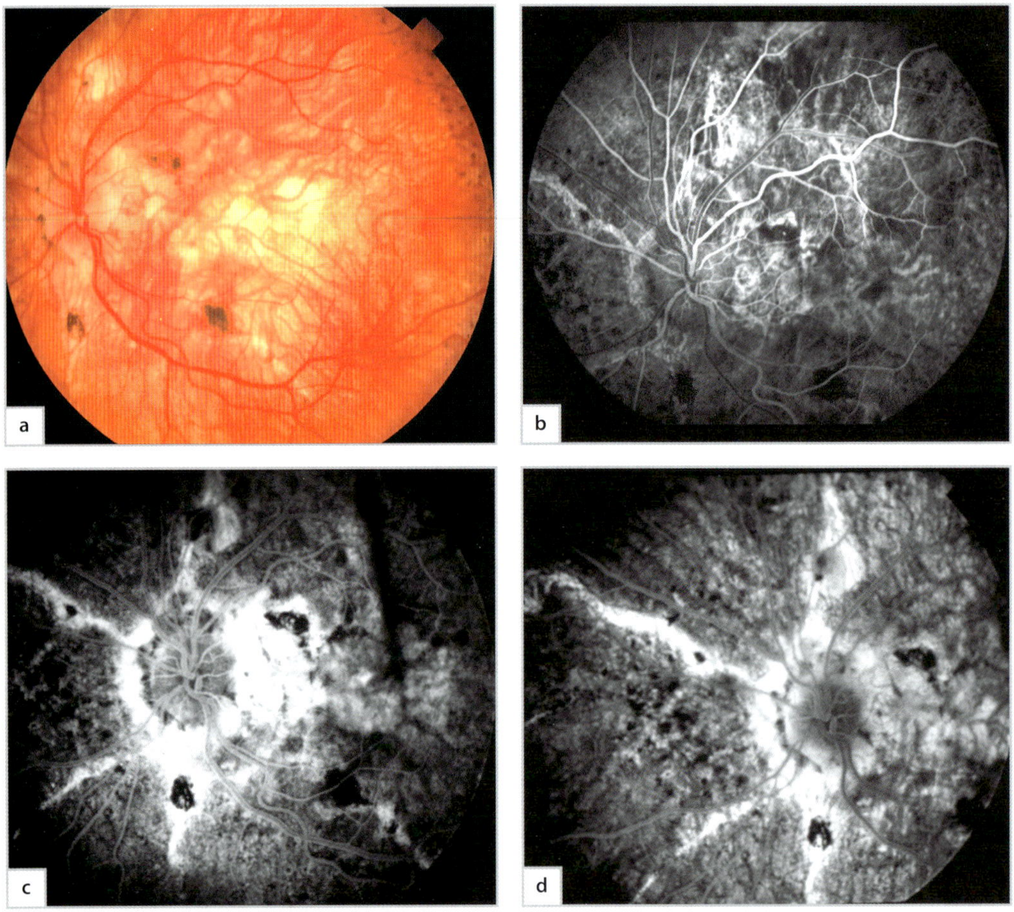

Figure 11.8 Angioid streaks. (a) The left eye shows advanced degenerative changes and some clumps of pigment in the posterior pole. (b) The arterial phase of the fluorescein angiogram shows patchy and linear hyperfluorescence affecting the choroid. (c) The late venous phase centered at the optic disc area shows radiating hyperfluorescence lines emanating from the outer edges of the optic disc. (d) The late phase shows marked staining of the exposed sclera along the angioid streaks and around the disc and macula. The hypofluorescent areas correspond to the clumps of retinal pigment epithelium.

VOGT–KOYANAGI–HARADA SYNDROME

Vogt–Koyanagi–Harada syndrome is combination of two disease entities: (1) Vogt–Koyanagi syndrome mainly presents with severe bilateral granulomatous panuveitis and meningoencephalitis, later developing poliosis, alopecia, and vitiligo; and (2) Harada's disease has limited skin changes but similar eye pathology, including extensive exudative retinal detachment and disc swelling. The disease is common in oriental and dark-skinned races, and is seen not infrequently in Caucasians. The disease may run a chronic stage and take several months to resolve (Moorthy et al. 1995, Arellanes-García et al. 2007).

Fluorescein angiography findings

Acute stage

During the acute stage of the disease, the transit shows masking of choroidal background due to exudative retinal detachment. Later phases of the transit show multiple irregular fluorescence dots scattered widely in the deeper layer of retina, probably at the level of RPE. During the late phase, the dye pools in the overlying serous detachment (**Figure 11.10**).

Recovery stage

The entire retina takes on a red glow, looking like a setting sun. Retinal pigment epithelial changes are seen at the posterior pole; most of these are probably the result of hyperfluorescence dots seen during the acute stage of angiography. The late phase shows minimal staining of the optic disc (**Figure 11.11**).

SERPIGINOUS CHOROIDOPATHY

Serpiginous choroidopathy is an uncommon disease affecting adults in their 50s. It is usually a bilateral disease but is very asymmetrical. Patients present with decreased vision without pain or redness of the eyes. There may be mild activity of the anterior chamber. The vitreous is often clear. Initial lesions begin near the optic disc and later extend towards the macular area to involve the entire posterior pole in due course. During the acute stage, the fundus examination shows yellow-gray areas of geographic lesions affecting the deeper layers with retinal edema. Such lesions may appear in crops as the healing process continues over the next few weeks. The inflammatory process destroys the RPE and underlying choroidal vessels. These lesions extend in a maplike or pseudopodial pattern, hence the disease is named serpiginous choroiditis (Laatikainen & Erkkla 1974, Lim et al. 2005).

Fluorescein angiography findings

During the acute phase of the disease, the early phase of fluorescein angiography shows masking of the background choroidal fluorescence; this is followed by patchy hyperfluorescence and leakage towards the late phase, often showing a typical geographic pattern. The healed lesions, on the other hand, show granular hyperfluorescence during the early phase due to atrophy of the RPE and a minor degree of staining toward the late phase (**Figure 11.12**).

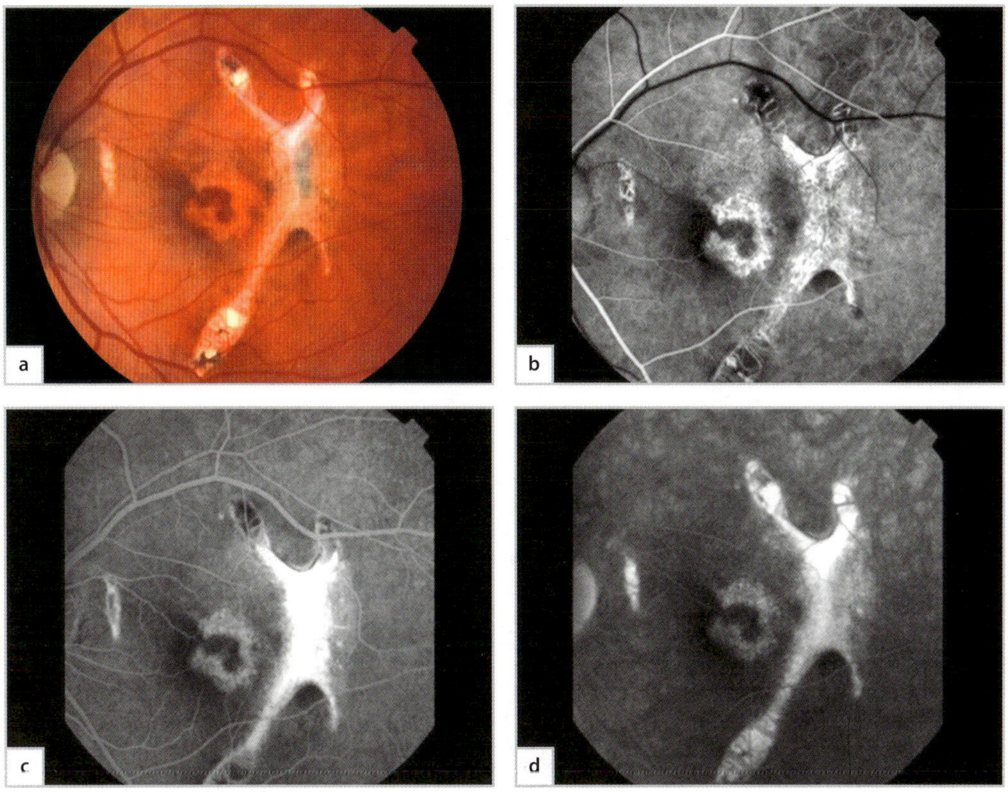

Figure 11.9 Choroidal rupture. (a) The left eye shows significant retinal pigment epithelial degenerative changes at the macula. Just lateral to the foveal area several large tears of the choroid are seen roughly concentric in relation to the optic disc. The two large tears are interconnected in an H shape with gray-green pigment at its center, possibly due to a subretinal neovascularization. There is a smaller tear just above the temporal border of the optic disc. (b) The arterial phase of the fluorescein angiogram shows mottled hyperfluorescence of the macular area, outlining the ruptures of the choroid. The rest of the fundus appears normal. (c) The late arteriovenous phase shows increased fluorescence from the ruptures. (d) The late phase shows staining of the ruptured areas.

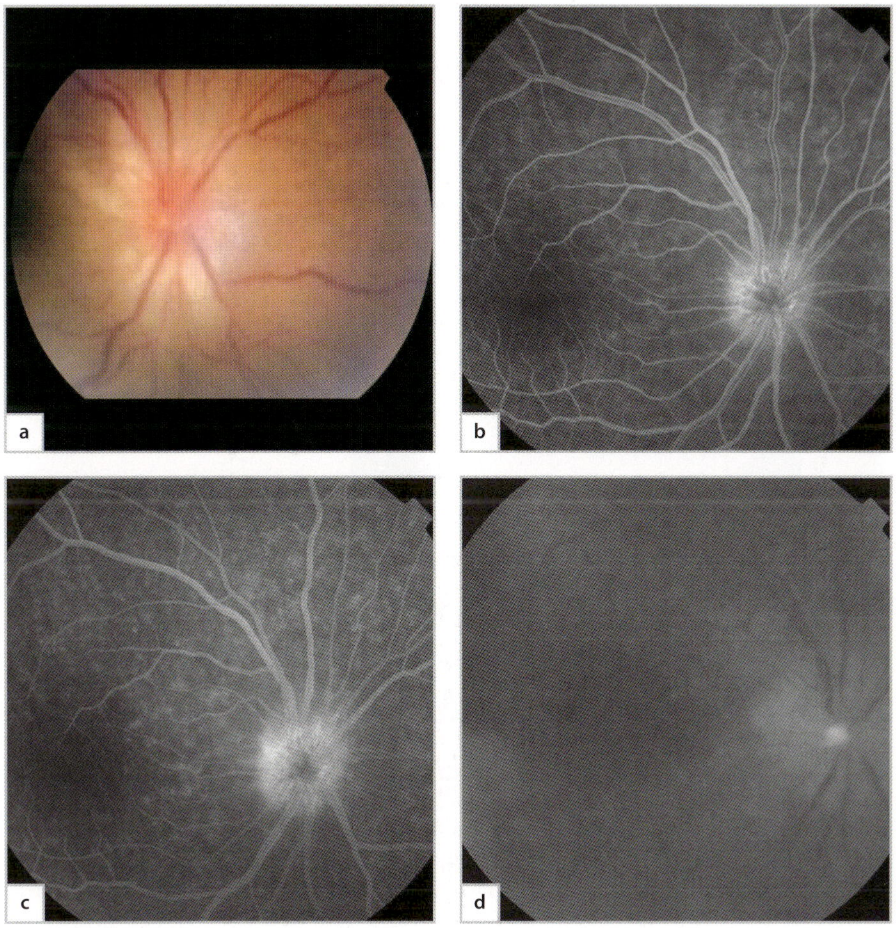

Figure 11.10 Vogt–Koyanagi–Harada syndrome: acute stage. (a) The right eye shows marked swelling of the optic disc with widespread serous retinal detachment. (b) The arteriovenous phase of the fluorescein angiogram shows masking of choroidal background fluorescence due to exudative retinal detachment. The disc margin is blurred due to leakage of dye from the swollen disc. The deeper layer of choroid and retina shows a number of bright dots scattered over the entire fundus. (c) The late arteriovenous phase shows marked leakage of dye from the optic disc and numerous hyperfluorescence dots in the deeper layer of the retina: these dots are typical of Vogt–Koyanagi–Harada syndrome. (d) The late phase shows considerable leakage from the disc and also leakage spreading into the subretinal space, saturating the subretinal fluid.

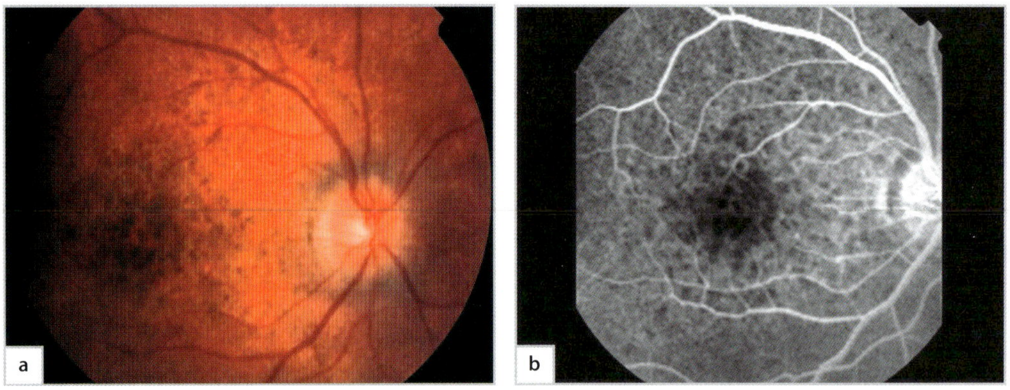

Figure 11.11 Vogt–Koyanagi–Harada syndrome: resolved stage. (a) The right eye shows a dark red glow similar to a setting sun's color. The optic disc swelling has now settled. There is mottling of the retinal pigment epithelium due to resolution of the deeper white dots seen during the acute stage of the disease. (b) The arteriovenous phase of the fluorescein angiogram shows punctate hypo- and hyperfluorescence in the posterior pole. Most of the hyperfluorescence spots seen in the acute stage are now hypofluorescent due to pigment proliferation.

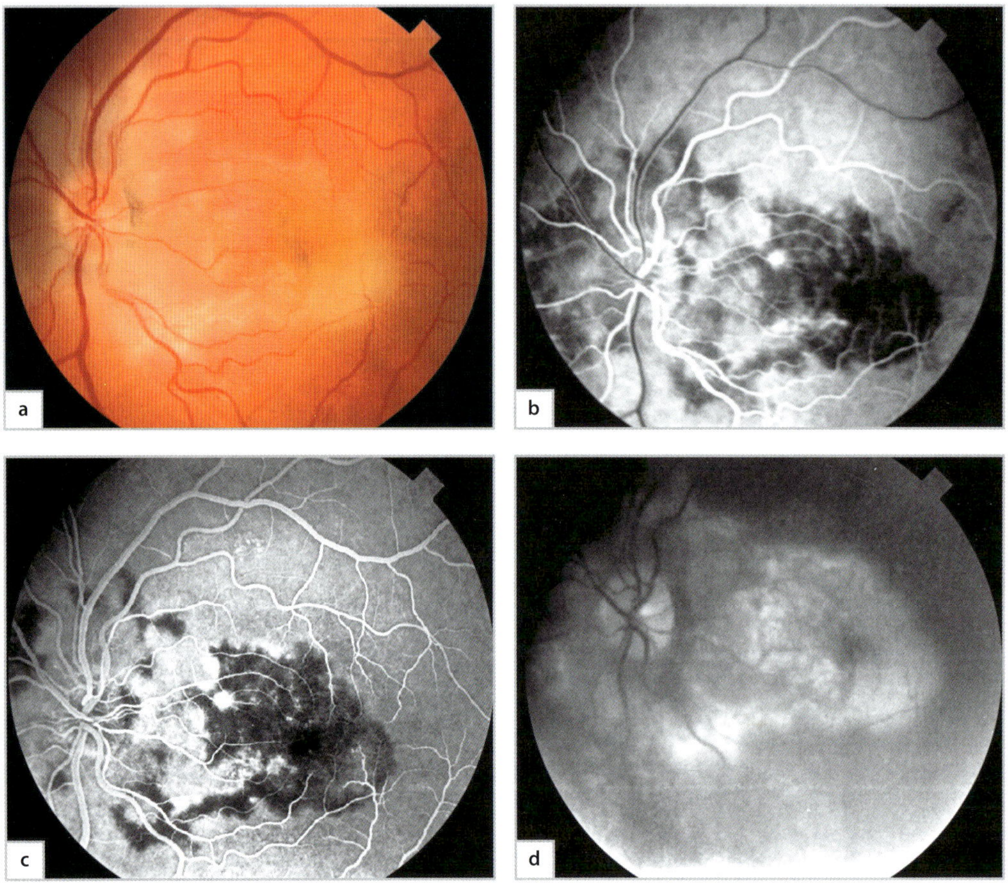

Figure 11.12 Serpiginous choroiditis: acute stage. (a) The left eye during an acute stage of disease shows deep-seated gray-white plaque-like lesions with slight alteration of retinal pigment epithelium and shallow serous retinal detachment of the posterior pole. (b) The arterial phase of the fluorescein angiogram shows a mixture of hypo- and hyperfluorescence of the choroid surrounding the optic disc and macular area. The darker hypofluorescence areas are due to masking of the choroidal background fluorescence, resulting from the gray-white lesions seen affecting the deeper layer of the choroid. (c) The arteriovenous phase shows continuing hypofluorescence from the deeper lesion but it is somewhat less intense due to filling of the overlying retinal capillaries. (d) The late phase shows a moderate degree of staining and leakage from the deeper choroidal lesions.

HYPERTROPHY OF RETINAL PIGMENT EPITHELIUM

Excessive accumulation of pigment within the retinal pigment epithelial cells is a frequently occurring congenital disorder. However, injury may stimulate a hypertrophy of the RPE that may be associated with pigment atrophy that extends some way beyond the demarcation of the hypertrophy zone. Jet-black round lesions are seen in the peripheral parts of the retina. These may be mistaken as choroidal nevus or malignant melanoma of the choroid. Melanocytic lesions are slate color, but hypertrophy of the RPE is jet-black. The pigment within the hypertrophic area may not be uniform and the borders are distinct and scalloped.

Fluorescein angiograph findings

Fluorescein angiography shows dense hypofluorescence due to total masking of choroidal background fluorescence. Occasionally a few hyperfluorescence spots may be seen within or overlying the lesion due to retinal pigment epithelial atrophy. The lesion remains hypofluorescence throughout the transit and late phases (**Figure 11.13**).

HELICOID DEGENERATION

This is a nonspecific choroidal degeneration sometimes appearing in several generations of the same family. The RPE atrophy mainly surrounds the disc and the nearby retina, often radiating in a fan-shaped manner resembling the propeller of an aircraft. Patients may remain symptom free, the degeneration being detected on routine examination. They are not to be confused with angioid streaks.

Fluorescein angiography findings

The color photograph usually shows the typical propeller-shaped RPE atrophy surrounding the optic disc. The fluorescein angiography does not add any further information except showing the typical hyperfluorescence lines emerging from the optic disc (**Figure 11.14**).

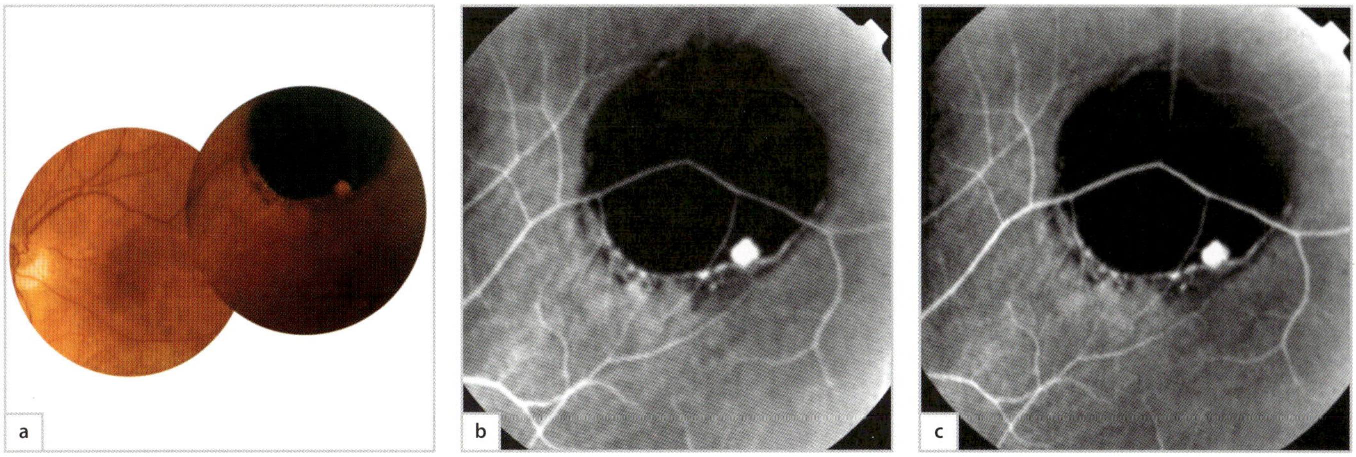

Figure 11.13 Hypertrophy of retinal pigment epithelium (RPE). (a) The composite photograph of the right eye shows a jet-black lesion with sharp borders seen at the superior temporal field. The lesion is flat and has a small retinal pigment epithelial atrophic spot at its lower border. (b) The early arteriovenous phase of the fluorescein angiogram shows the dense hypofluorescence totally masking the choroidal details. The hyperfluorescence seen at the lower border is due to the retinal pigment epithelial atrophy spot seen in the composite photograph. (c) The late arteriovenous phase shows consistent hypofluorescence of the lesion. The intensity of hyperfluorescence from the RPE defect has now reduced. The late phase shows total hypofluorescence of the lesion but only mild staining from the RPE defect.

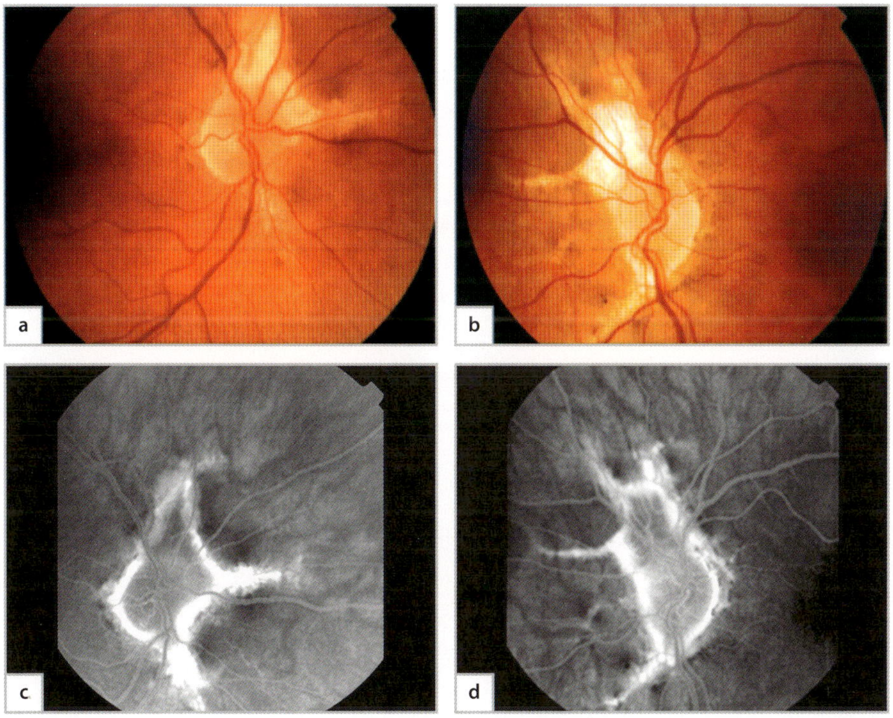

Figure 11.14 Helicoid degeneration. (a) The right eye shows choroidal degenerative changes surrounding the optic disc. The degenerative changes extend in a radial direction from the border of the optic disc to the nearby retina. (b) The left eye shows similar choroidal denegation affecting round and nearby retinal area. (c and d) The late phase of the fluorescein angiogram shows choroidal changes around the optic disc extending to the nearby retina in a radial fashion resembling a propeller of an aeroplane.

REFERENCES

Arellanes-García L, Hernández-Barrios M, Fromow-Guerra J, Cervantes-Fanning P. Fluorescein fundus angiographic findings in Vogt-Koyanagi Harada syndrome. *Int Ophthalmol* 2007; **27**:166–161.

Cangemi FE, Trempe CL, Walsh JB. Choroidal folds. *Am J Ophthalmol* 1978; **86**:380–387.

Chopdar A. A variant of central areolar choroidal dystrophy. *Ophthalmic Paediatr Genet* 1993; **14**:151–164.

Clarkson JG, Altman RD. Angioid streaks. *Surv Ophthalmol* 1982; **26**:235–246.

Cohen SM, Gass JD. Bilateral radial chorioretinal folds. *Int Ophthalmol* 1994–1995; **18**:243–245.

Federman JL, Shields JA, Tomer TL. Angioid streaks. II. Fluorescein angiographic features. *Arch Ophthalmol* 1975; **93**:951–962.

Gemenetzi M, De Salvo G, Lotery AJ. Central serous chorioretinopathy: an update on pathogenesis and treatment. *Eye* 2010; **24**:1743–1756.

Laatikainen L, Erkkila H. Serpiginous choroiditis. *Br J Ophthalmol* 1974; **58**:777–783.

Lim WK, Buggage RR, Nussenblatt RB. Serpiginous choroiditis. *Surv Ophthalmol* 2005; 50 231–244.

Luxenberg MN. Subretinal neovascularization associated with rupture of the choroid. *Arch Ophthalmol* 1986; **104**:1233.

Moorthy RS, Inomata H, Rao NA. Vogt-Koyanagi-Harada syndrome. *Surv Ophthalmol* 1995; **39**:265–292.

Noble KG. Central areolar choroidal dystrophy. *Am J Ophthalmol* 1977; **84**:310–318.

Noble KG, Carr RE, Siegel IM. Fluorescein angiography of the hereditary choroidal dystrophies. *B J Ophthalmol* 1977; **61**:43–53.

Perkins ES. Ocular toxoplasmosis. *Br J Ophthalmol* 1973; 57:1–17.

Smith JL, Gass JDM, Justice, J. Fluorescein fundus photography of angioid streaks. *Br J Ophthalmol* 1964; **48**:517–521.

Yoshioka H, Sugita T. Fluorescein fundus photographic studies on central serous retinopathy. IV. *Acta Soc. Path. Jap.,* 1970; **74**:268–272.

Chapter 12 Diseases of the optic nerve head

Amresh Chopdar

INTRODUCTION

To understand pathological changes of the optic nerve head, a thorough knowledge of its blood supply is essential. The main blood supply is from the short posterior ciliary arteries, except for the surface layer, which derives from the branches of the retinal arterioles. Venous drainage is through the central retinal vein (see Chapter 1).

ANTERIOR ISCHEMIC OPTIC NEUROPATHY

There are two types of anterior ischemic optic neuropathy: one involving posterior ciliary artery system (arteritic) and the other nonarteritic involving the retinal arteriolar system (nonarteritic).

Arteritic type

Anterior ischaemic optic neuropathy (AION) secondary to giant cell arteritis is referred to as arteritic type. Here the posterior ciliary artery is the main source of inflammation and occlusion. If a cilioretinal artery is present, both the choroid and the retinal segment supplied by the cilioretinal artery are affected. The color of the optic disc varies from pale pink to chalky white. A stereoscopic examination of the optic disc reveals a deep-seated infarct, affecting the prelamina and the region beyond. The superficial nerve fiber layer may remain transparent during the early stage of the development of the disease. Soon the edema extends to the peripapillary region. Following resolution the optic disc becomes pale due to atrophic changes (Hayreh 1974a, Eagling et al. 1974).

Fluorescein angiography findings

Acute stage

In the first week, during the transit phase, the choroidal filling is slow and patchy, and the choroid may remain unfilled throughout the period of angiography, especially along the watershed region passing across the optic disc. The infarcted part of the optic disc shows marked hypofluorescence. The retinal blood vessels may fill in the usual manner (Hayreh 1974b) (**Figure 12.1**).

Recovery stage

Following the onset of the acute infarction, recovery takes place over several weeks. During the first 2 weeks, the choroidal circulation begins to recover. The paleness of the optic disc increases, but the initial swelling slowly diminishes.

During the second week, fluorescein angiography still shows a delay in choroidal filling. As the choriocapillaris begins to recover, the lobular pattern becomes apparent during the mid venous phase of the transit. The optic disc remains hypofluorescent during the transit, leading to hyperfluorescence towards the late phase as the leaked dye impregnates the swollen optic disc (**Figure 12.2**).

Resolved stage

The optic disc appears very pale and atrophic. The cup of the disc may show a minimal degree of increased cupping, though it is characteristically different to that seen in cases of advanced glaucoma.

On fluoroscein angiography it is seen that choroidal circulation begins to improve and filling may be completed during the arteriovenous phase. The disc begins to show some fluorescence and produces a mild staining during the late phase of the angiography (**Figure 12.3**).

Nonarteritic type

Frequently the nonarteritic form of AION is seen in association with hypertension, arteriosclerosis, diabetes, and other forms of collagen vascular diseases. In nonarteritic AION the disc, though swollen, may show normal color or even be slightly pink. Flame-shaped hemorrhages near the optic disc are frequently seen in nonarteritic AION. The retinal blood vessels show a degree of narrowing and arteriosclerotic changes. The disc swelling begins to subside about 7–10 days after the onset, and by about 6 weeks the optic disc becomes pale and atrophic.

Fluorescein angiography findings

The choroidal circulation largely remains unaffected. Most of the changes are associated with the retinal vascular tree. The prepapillary capillaries show a variable degree of occlusion and congestion, depending on the area of involvement and passive congestion. Similarly, leakage of dye extends to the affected area during the late phase (**Figure 12.4**).

PAPILLEDEMA

Optic disc edema due to raised intracranial pressure is known as papilledema. It is of significant importance to neurologists, neurosurgeons, ophthalmologists, and general physicians because of its role as a classic sign of increased intracranial pressure. Therefore, it is important that the ophthalmologist gives an unambiguous opinion and differentiates from other causes of optic disc swelling.

The swelling begins at the inferior pole of the optic disc, followed by the superior, nasal, and finally the temporal quadrant. Striation of the optic nerve fiber in the peripapillary area is a consistent finding, best detected when examined utilizing a red-free fundus photographic technique. Microvascular changes such as capillary dilatation and microaneurysm around the optic disc are seen in long-standing cases of papilledema (Hayreh 1977, Hayreh & Hayreh 1977a).

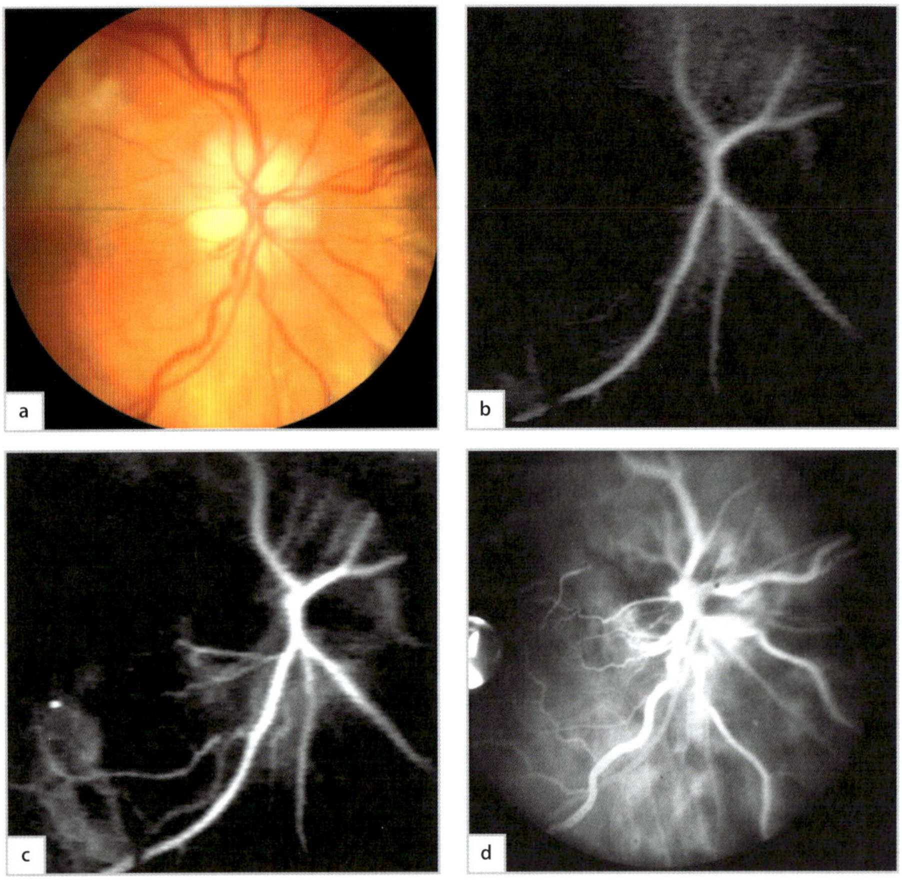

Figure 12.1 Arteritic anterior ischemic optic neuropathy: acute stage. (a) The right eye shows a very pale swollen optic disc. A cilioretinal artery emerges from a 10 o'clock position and is also occluded, resulting in the cloudy swelling along its course from the lateral border of the optic disc towards the posterior pole arching over the macular area. (b) The arterial phase of the fluorescein angiogram shows a very dark background due to almost total obstruction of choroidal circulation. A faint glow can be seen at inferior temporal edge of the frame. (c) The mid transit phase shows the retinal artery filling but the choroid remains hypofluorescent. There is still no visible circulation on or around the optic disc. (d) The late venous phase shows the retinal veins are full, yet there is no evidence of retinal capillaries or disc vessels filling. The disc remains avascular due to severe infarction. There is no evidence of leakage from the disc, as no dye is percolating into the disc.

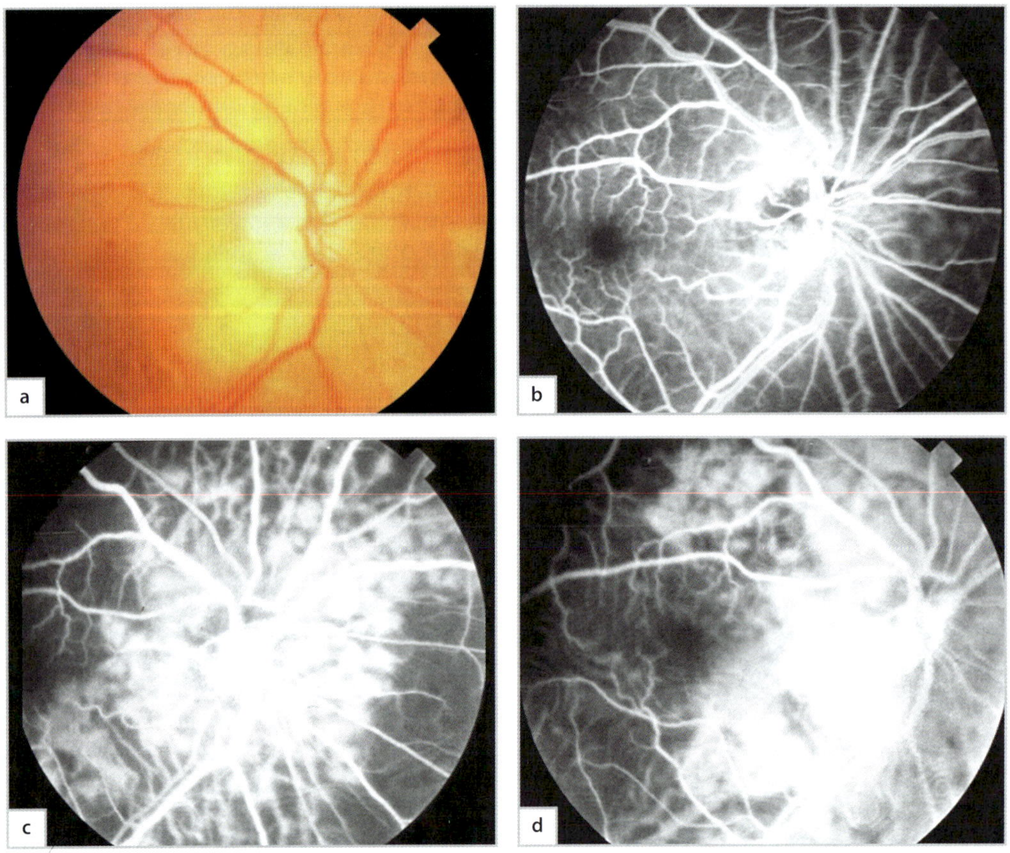

Figure 12.2 Arteritic anterior ischemic optic neuropathy (AION): recovery stage. (a) In AION of 2 weeks' duration, the right eye shows moderate recovery of the swelling of the optic disc. There are several gray infarcted lesions on the temporal side of the optic disc, possibly due to the presence of small cilioretinal vessels. (b) The arteriovenous phase of the fluorescein angiogram shows complete filling of the retinal circulation, yet the choroid largely remains unfilled and hypofluorescent. There is some leakage from the margin of the optic disc. (c) The late venous phase shows the dye has passed out of the retinal arteriolar circulation, leaving the veins fully filled. Now the choroidal lobules around the optic disc seem to make some attempts to fill. The hexagonal lobular pattern of the choriocapillaris can be easily made out due to lower perfusion pressure in the choroid. (d) This frame shows the disc and the macular area. Note that the circulation around the optic disc and medial part of the fundus is supplied by the medial posterior ciliary artery and is filling with and already producing some leakage; however, the choroid in the submacular area and temporal field supplied by the lateral posterior ciliary artery remain unfilled.

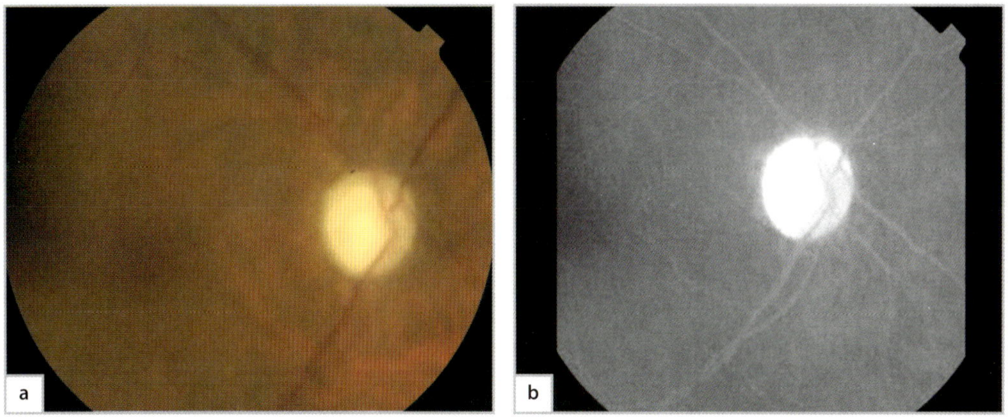

Figure 12.3 Resolved arteritic anterior ischemic optic neuropathy. (a) The right eye several weeks later shows a pale and atrophic optic disc following full resolution. (b) The same eye during the late phase of the fluorescein angiogram shows mild staining of the optic disc.

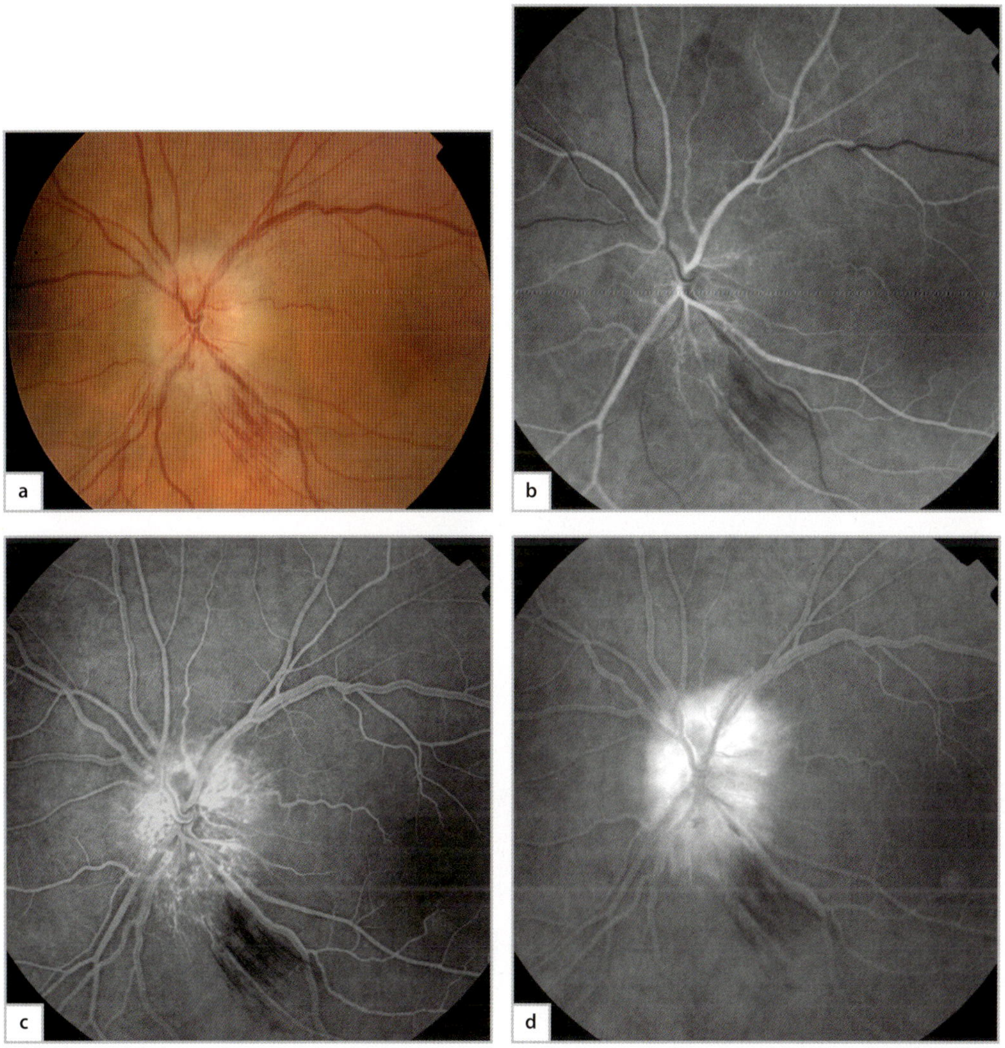

Figure 12.4 Nonarteritic anterior ischemic optic neuropathy (AION). (a) The left eye shows a nonarteritic type of AION with a congested, pink looking, moderately swollen optic disc. There is some degree of narrowing of retinal arterioles, involving the inferior part of the optic disc and nearby retina. There are many splinter-shaped hemorrhages in the affected area. The retinal veins show a mild degree of congestion. (b) The arterial phase of the fluorescein angiogram shows marked narrowing of a branch of the retinal arteriole in the lower part of the disc, extending some distance along its course. There is some loss of prepapillary capillaries affecting the whole of the disc surface, an indication of a moderate degree of ischemia of the optic disc. (c) The arteriovenous phase shows severe ischemia of the inferior part of the optic disc and the area served by the severe arteriosclerosis of the branch of the retinal arteriole. The retinal hemorrhages remain hypofluorescent. The upper part of the optic disc shows a moderate degree of passive congestion with dilated vessels. (d) The late phase shows profuse leakage from the upper part of the optic disc, less so from the inferior part. The retinal hemorrhages remain hypofluorescent.

Fluorescein angiography findings

Evolutionary papilledema

During the very early stages of papilledema, there may no positive finding detected through fundus fluorescein angiography. As the papilledema progresses microvascular changes on the disc become visible during the transit phase of angiography. The late phase of angiography leads to hyperfluorescence due to the leakage of dye from the optic disc. The pattern of leakage follows the development of edema, as described above. The final hyperfluorescent appearance of the disc takes an oval shape, longest in its vertical axis, with a concavity toward the macular area (Hayreh & Hayreh 1977b).

Fully developed papilledema

Masking of the background choroidal fluorescence is seen around the optic disc during the early phase of angiography, due to the swelling of the peripapillary retina. Soon the angiography reveals dilated capillaries on and around the optic disc and laden with microaneurysms. The pre- and peripapillary capillaries show marked dilatation. The veins may show a variable degree of congestion. The late phase shows a substantial degree of leakage of dye. The shape of the leakage is often oval, as described earlier (**Figure 12.5**).

Chronic papilledema

Papilledema undergoing resolution is also known as vintage papilledema. The secondary vascular changes such as microaneurysm and dilatation also gradually reduce. The typical oval configuration of disc swelling seen in recently developed papilledema also subsides due to continuing atrophy of the disc (**Figure 12.6**).

DRUSEN OF THE OPTIC DISC

This is optic disc swelling due to the deposition of hyaline materials at the level of Bruch's membrane and it may be a hereditary condition. It may lead to visual field defects and needs to be distinguished from papilledema. Secondary macular changes similar to disciform macular degeneration may also be associated with optic disc drusen. The disc margin appears blurred and irregular. Frequently, glistening particles can be seen on the disc surface.

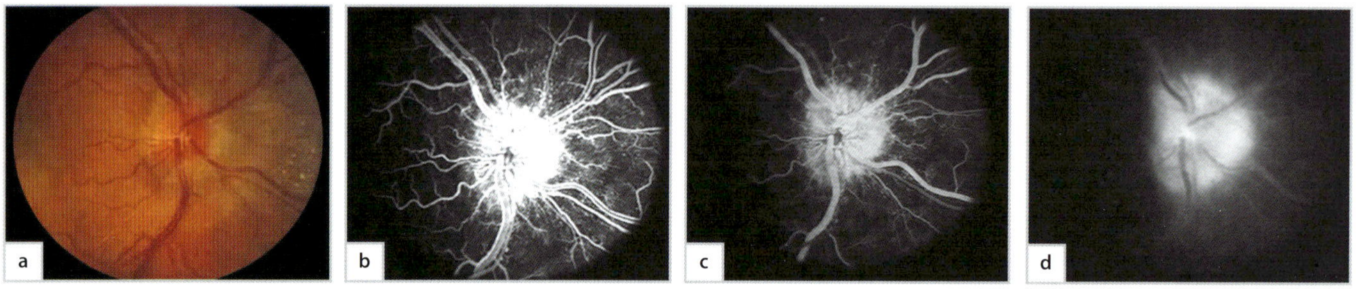

Figure 12.5 Fully developed papilledema. (a) The optic disc is moderately swollen, with capillary dilatation and microaneurysm formation on the disc surface. The pattern of swelling is much more pronounced in the vertical direction than the horizontal. The retinal veins show moderate dilatation. (b) The early arteriovenous phase of the fluorescein angiogram shows the microaneurysms, and capillary dilatation on and around the optic disc following the epipapillary and peripapillary capillaries. Note that the pathological changes obey the inferior, superior nasal, and temporal (ISNT) rule. (c) The late venous phase shows dilated retinal veins and commencement of leakage from the optic disc and surrounding areas. The leakage is consistent with the ISNT rule. (d) The late phase shows profuse leakage of dye closely following the pattern of the disc swelling.

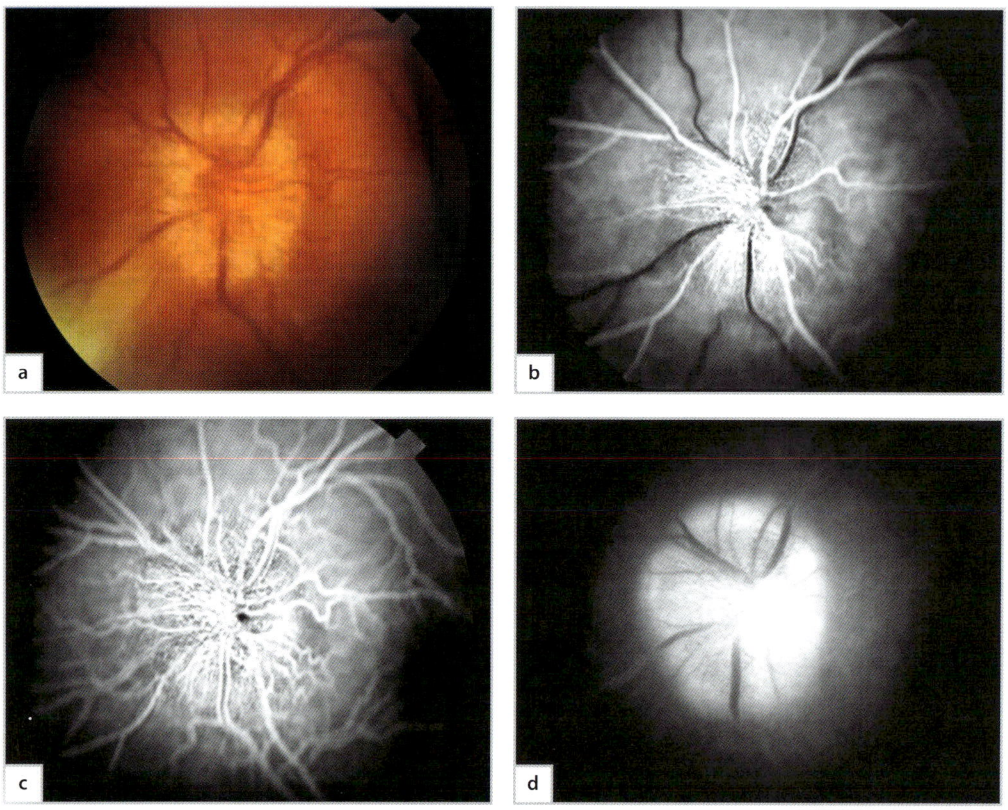

Figure 12.6 Chronic ('vintage') papilledema. (a) The left eye shows a slowly subsiding long-standing papilledema and regressing microvascular changes from the disc surface and surrounding areas. (b) The arterial phase of the fluorescein angiogram shows capillary dilatation and microaneurysm on the disc surface and surrounding area. (c) The arteriovenous phase shows the full architecture of the capillary dilatation and microaneurysms but no evidence of leakage or staining, due to maturation of walls of the capillaries to maintain the natural blood-retinal barrier. The inferior, superior nasal, and temporal rule no longer holds true. (d) The late phase shows no evidence of leakage and only moderate degree of staining involving the entire swollen optic disc.

Fluorescein angiography findings

The preinjection frame with green and blue filters in position shows strong autofluorescence. (Kelley 1974) No abnormalities are seen during the early phase of the angiography. Once the retinal capillaries are filled, the autofluorescence is lost and the optic disc appears normal. During the late venous phase of angiography, the disc margin becomes hyperfluorescent. This continues through the transit producing staining of the underlying drusen. The margin of the disc is crenated owing to irregular deposit of hyaline materials. When disciform changes occur, a subretinal neovascular membrane may be seen to leak (Miller et al. 1965) Sanders & Ffytche 1967, Mustonen & Nieminen 1982a, b] (**Figure 12.7**).

OPTIC NEURITIS

The main clinical picture of this disease is marked swelling of the disc with severe loss of vision. The cause of the disc swelling is not clearly understood, but it is commonly believed to be due to axonal swelling arising from axoplasmic flow block as a result of demyelination.

Fluorescein angiography findings

During the prearterial phase, there is some degree of masking of choroidal background fluorescence, especially around the optic disc. The lesions around the optic disc may show loss of vascularity. In severe cases, choroidal folds may be seen around the optic disc. The late phase produces a moderate degree of leakage from the optic disc. Seldom does the leakage extend to the retina (Walsh & Blair 1969) (**Figure 12.8**).

OPTIC ATROPHY

Optic atrophy results from a wide variety of causes; many of them have been described above. All cases of optic atrophy are associated with moderate-to-severe loss of vision and visual field. When the light is shown to the affected eye, the pupil usually shows a typical relative afferent pupillary defect. Retinal examination reveals a pale optic disc and attenuated retinal blood vessels on and around the optic disc.

Fluorescein angiography findings

The prearterial phase shows no abnormality, but the retinal phases show only a few blood vessels on the disc surface during the transit, and staining toward the late phase (**Figure 12.3**).

COLOBOMA OF THE OPTIC DISC

Coloboma is due to nonunion of the most posterior part of the embryonic ocular fissure, affecting the optic cup, and peripapillary retina, commonly affecting the inferior temporal part of the optic disc. Pigment clumping at the border of the normal and abnormal retina is usual. The retinal blood vessels pass around the edges of the coloboma.

Fluorescein angiography findings

The fluorescein angiogram shows an empty space within the optic disc, which looks dark due to hypofluorescence. The retinal blood vessels emerge from the edges of the optic disc. The typical branching pattern is no longer visible. The choroidal and retinal circulation may remain normal appearance (**Figure 12.9**).

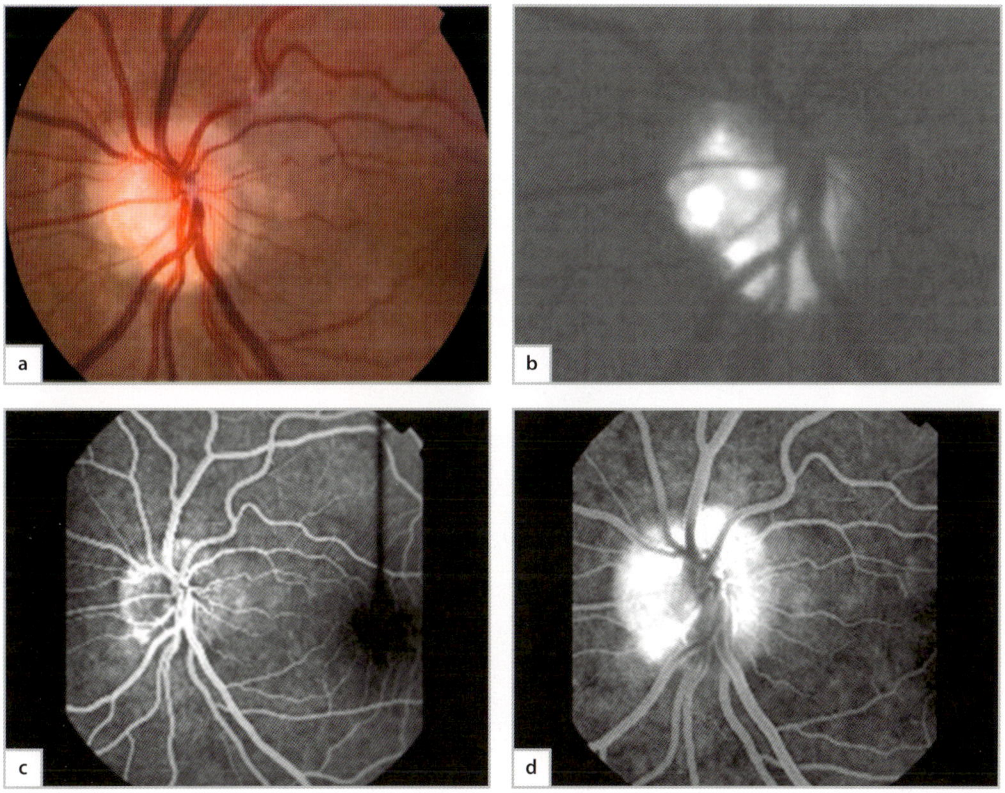

Figure 12.7 Disc drusen. (a) The left eye shows slightly pale swollen optic disc with an irregular border, especially in the inferior nasal quadrant. (b) The black and white photograph of the optic disc with green and blue filters in position prior to injection of fluorescein dye shows the autofluorescence of the hyaline materials, mainly of the nasal part of the optic disc. (c) The arteriovenous phase of the fluorescein angiogram shows normal filling of the disc and retina. The nasal part where the hyaline materials deposition appears normal. (d) The late phase of FFA shows intense staining of the entire optic disc with an irregular disc margin, suggesting more extensive deposit of hyaline materials than seen on the autofluorescence frame.

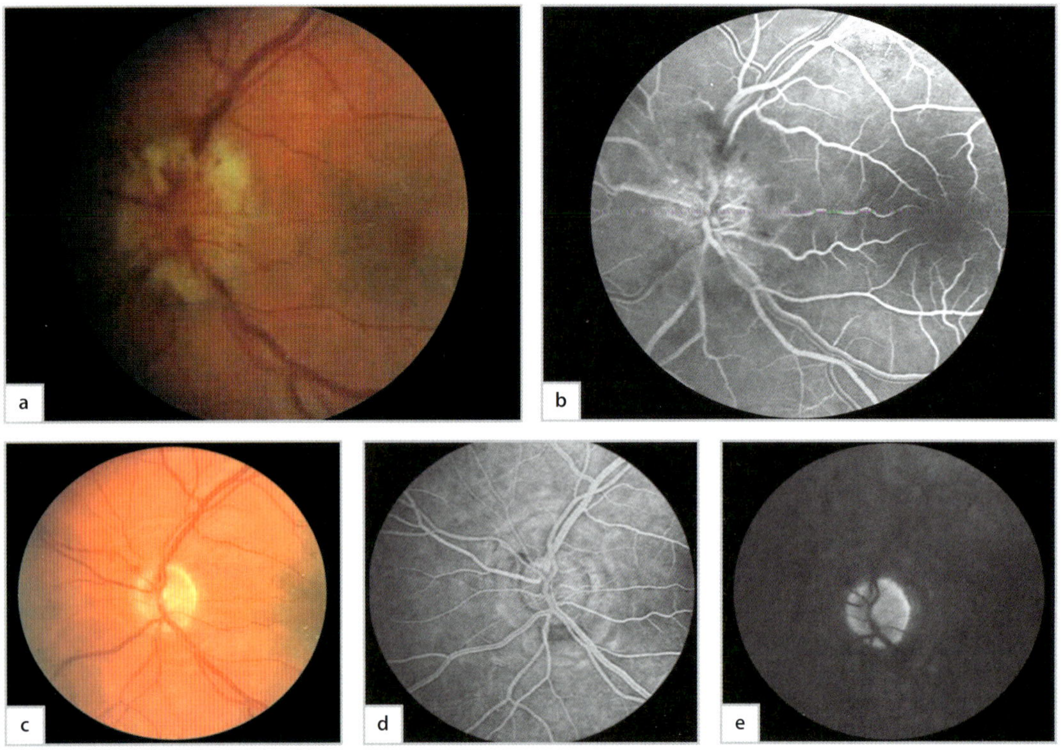

Figure 12.8 Optic neuritis. (a) The left eye during the acute stage of optic neuritis shows the entire optic disc to be swollen with gray-white patches similar to cotton-wool spots surrounding the optic disc. There is a considerable degree of dilatation of the retinal veins. There are a few splinter-shaped hemorrhages on the surface of the optic disc. (b) The arteriovenous phase of the fluorescein angiogram shows some loss of vascularity around the superior and inferior polar region of the optic disc associated with mild congestion on the nasal and temporal aspect. The retinal vessels appear normal. (c) The same eye during the resolved stage shows complete resolution of the swelling of the optic disc. The retinal blood vessels also have resolved and now show comparatively normal configuration. The concentric rings around the optic disc, due to choroidal folds, are visible. There are also several hard exudates seen near the macular area. (d) The arteriovenous phase shows normal optic disc vasculature, yet the concentric rings of choroidal folds are clearly noticeable. (e) The late phase shows mild staining of the partly atrophic optic disc.

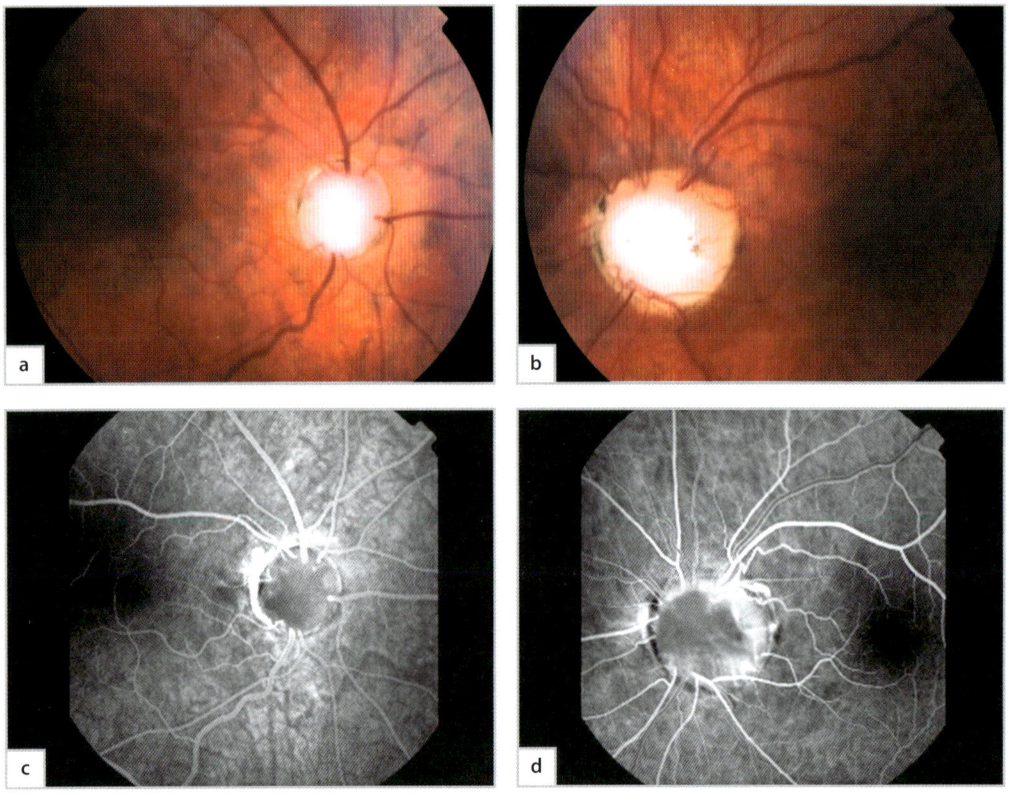

Figure 12.9 Coloboma of the optic disc. (a) The right eye has a large empty space at the center of the optic disc. The retinal blood vessels emerge from the edges of the optic disc. The conventional branching pattern of the retinal blood vessels is no longer applicable. (b) The left eye of the same person has almost identical changes at the optic disc. (c) The late phase of the fluorescein angiogram shows the excavation of the center of the optic disc. There is no evidence of leakage. (d) The late phase of the left eye shows almost identical fluorescein angiographic finding.

PIT ON THE DISC

This is a form of coloboma of the disc but is smaller in size. It is usually seen in the inferior part of the optic disc. Ophthalmoscopy shows a small round to oval bluish depression on the disc. Very often this is associated with serous detachment of the retina at the macula (Johnson et al. 1963).

Fluorescein angiography findings

The early part of the angiography shows an empty area on the disc. During progression of the transit, the same area remains virtually unchanged. The dye may leak to the macular area if there is associated macular edema. The pit area may show a limited degree of staining (**Figure 12.10**).

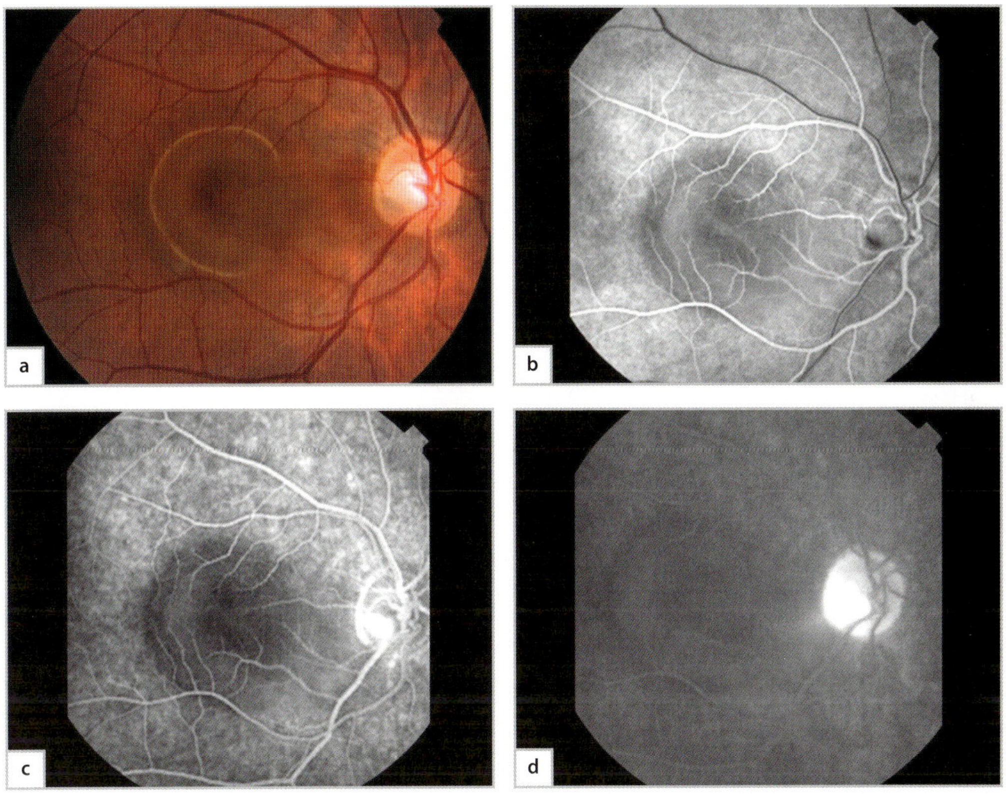

Figure 12.10 Pit on the optic disc. (a) The right eye shows a localized area of oval dark empty space at the inferior temporal border of the optic disc. The macular area shows serous retinal detachment similar to that seen in central serous choroidopathy. (b) The early arterial phase of the fluorescein angiogram shows an oval boat-shaped dark hypofluorescent area at the inferior temporal part of the optic disc. The serous detachment of the macular area is already showing a limited amount of hyperfluorescence due to leakage of dye into the serous detachment. (c) The late venous phase shows moderate degree of hyperfluorescence due to staining of the pit area. (d) The late phase shows intense staining of the pit and also limited leakage into the serous detachment of the macula.

REFERENCES

Eagling E M, Sanders MD, Miller SJH. Ischaemic papillopathy. A clinical and fluorescein angiographic review of forty cases. *Br J Ophthalmol* 1974; ii:990–1008.

Hayreh MS, Hayreh SS. Optic disc edema in raised intracranial pressure. I. Evolution and resolution. *Arch Ophthalmol* 1977a; **95**:1237–1244.

Hayreh MS, Hayreh MS. Optic disc edema in raised intracranial pressure. II. Early detection with fluorescein fundus angiography and stereoscopic color photography. *Arch Ophthalmol* 1977b; **95**:1245–1254.

Hayreh SS. Anterior ischaemic optic neuropathy. I. Terminology and pathogenesis. *Br J Ophthalmol* 1974a; **58**:955.

Hayreh SS. Anterior ischaemic optic neuropathy. II. Fundus on ophthalmoscopy and fluorescein angiography. *Br J Ophthalmol* 1974b; **58**:964–980.

Hayreh SS. Optic disc edema in raised intracranial pressure. III. Pathogenesis. *Arch Ophthalmol* 1977; **95**:1553–1565.

Johnson AW, Smith JL, Hart ML. Macular changes with pit of the disc. Fluorescein photography. *Am J Ophthalmol* 1963; **55**:1070–1072.

Kelley J. Autofluorescence of drusen of optic nerve head. *Arch Ophthalmol* 1974; **92**:263–264.

Miller SJ H, Sanders MD, Ffytche TJ. Fluorescein fundus photography in the detection of papilloedema and its differentiation from pseudopapilloedema. *Lancet* 1965; ii:651–654.

Mustonen E, Nieminen H. Optic disc drusen—a photographic study. I. Autofluorescence pictures and fluorescein angiography. *Acta Ophthalmol (Copen)* 1982a; **60**:849–858.

Mustonen E, Nieminen H. Optic disc drusen—a photographic study. II. Retinal nerve fibre layer photography. *Acta Ophthalmol* 1982b; **60**:859–872.

Sanders MD, Ffytche TJ. Fluorescein angiography in the diagnosis of drusen of the optic disc. *Trans Ophthalmol Soc UK* 1967; **87**:457–468.

Walsh FB, Blair CJ. Papilloedema, optic neuritis, and pseudo-papilloedema. The use of fluorescein angiography in differential diagnosis. *Trans Am Acad Ophthalmol Otolaryngol* 1969; **73**:914–928.

Chapter 13 Intraocular neoplasms

Amresh Chopdar

INTRODUCTION

The most commonly occurring neoplasm of the posterior segment involves the choroid, followed by the optic nerve head and retinal vessels. Clinical examination points to the nature of the tumor's pathology. However, retinal angiography is helpful to confirm the diagnosis and plan the treatment. There is a wide variation in angiographic findings; hence, it is wise to exercise caution in the interpretation.

CHOROIDAL NEVUS

Choroidal nevi are flat-pigmented lesions situated within the choroid. They appear slate gray in color and may be oval or circular in configuration, with borders that are either feathery or well defined (but not always sharply defined). They may hide the choroidal vessels and are avascular. The overlying retina occasionally may show a few drusen-like deposits, otherwise it remains normal.

Fluorescein angiography findings

The nevi remain hypofluorescent throughout the transit and the late phase of fluorescein angiography. During the mid-transit phase, when the retinal capillaries are fully filled, dye may obscure the view of the nevus, but once the dye empties from the retinal circulation, the hypofluorescent nevus is revealed again. These lesions do not show any evidence of tumor blood vessels or leakage of dye (**Figure 13.1a** and **b**).

ICG angiography findings

The area of hypofluorescence is often wider than is apparent on fluorescein angiography. The border of the nevus may be better defined and shows no abnormal choroidal blood vessels. The choroidal vessels may travel across the nevus uninterrupted. The late phase of indocyanine green (ICG) angiography shows a well-defined area of hypofluorescence within the choroid (**Figure 13.1c** and **d**).

MALIGNANT MELANOMA OF THE CHOROID

Malignant melanoma of the choroid is the most commonly occurring intraocular malignancy. It affects men and women equally and can occur in any age, although it is most frequently seen in older age group. Malignant melanoma varies in its presentation with regard to the degree of pigmentation, size, and associated exudative retinal detachment. Occasionally, retinal and vitreous hemorrhages may be

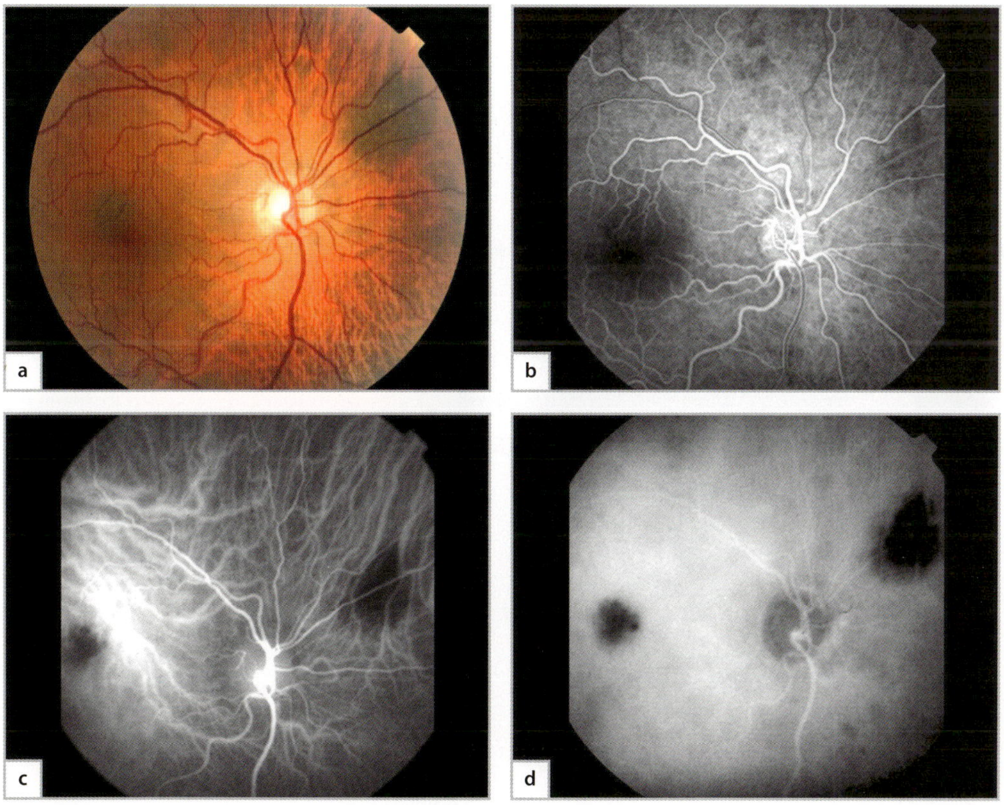

Figure 13.1 Choroidal nevus. (a) The right eye shows at least two choroidal nevi seen: one at the macula and the other nasal to the optic disc. (b) The early arteriovenous phase of the fluorescein angiogram shows two hypofluorescent areas: one near the macula and the other nasal to the optic disc. (c) The mid transit phase of the indocyanine green (ICG) angiogram shows well-circumscribed hypofluorescent lesions at the macula and superior nasal quadrant. The choroidal vasculature traverses normally over the lesions. (d) The late phase of the ICG angiogram shows persistent hypofluorescence of both the lesions without any evidence of staining or leakage.

seen. Lipofuscin, an accumulation of orange pigment, is frequently seen on the surface of the tumor, but it is not a diagnostic feature. A diffuse flat malignant melanoma may prove difficult to differentiate from a choroidal nevus. The gross pathological appearance is a typical collar button or mushroom-shaped lesion arising from the choroid and growing into the vitreous cavity, lifting the overlying retina. Histopathological sections show densely packed tumor cells with a few vascular channels with anastomoses (Hayreh 1970, Cantrill et al. 1984).

Fluorescein angiography findings

There is no single pathognomonic feature that can positively diagnose malignant melanoma with complete accuracy. The fluorescein angiogram mainly shows two different patterns. Firstly, the commonest angiographic findings are a short-lived period of hypofluorescence during the prearterial phase, followed by an increased patchy fluorescence on the tumor surface. The tumor surface may also show the architecture of the tumor blood vessels. Most of the retinal capillaries overlying the tumor surface may already have been destroyed, leaving only the main vessels to fill during the arteriovenous phase. However, on the periphery of the tumor mass the retinal capillaries may remain and become engorged. These engorged capillaries fill during the venous phase to reveal a prominent network surrounding the tumor mass. The two sets of vascular networks, as seen on fluorescein angiography, are referred to as dual circulation. This is often a misnomes. During angiography, the dye not only leaks profusely into the tumor mass but also spreads to fill the subretinal space (**Figure 13.2**).

A second type of leakage, called a focal leakage, has been described in cases where the tumor is in close contact with the overlying necrotizing retina without any significant retinal detachment at the apical region. In this case, the tumor surface shows large tumor vessels, which produce localized leakage of the fluorescein dye on the tumor surface but pooling at the base of the tumor (**Figure 13.3**).

In the case of a flat tumor, the retinal pigment epithelium often shows some degree of degenerative change producing punctate hyperfluorescence during the prearterial phase due to a window defect. Thus, a combination of hyper- and hypofluorescence is seen, leading to a gradual and steady increase in fluorescence, and eventually mild leakage of dye during the late phase (Edwards et al. 1969, Suckling 1969, Petti 1970, Fishman 1977).

ICG angiography findings

The pattern of abnormalities seen on ICG angiography in cases of malignant melanoma of the choroid depends on the amount of pigmentation and the vascularity of tumor mass. Generally, the tumor appears larger than on ophthalmoscopy or fluorescein angiography. During the early phase of angiography, a large portion of the tumor shows extensive hypofluorescence. Progressively the intrinsic vascular pattern becomes visible during the progress of the transit. The tumor vessels appear before the retinal vessels; therefore, it is necessary to capture early photographs lest these features are lost to view. The tumor vessels are often dilated, with a tortuous corkscrew appearance, and may show cross anastomotic channels, which can lead to significant leakage toward the late phase (**Figure 13.4**).

CHOROIDAL METASTASES

The most common metastatic tumors are from the breast, lungs, and prostate. They commonly affect the posterior polar region of the fundus. They are flat or mildly elevated, gray-yellow looking lesions affecting a wider area of the choroid and retina, and they are associated with shallow exudative retinal detachment. The tumor often has a lobular pattern, indicating the multiple nature of the deposits. Occasionally, a marked metastatic tumor may resemble a choroidal osteoma, being a gray-looking lesion in the deeper layer of the retina (Shields et al. 1997).

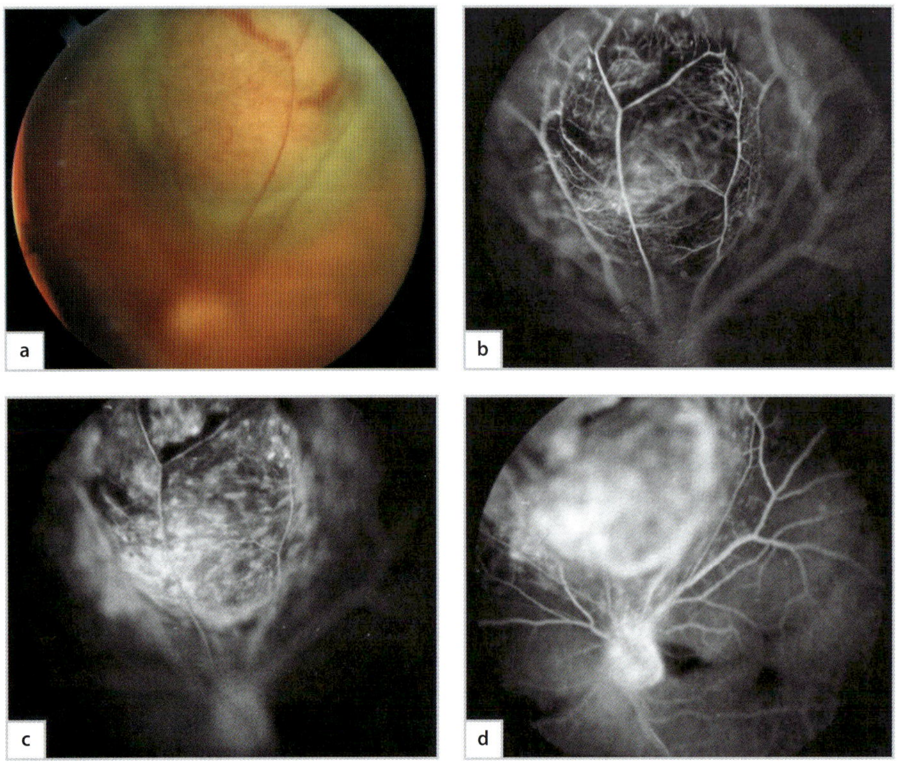

Figure 13.2 Malignant melanoma of the choroid. (a) There is a choroidal melanoma above the optic disc under a large area of serous retinal detachment. There are several small areas of hemorrhages on the retina and the tumor. (b) The arteriovenous phase of the fluorescein angiogram shows relative hypofluorescence from the tumor, yet several tumor blood vessels are filling up on the tumor surface. The superficial thinner retinal vessels fill gradually, with some degree of engorgement. The appearance of these two separate sets of vascular pattern is sometime described as dual circulation, which is a misnomer. (c) The late transit phase shows moderate degree of leakage from the tumor vessels slowly spreading into the serous retinal detachment area. (d) The late phase shows profuse leakage into the tumor, outlining the tumor contour, and patchy leakage from the surface. The overlying extensive serous detachment area involving the posterior pole of the fundus is outlined due to the saturated subretinal fluid.

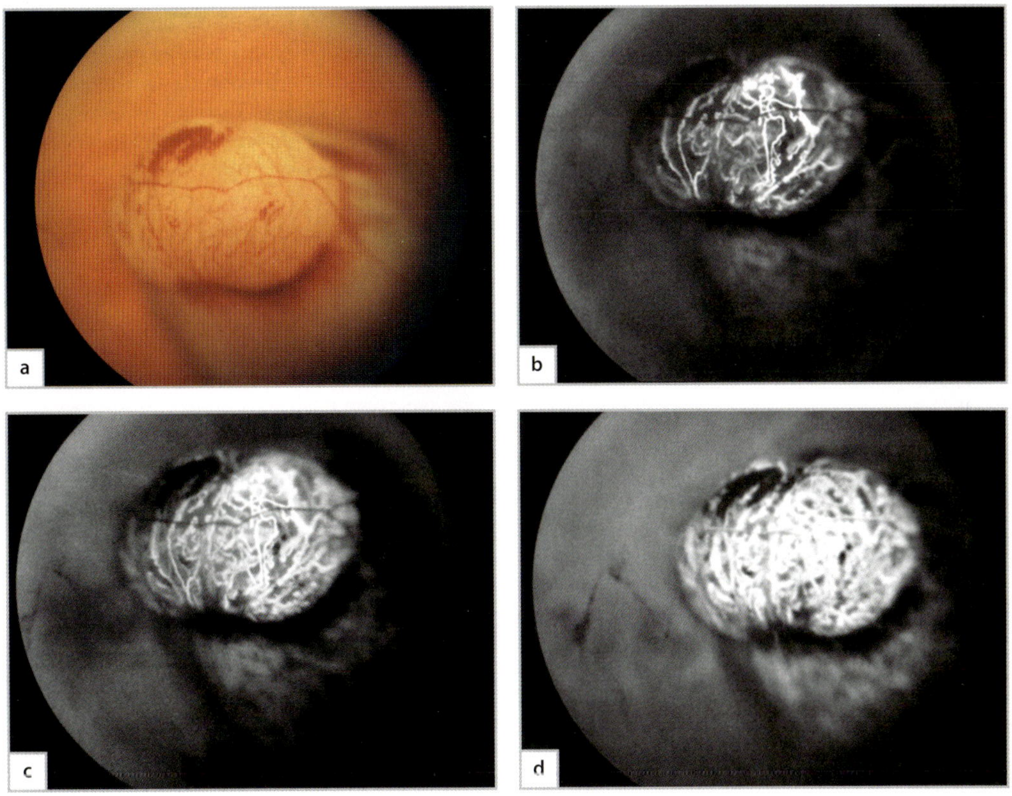

Figure 13.3 Malignant melanoma of the choroid with focal leakage. (a) There is a typical collar button type of lesion protruding into the vitreous associated with serous retinal detachment and hemorrhages. (b) The prearterial phase of the fluorescein angiogram shows the complex architecture of tumor vessels, seen crisscrossing with cross anastomoses on the tumor surface. (c) The later frame shows there is still no dye on the retinal vessel that is crossing the tumor. The underlying tumor vessels are seen to be leaking, beginning to spread into the subretinal space. (d) The late phase shows a moderate degree of leakage of dye from the tumor vessels, staining the tumor, and dye spreading into the subretinal space.

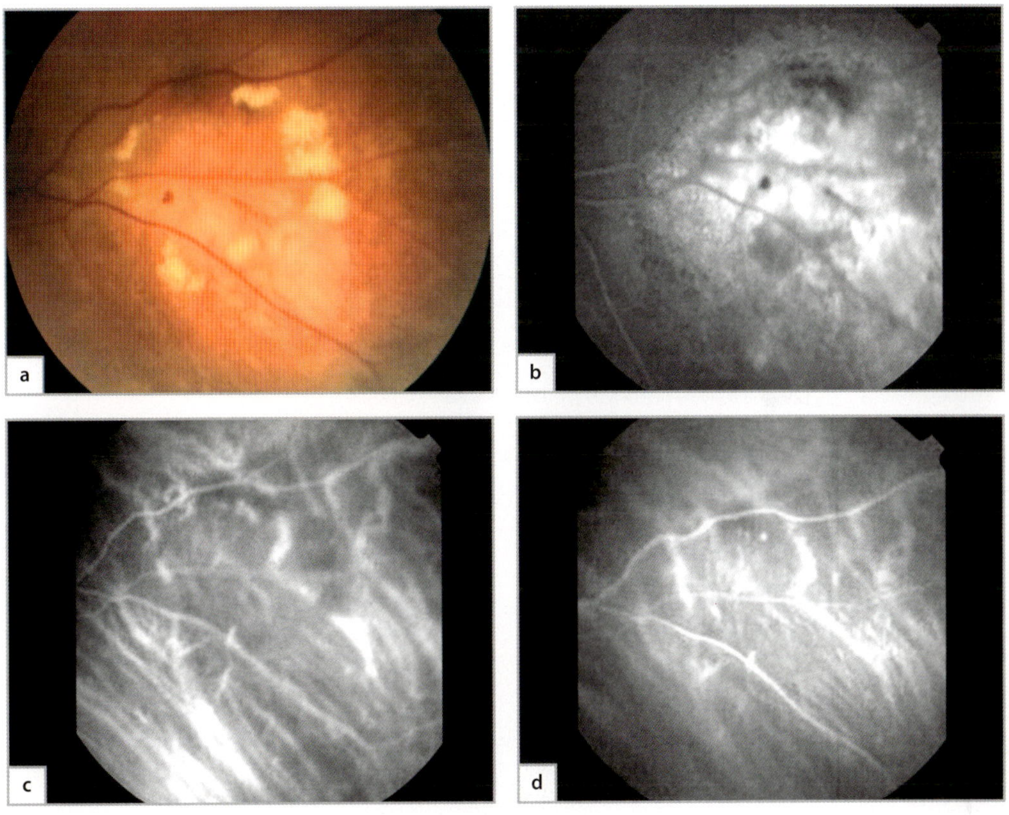

Figure 13.4 A flat amelanotic malignant melanoma of the choroid. (a) The peripheral part of the fundus shows a flat lesion, which has been increasing in size for the past 6 months, with associated exudative changes around the base. (b) The late phase of the fluorescein angiogram shows staining of the tumor but no definite leakage. (c) The late transit phase of the indocyanine green (ICG) angiogram shows increasing tortuosity of the tumor vessels and cross linkage, an indication of growing tumor. (d) The late phase of the ICG angiogram shows minimal leakage, especially near the tumor vessels.

Fluorescein angiography findings

Metastatic lesions show several different varieties of leaking pattern, depending on the cellular content. Adenocarcinoma mainly consists of a cellular structure, whereas other types may contain variable amounts of fibrous tissue and may even show osseous changes.

Commonly, fluorescein angiography shows a short-lived hypofluorescence during the prearterial phase. During the arterial phase, localized areas of patchy hyperfluorescence appear in a widespread area; these increase in fluorescence during the venous phase of the transit and tend to coalesce to form larger area covering the entire region of involvement. During the late phase, the hyperfluorescence spreads to include the entire area with moderate leakage (**Figure 13.5**) (Davis & Robertson 1973).

In a second pattern, when they are more localized and elevated, the tumors appear yellow and brown with limited serous detachment of the retina. In these atypical appearances, the tumor masks the choroidal background fluorescence, either densely or partly silhouetting its entire surface during the early phases, leading to a localized area of leakage towards the late phase (**Figure 13.6**).

The third type of fluorescein pattern shows evidence of transition toward a choroidal osteoma-like appearance, fluorescein angiography shows extensive masking of background fluorescence during the early phase, leading to patchy leakage in the mid-transit phase, resulting in staining and hyperfluorescence towards the late phase (**Figure 13.7**).

CHOROIDAL HEMANGIOMA

Choroidal hemangioma is an exceedingly slow-growing benign rare tumor of congenital origin. The lesion is a cavernous hemangioma, commonly situated in the posterior pole near the optic disc. The tumor appears as a subtle localized domed-shaped dark-red lesion. The visual symptoms, such as field defect and reduced acuity, often follow a period of worsening of the lesion. Ultrasonography is the most helpful way to diagnose choroidal hemangioma (MacLean & Maumenee 1960, Norton & Gutman 1968, Witschel 1976).

Fluorescein angiography findings

Fluorescein angiography is helpful in differentiating choroidal hemangioma from malignant melanoma of the choroid. It is essential to acquire images in the very early prearterial circulation phase these show ill-defined lacunae and linear hyperfluorescence within a hypofluorescent area, like a river in an atlas. Soon the entire area becomes hyperfluorescent as vessels coalesce to cover the whole tumor. Punctate fluorescence overlying the tumor indicates retinal pigment epithelial degeneration. During the late phase, the dye concentrates on the tumor and shows a localized area of moderately intense hyperfluorescence due to leakage of dye (**Figure 13.8**).

ICG angiography findings

The vascular arrangement of choroidal hemangioma is best demonstrated during the early phase of angiography. It is important that recording of the angiogram is started well before the dye becomes visible in the choroidal circulation. During the transit phase, more and more blood vessels fill a larger area, showing typical hyperfluorescence like a fisherman's bag of earthworms. ICG angiography shows these vascular patterns much more clearly than fluorescein angiography. The late phase shows a localized area of leakage from the tumor mass.

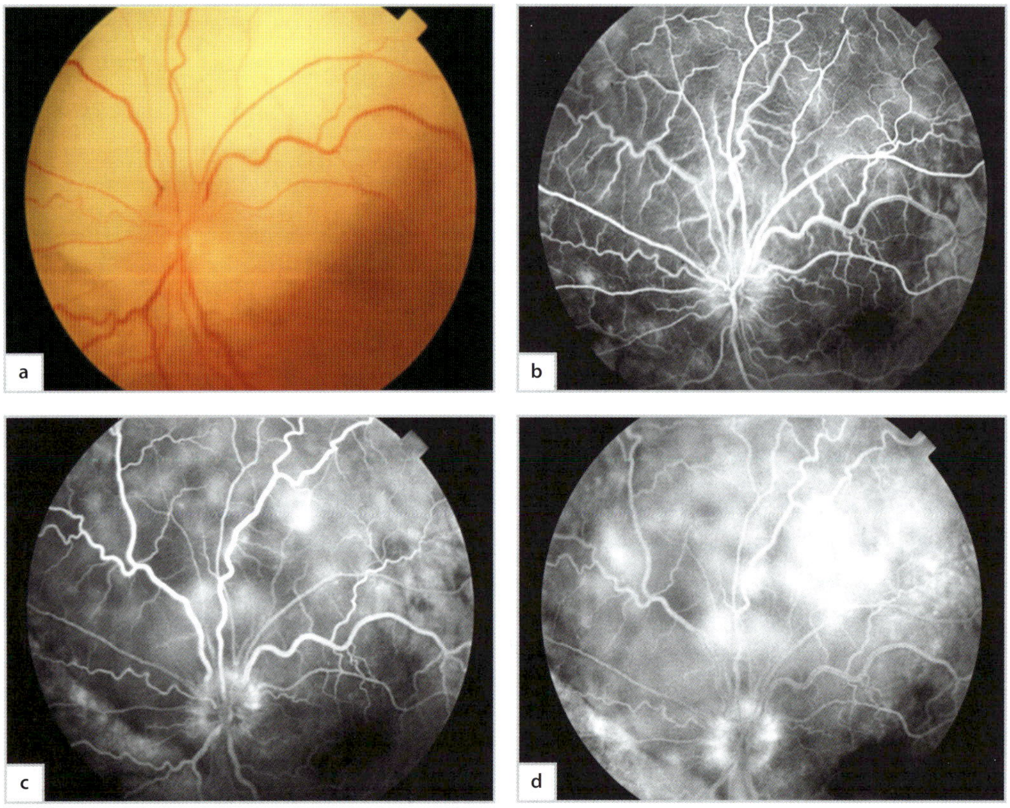

Figure 13.5 Metastatic adenocarcinoma of the breast. (a) The left eye has a large area of gray-yellow lesions, affecting the whole of the superior half of the retina. The retinal arterioles appear slightly narrowed and veins slightly congested. The optic disc margin is also swollen and blurred. (b) The early arteriovenous phase of the fluorescein angiogram shows good filling of the retinal circulation but shows patchy masking of the choroidal background fluorescence. (c) The venous phase shows patchy hypo- and hyperfluorescence in the deeper layer. There is some evidence of commencement of leakage from the upper border of the optic disc. (d) The late phase shows coalescing of the patchy hyperfluorescence area to form wider areas of leakage extending to the whole of the superior half of the fundus. There is also a moderate amount of leakage from the optic disc margin.

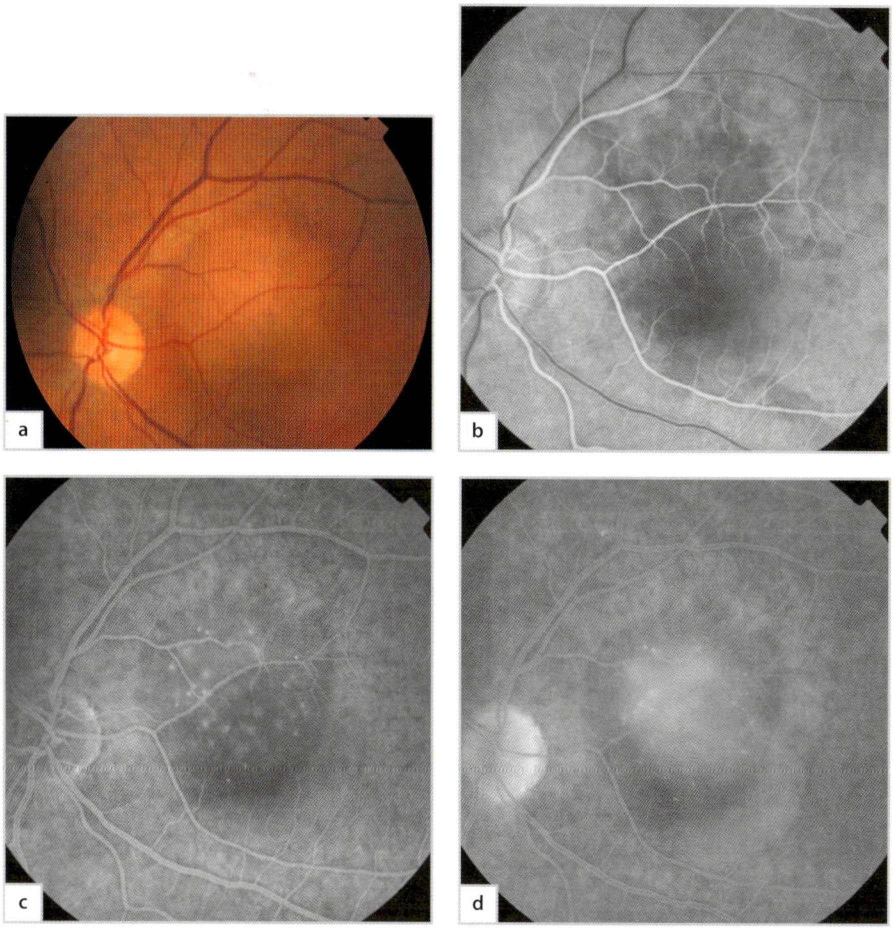

Figure 13.6 Metastatic carcinoma of the breast. (a) The left eye of a woman suffering from carcinoma of the breast shows a large moderately elevated lesion in the posterior pole including the macular area, associated with some visual loss. (b) The arterial phase of the fluroscein angiogram shows a patchy hypo- and hyperfluorescence within the area of the elevated lesion seen in part (a). (c) The late venous phase shows a well-defined border and an increased number of fluorescence spots within the lesion. (d) The late phase shows a moderate degree of lobular–patterned leakage filling the tumor site.

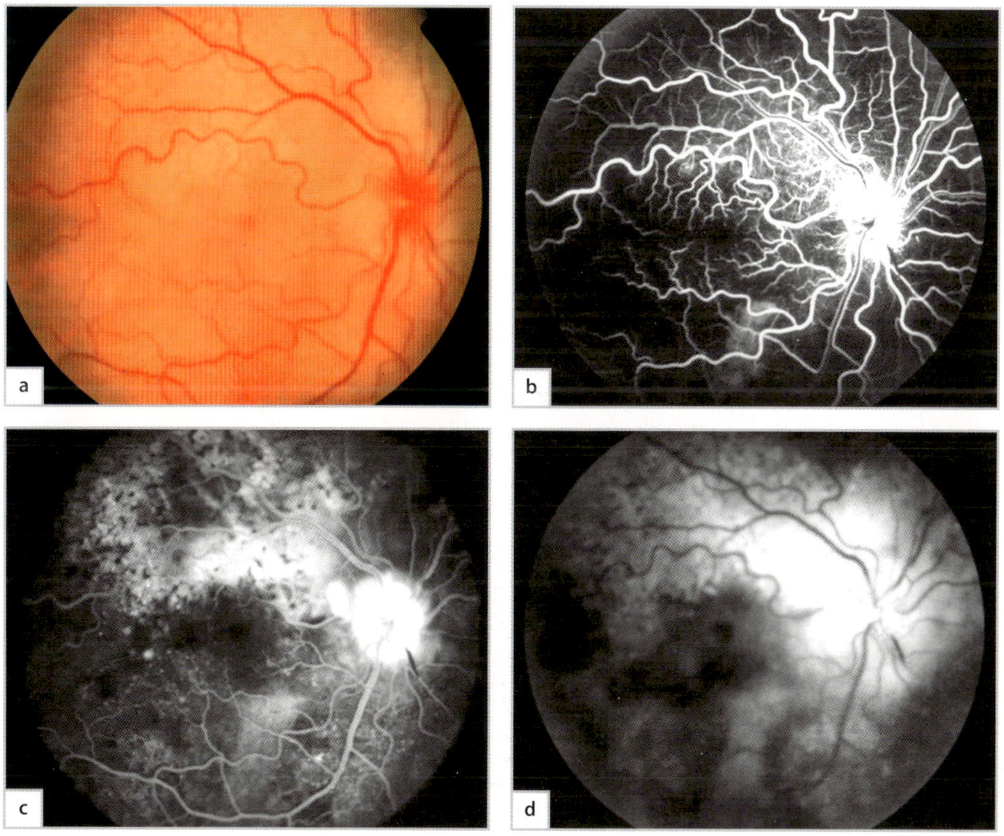

Figure 13.7 Metastatic carcinoma from the breast with transition towards an osteoma-like appearance. (a) The right eye of a patient with carcinoma of the breast shows deep-seated gray-white lesions, affecting the whole of the posterior pole. There is virtually no exudative detachment. The tortuosity of the retinal arterioles is probably a congenital anomaly. The optic disc is pink and slightly swollen and shows some hemorrhages. (b) The arteriovenous phase of the fluorescein angiogram shows marked hypofluorescence of the choroid due to intense masking of the background fluorescence. The optic disc is already showing some evidence of leakage. (c) The late venous phase shows mixture of patchy hyper- and hypofluorescence of the posterior pole with leakage from the optic disc. The hypofluorescence patches look like bone spicules. (d) The late phase shows intense staining of the deep choroidal lesion.

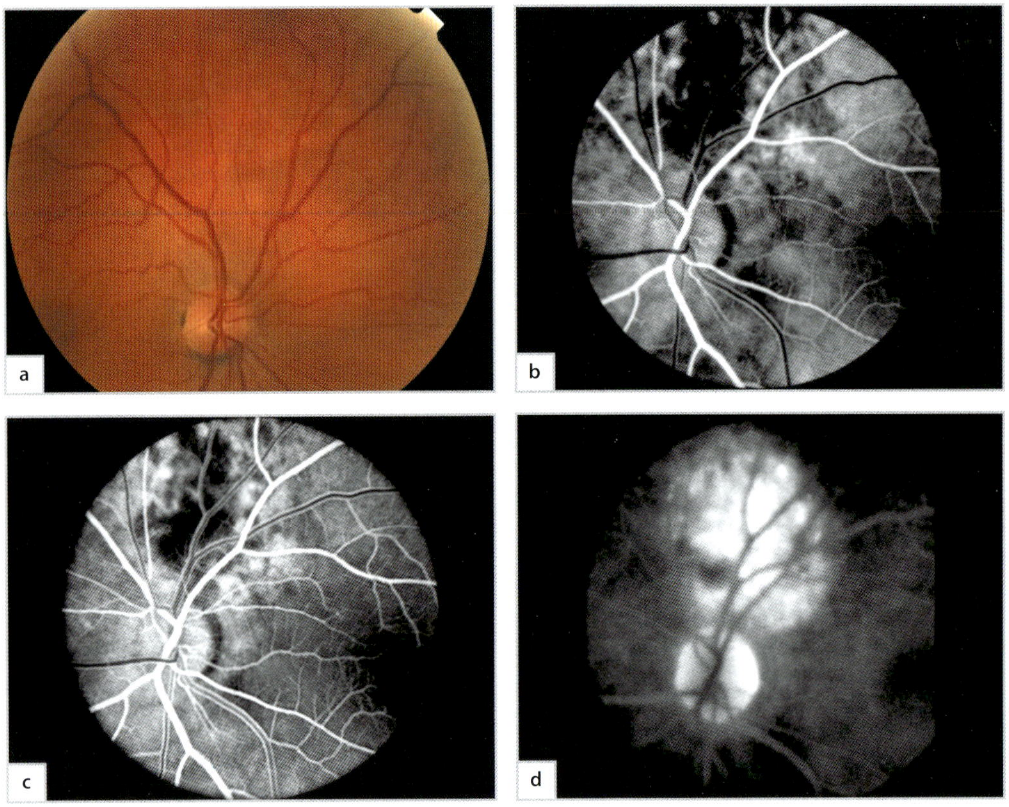

Figure 13.8 Choroidal hemangioma. (a) The left eye shows an ill-defined dusky-red raised lesion above the optic disc. (b) The early arterial phase of the fluorescein angiogram shows few areas of hyperfluorescence in the choroid. (c) The early arteriovenous phase shows numerous hyperfluorescence areas of different shapes and sizes, some linear and other as lacunae. (d) The late phase shows concentration of dye in a localized area delineating the tumor.

HEMANGIOMA (HEMANGIOBLASTOMA) OF THE OPTIC NERVE HEAD

Juxtapapillary capillary hemangioblastomas are vascular lesions, that occur on the optic nerve head or immediately adjacent to the optic disc. Although juxtapapillary capillary hemangioblastoma may appear as an isolated clinical entity, it is more likely to be a precursor to the diagnosis of von Hippel–Lindau (VHL) disease. When associated with VHL disease, the ocular complications from a hemangioblastoma are generally greater, and subsequently the prognosis is poorer than an isolated entity. Clinically, a group of dilated tortuous capillaries with microaneurysmal changes is seen next to the optic disc. In chronic cases, a moderate degree of exudation and lipid deposits are found surrounding the tumor (Schindler et al. 1975 McCabe et al. 2000, Hoobyar et al. 2002).

Fluorescein angiography findings

During the early phase of the angiography, the tumor area shows bunches of dilated tortuous blood vessels with microaneurysmal changes. During the progress of the transit, a moderate amount of dye may leak around the optic disc and spread to the nearby retina. The fluorescein angiogram shows steadily increasing dilatation and capillary changes at the optic disc, progressing to moderate leakage during the late phase (Male et al. 1984) (**Figure 13.9**).

ANGIOMATOSIS RETINAE

VHL disease is generally recognized as a phacomatosis of the retina. Phacomatoses are a group of diseases that characteristically affect the skin, eyes, central nervous system, and the viscera. The commonest ones are tuberous sclerosis, neurofibromatosis, and the Sturge–Weber syndrome. VHL disease is transmitted as an autosomal dominant trait with incomplete penetrance. It may affect the central nervous system, for example the medulla, pons, and spinal cord. Cysts of the pancreas and kidney are also commonly associated with VHL disease. The disease affects both sexes, and symptoms appear during the early teens. The fundal changes can be described in three different stages.
Stage 1. Development of feeder vessels: The afferent feeder vessel is an arteriole and the efferent is a venule. A large angioma is often accompanied by several smaller ones, affecting a wider area of the mid-periphery of the retina.
Stage 2. Exudation, hemorrhage, and retinal detachment: The tumor leads to massive outpouring of serum and lipids into the subretinal space. These may deposit at a remote site such as the macular area.
Stage 3. Destruction of the eye: Retinal detachment, secondary glaucoma, and phthisis bulbi are the end stage of the effects of the disease on the eye.

Fluorescein angiography findings

It is essential to capture the early arterial phase of the angiogram to demonstrate the arterial feeder vessel; this helps in planning the treatment. During the progress of the transit, further microvascular

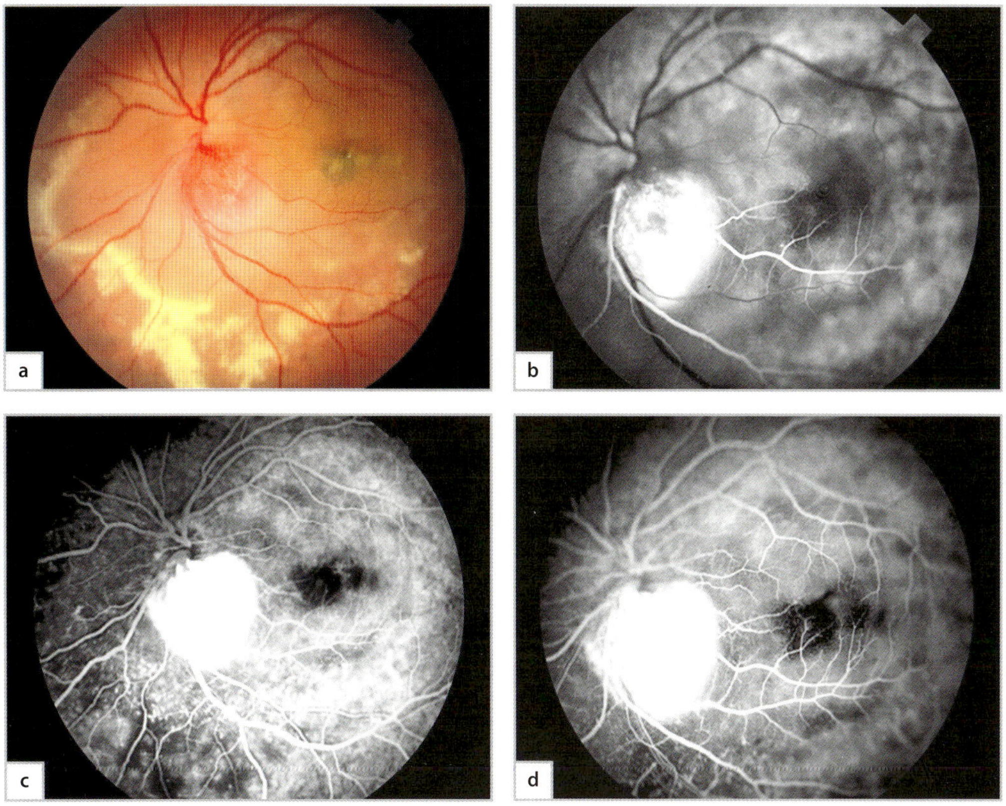

Figure 13.9 Juxtapapillary hemangioblastoma. (a) The left eye shows a large juxtapapillary optic disc hemangioblastoma, occupying the lower part of the optic disc associated with widespread exudative retinal detachment and lipid exudation. (b) The arterial phase of the fluorescein angiogram shows patchy filling of the choroid. A large area of spade-shaped hyperfluorescence lesion is seen at the inferior part of the optic disc. The deeper retina shows patchy hyperfluorescence within the exudative detachment area. (c) The arteriovenous phase shows the spade-shaped hyperfluorescence from the lower part of the optic disc. The nearby retina shows some capillary dilatation and microaneurysm formation. The deeper layer shows coalescing of hyperfluorescent patchy areas to form a more confluent zone of leakage. (d) The late phase shows intense staining of the tumor and heavy concentration of dye within the tumor. There is a moderate amount of leakage of dye into the subretinal surface.

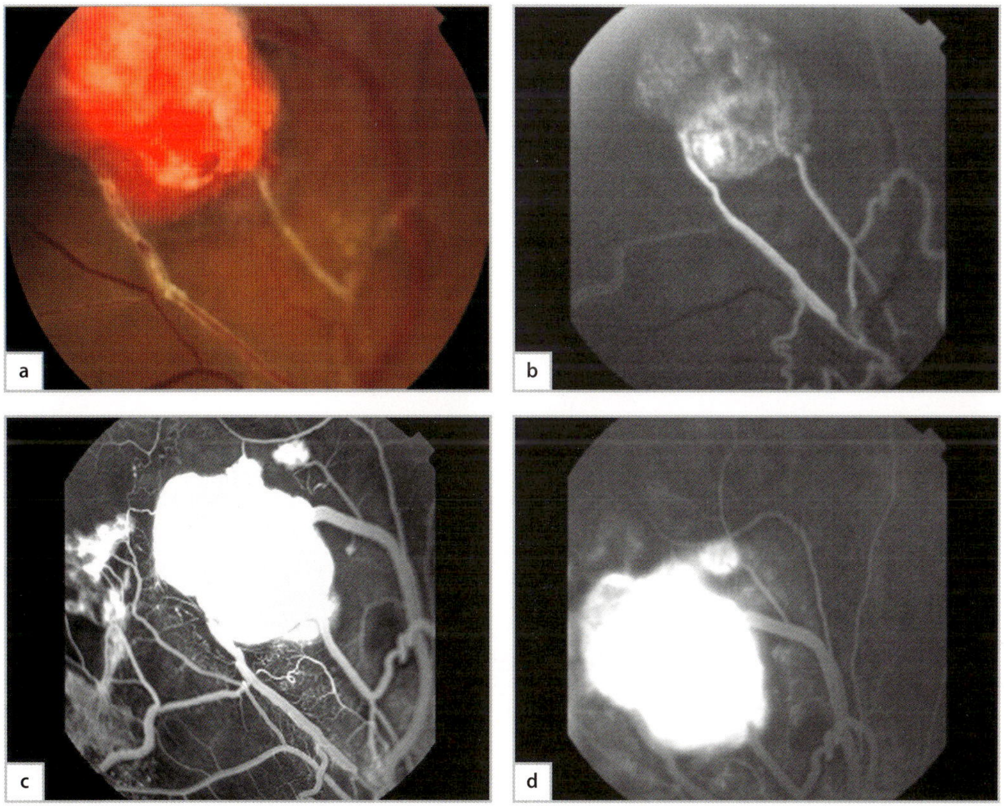

Figure 13.10 Angiomatosis retinae (von Hippel–Lindau disease). (a) The peripheral part of the retina shows a large angiomatous lesion with feeder and drainage vessels. (b) The early arterial phase of the fluorescein angiogram shows two feeder vessels into the angioma, which is beginning to fill. (c) The arteriovenous phase shows almost a fully filled angioma and several satellite, smaller angiomatous lesions. (d) The late phase shows intense staining but no significant leakage.

abnormalities become apparent, showing satellite aneurysms. During the venous phase, the efferent venous channel fills from within the tumor. The late phase of the angiogram shows leakage of dye from both the tumor and the surrounding microvascular angiopathy (Haining & Zweifach 1967) (**Figure 13.10**).

RACEMOSE HEMANGIOMA (WYBURN–MASON SYNDROME)

Hemangioma of the retina often affecting one eye only and associated with similar vascular changes in the midbrain was first recognized by Wyburn-Mason in 1943. Clinically, a complex arteriovenous communication is seen, with grossly dilated and tortuous blood vessels, at times associated with aneurysmal dilatation.

Fluorescein angiography findings

Fluorescein angiography reveals the complex vascular arrangement, most prominent during the arteriovenous phase. Normally, the dye does not leak out of the blood vessels. However, in long-standing cases where there have been secondary changes, a minimal focal leakage may be expected (**Figure 13.11**).

CHOROIDAL OSTEOMA

Choroidal osteoma is commonly seen in older females, affecting the posterior pole of the fundus. The etiology is uncertain. The vision is affected if the macular area has been involved. The lesion appears as a deep-seated gray-white lesion with minimal elevation. There may be some pigment clumping on the surface of the lesion. Ultrasonography and computed tomography show evidence of calcification in the choroid (Gass et al. 1978, Gass 1979, Shields et al. 1988, Bloom et al. 1992).

Fluorescein angiography findings

The fluorescein angiogram shows a mixture of hypo- and hyperfluorescence during early phase of angiography due to a window defect. During the progress of transit, areas of hyperfluorescence increase and tend to coalesce to form larger areas of hyperfluorescence. The late phase shows a moderate degree of staining (**Figure 13.12**).

MELANOCYTOMA

This is a benign tumor commonly arising from the optic nerve head area. It is derived from uveal dendritic melanocytes. It equally common in all races. Occasionally, the tumor may be slightly elevated and extend to involve the nearby retina. Often a variable amount of retinal pigment epithelial degeneration is seen around the lesion. There is no evidence of serous retinal detachment. These tumors do not become malignant (Shields 1978).

Fluorescein angiography findings

Fluorescein angiography shows extensive masking of not only the choroid but also the retinal vessels at and near the optic disc. The masking continues throughout the transit period and may produce a minimum degree of staining toward the late phase, where there is retinal pigment epithelial degeneration (**Figure 13.13**).

RETINAL ASTROCYTOMA

This is a benign tumor seen in tuberous sclerosis and neurofibromatosis but it may also be seen in isolation. It is often discovered accidentally on routine examination. Ophthalmoscopy shows a yellow-white mass resembling a mound of sago grains. Histological examination shows densely packed retinal astrocytes (Ikeda et al. 1995).

Fluorescein angiography findings

These tumors are highly autofluorescence; hence it is essential to take preinjection photographs with the appropriate filter combination. During the early phase of the transit, very little is seen owing to the masking of the background choroidal fluorescence. During the mid -transit phase, the tumor increases in fluorescence and often has some vascular change around it. The late phase shows marked staining of the entire tumor (**Figure 13.14**).

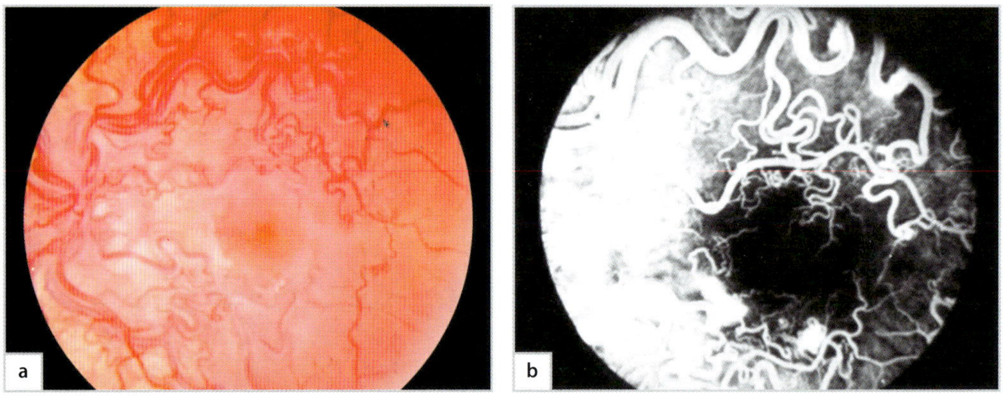

Figure 13.11 Wyburn–Mason's syndrome. (a) The left eye shows complex arteriovenous anastomoses with markedly tortuous blood vessels both arteries and veins. (b) The late transit of the fluorescein angiogram shows the dilated tortuous blood vessels in all areas, but there is no evidence of any significant leakage. The plaques of hyperfluorescent lesions are due to retinal pigment epithelial atrophy.

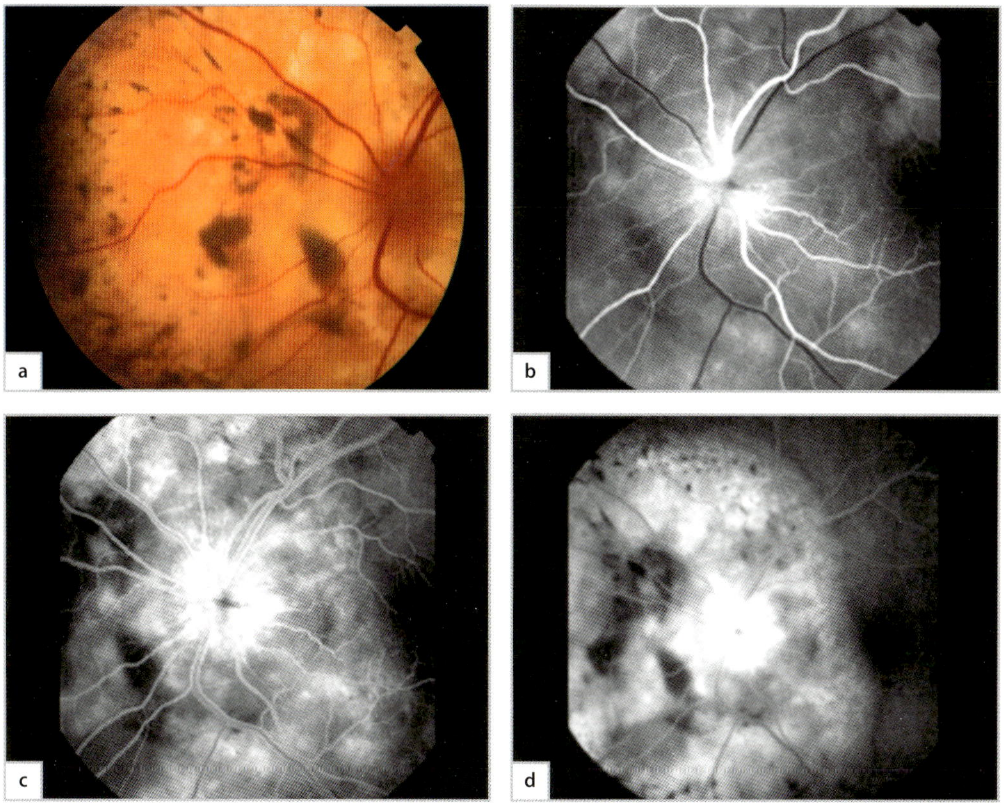

Figure 13.12 Choroidal osteoma. (a) The left eye shows a large area of deep-seated gray-yellow lesion with overlying mottling of retinal pigment epithelium The optic disc shows some degree of swelling. (b) The early phase of the fluorescein angiogram shows severe masking of choroid. The optic disc shows some dilated disc vessels. (c) The late venous phase shows patchy hyperfluorescence of the choroid and increases dilatation and commencement of leakage from the optic disc. (d) The late phase shows mottled hyperfluorescence of choroid and leakage from the optic disc.

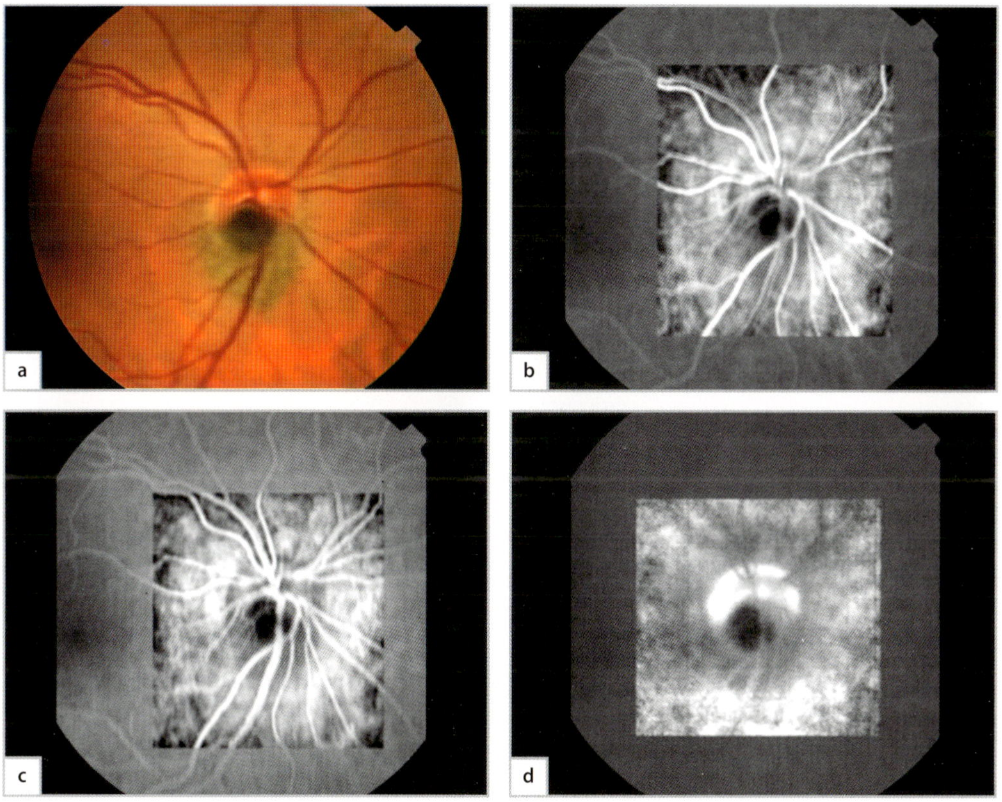

Figure 13.13 Melanocytoma of optic disc. (a) The right eye shows a jet-black slightly elevated lesion arising from the optic disc, extending in a downward direction. The lesion beyond the optic disc margin shows slate-gray coloration due to deep-seated nature of the lesion. (b) The enhanced optic disc area during the arterial phase of the fluorescein angiogram shows masking of the disc vasculature from the center downwards. (c) The arteriovenous phase continues to show hypofluorescence of the optic disc. (d) The late phase shows mild degree of staining of the upper part of the optic disc, while the lower part remains hypofluorescent.

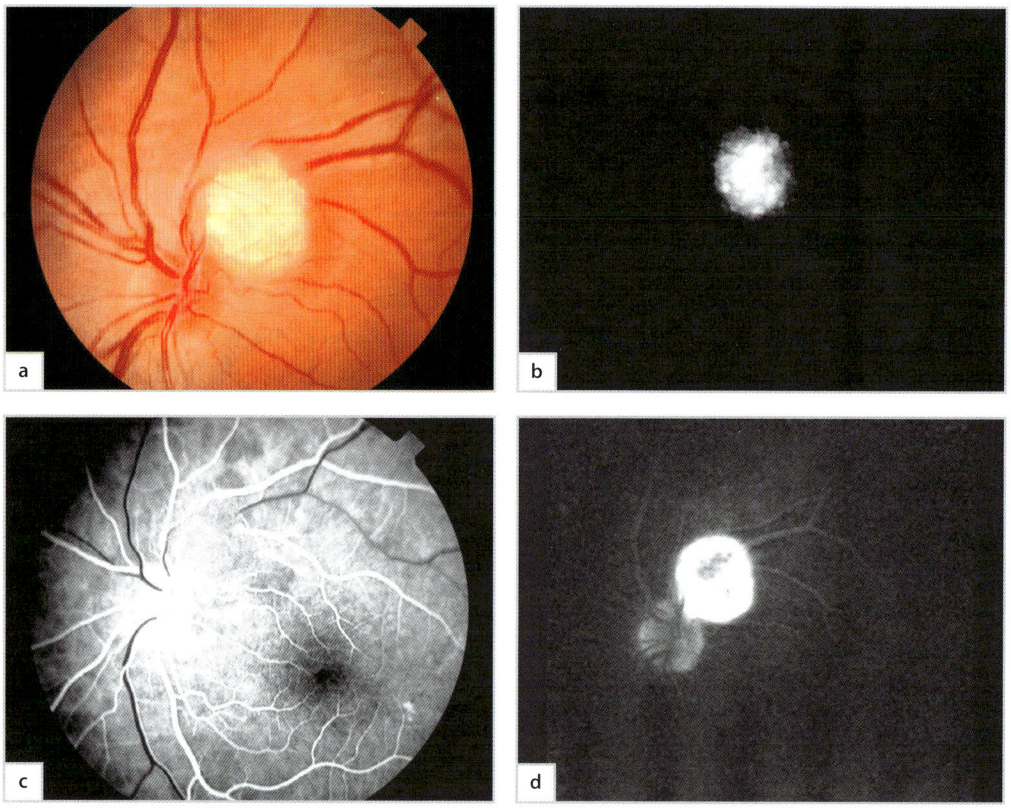

Figure 13.14 Retinal astrocytoma. (a) The left eye shows a dense mulberry-like white lesion upper temporal to the optic disc. (b) The preinjection photograph with green and yellow filters shows intense autofluorescence of the astrocytoma lesion. (c) The early transit phase of the fluorescein angiogram shows normal fillings of all the retinal arterioles and the capillaries. The capillaries over the astrocytoma look slightly more prominent. (d) The late phase shows intense fluorescence due to staining. It produces no real leakage.

REFERENCES

Bloom PA, Ferris JD, Laidlaw A. Appearance of choroidal osteoma with diagnostic imaging. *Br J Radiol* 1992; **65**:845–848.

Cantrill HL, Cameron JD, Ramsay RC, Knobloch WH. Retinal vascular changes in malignant melanoma of the choroid. *Am J Ophthalmol* 1984; **97**:411–418.

Davis DL, Robertson DM. Fluorescein angiography of metastatic choroidal tumours. *Arch Ophthalmol* 1973; **89**:97–99.

Edwards WC, Layden WE, McDonald R Jr. Fluorescein angiography of malignant melanoma of the choroid. *Am J Ophthalmol* 1969; **68**:797–808.

Fishman G A. The value of fluorescein angiography in the differential diagnosis of choroidal melanomas. In: Peyman GA, et al. (eds.), Intraocular tumours. New York: Appleton/Century/Crofts, WW 1491611976, 1977:9–34.

Gass JD. New observations concerning choroidal osteomas. *Int Ophthalmol* 1979; **1**:71–84.

Gass JD, Guerry RK, Jack RL, Harris G. Choroidal osteoma. *Arch Ophthalmol* 1978; **96**:428–435.

Haining W M, Zweifach PH. Fluorescein angiography in von Hippel-Lindau disease. *Arch Ophthalmol* 1967; **78**:475–479.

Hayreh SS. Choroidal melanomata. Fluorescein angiographic and histopathologic study. *Br J Ophthalmol* 1970; **54**:145–160.

Hoobyar AR, Ferrucci S, Anderson SF, Townsend JC. Juxtapapillary capillary hemangioblastoma. *Optom Vis Sci* 2002; **79**:346–352.

Ikeda T, Ogawa K, Kitanishi K. A case of uncomplicated retinal astrocytoma Nippon Ganka Gakkai zasshi 99. 1995; **9**:1052–1055.

MacLean AL, Maumenee AE. Hemangioma of the choroid. *Am J Ophthalmol* 1960; **50**:3–11.

McCabe CM, Flynn HW Jr, Shields CL, et al. Juxtapapillary capillary hemangiomas. Clinical features and visual acuity outcomes. *Ophthalmology* 2000; **107**:2240–2248.

Mele A, Cennamo G, Sorrentino V, Capobianco S. Fluoroangiographic and echographic study on a juxtapapillary hamartoma of retinal pigment epithelium. *Ophthalmologica* 1984; **189**:180–185.

Norton EW, Gutman F. Fluorescein angiography of hemangiomas. *Ophtalmologica* 1968; **150**:5–17.

Pettit TH, Barton A, Foos RY, Christensen RE. Fluorescein angiography of choroidal melanomas. *Arch Ophthalmol* 1970; **83**:27–38.

Schindler RF, Sarin LK, McDonald PR. Haemangiomata of optic disc. *Can J Ophthalmol* 1975; **10**:305–318.

Shields CL, Shields JA, Augsburger J J. Choroidal osteoma. *Surv Ophthalmol* 1988; **33**:17–27.

Shields CL, Shields JA, Gross NE, et al. Survey of 520 eyes with uveal metastases. *Ophthalmology* 1997; **104**:1265–1276.

Shields JA. Melanocytoma of the optic nerve head: a review. *Int Ophthalmol* 1978; **1**:31–37.

Suckling RD, Donaldson KA. The differential diagnosis of benign and malignant choroidal melanomata using fluorescein angiography. *Trans Ophthalmol Soc NZ* 1969; **21**:85–88.

Witschel H, Font RL. Hemangioma of the choroid: a clinicopathologic study a study of 71 cases and review of the literature. *Surv Ophthalmol* 1976; **20**:415–431.

Wyburn-Mason R. Arteriovenous aneurysm of midbrain and retina: facial nevi and mental changes. *Brain* 1943; **66**:163–203.

Chapter 14 Diabetic retinopathy and maculopathy

Sushma Dhar-Munshi

INTRODUCTION

Diabetes mellitus is a disorder of carbohydrate metabolism, which is characterized by hyperglycemia due to etiological factors ranging from lack of insulin to decreased sensitivity. Mainly there are two types of diabetes. In type 1 or insulin-dependent diabetes mellitus there is failure of production of insulin due to malfunctioning beta-cells in the islets of Langerhans in the pancreas. Type 2 or noninsulin-dependent diabetes is due to insufficient insulin production to meet the body's requirement.

PATHOGENESIS

Diabetic retinopathy is essentially a microvascular angiopathy that affects the precapillary arterioles, capillaries, and venules. Altered blood rheology leads to thickening of the basement membrane of the capillaries and damaged endothelial cells that in turn lead to platelet aggregation and microvascular occlusion in the venous circulation. Occlusion of microvascular circulation causes focal retinal ischemia, resulting in the formation of arteriovenous anastomosis and production of cytokines such as vascular endothelial growth factors (VEGFs). The VEGFs are a major stimulus for the formation and proliferation of retinal new vessels, which tend to bleed and cause fibrosis. Loss of pericytes leads to weakening of the capillary wall, decompensation of the tight junctions between endothelial cells increases vascular permeability, and leakage of fluid, particulates, and blood leads to retinal edema, lipid exudation, and retinal hemorrhages. The weakness in the capillary wall causes saccular out-pouching, leading to the formation of microaneurysms (Ashton 1949, 1953).

The imaging modalities for detection of diabetic retinopathy have undergone great advances over the last five decades, and these have helped greatly to understand the sequence of changes in the pathogenesis of diabetic retinopathy.

CLASSIFICATION OF DIABETIC RETINOPATHY

There are several classifications of diabetic retinopathy that have been proposed, but the most commonly used is developed from the Diabetic Retinopathy Study (DRS) and Early Treatment of Diabetic Retinopathy Study (ETDRS) (ETDRS Reports 4 and 11). Currently several newer classifications are being developed, but for practical purposes and for simplicity of use in a clinical setting, this chapter will adhere to the above-mentioned classification.

Diabetic retinopathy is broadly classified into nonproliferative and proliferative retinopathy and is associated with macular edema recognized as diabetic maculopathy of different grades, depending on the severity and type of changes. The hallmark of nonproliferative diabetic retinopathy is the microaneurysm, which appears as a red dot near a capillary or arteriole. The other changes seen are dot and blot hemorrhages, flame-shaped superficial hemorrhages, vascular dilatation, cotton wool spots, and retinal edema. Nonproliferative diabetic retinopathy is classified as minimal, mild, moderate, and severe also known as preproliferative retinopathy (parentheses).

Proliferative diabetic retinopathy ensues when new blood vessels arise from the edges of the ischemic part of the retina. These vessels are immature and fragile and prone to leakage of fluid and blood. They may also be associated with growth of fibrous tissue, resulting in retinal and vitreous hemorrhages, and traction retinal detachment. Diabetic maculopathy is a term used when changes like microaneurysms, hemorrhages, hard exudates, and retinal edema are seen in the macular area. In recent years, diabetic maculopathy has been referred as diabetic macular edema (DME).

All these changes can be demonstrated by fundus fluorescein angiography (FFA) and ocular coherence tomography (OCT), which have revolutionized retinal imaging. These two modalities used jointly form the basic armamentaria for diagnosing and managing diabetic retinopathy.

Microaneurysms

These are the earliest clinical sign of diabetic retinopathy, distributed in clumps or widely scattered over the fundus. They are present in the inner nuclear layer of the retina and seen as red dots with or without a central reflex. Clinically, they may be indistinguishable from fine dot hemorrhages. They may exhibit a central reflex or a capsular halo and which is seen connected to a fine retinal vessel (Norton & Gutman 1965). Fluorescein angiography shows hyperfluorescence during the early venous phase and some leakage toward the late phase.

Vascular abnormalities

The early changes seen are venous caliber changes like dilatation and beading, and later there occurs segmental narrowing causing string of sausage appearance. Sometimes branch retinal vein occlusions can occur. These changes are highlighted in the venous phase of FFA, and the vessel wall may show some staining and leakage in the late phase (Cogan et al. 1961).

Intraretinal hemorrhages

There are two types of hemorrhages seen in diabetic retinopathy. The dot and blot hemorrhages that are in the deeper layers of the retina and the superficial flame shaped ones that lie in the nerve fiber layer (Scott et al. 1963). Masking of background fluorescence is hallmark of all types of retinal hemorrhages. There may be some late staining seen around the hemorrhages.

Hard exudates

These consist of residual protein and lipid in the plexiform layer after the exudate fluid has been reabsorbed. They may be seen in isolation or grouped in clumps around a leaking microaneurysm in a circinate pattern. Hard exudates are waxy yellow in appearance with a sharp margin and mask fluorescence through all phases of the angiogram (Cogan et al. 1961).

Cotton wool spots

These appear as fluffy white areas with soft margins in the superficial layers of the retina. They are nerve fiber layer infarcts due to occlusion of small arterioles and they indicate ischemia. On fluorescein angiography, these appear as homogenous gray areas masking fluorescence with some late staining of their margins (Kohner 1969).

Retinal edema

The leakage of fluid from dilated capillaries and microaneurysms causes the retina to lose its transparency and appear gray and thickened. Initially the edema is limited to the deeper layers of the retina, but in later stages it moves to the superficial layers including the nerve fiber layer. Fluorescein angiography shows hypofluorescence during the early phase and leakage during the late phase. On the OCT, retinal edema is seen initially as initial thickening of the retina and later as small intraretinal cysts (Yamana 1983). These cysts enlarge and coalesce in time into larger ones. Sometimes the fluid may cause serous retinal detachments.

Ischemia

Fluorescein angiography shows featureless areas of capillary dropout or blunting of arterioles with pruning of their perpendicular branches (ETDRS Report 11).

Retinal new vessels

These are seen in proliferative diabetic eye disease and show increasing leakage of fluorescein due to deficiency of the tight endothelial junctions. These may remain flat on the disc and retina later growing toward the vitreous. They are fragile and may lead to retinal, subhyaloid, and vitreous hemorrhages.

NONPROLIFERATIVE DIABETIC RETINOPATHY

Minimal nonproliferative diabetic retinopathy

In this earliest stage of nonproliferative diabetic retinopathy, patients are asymptomatic. Clinically a few red dots, due to microaneurysms, are seen at the posterior pole and there may be a minimal degree of venous dilatation. Fluorescein angiography shows a few hyperfluorescent spots, corresponding to the microaneurysms, with or without minimal leakage (**Figure 14.1**).

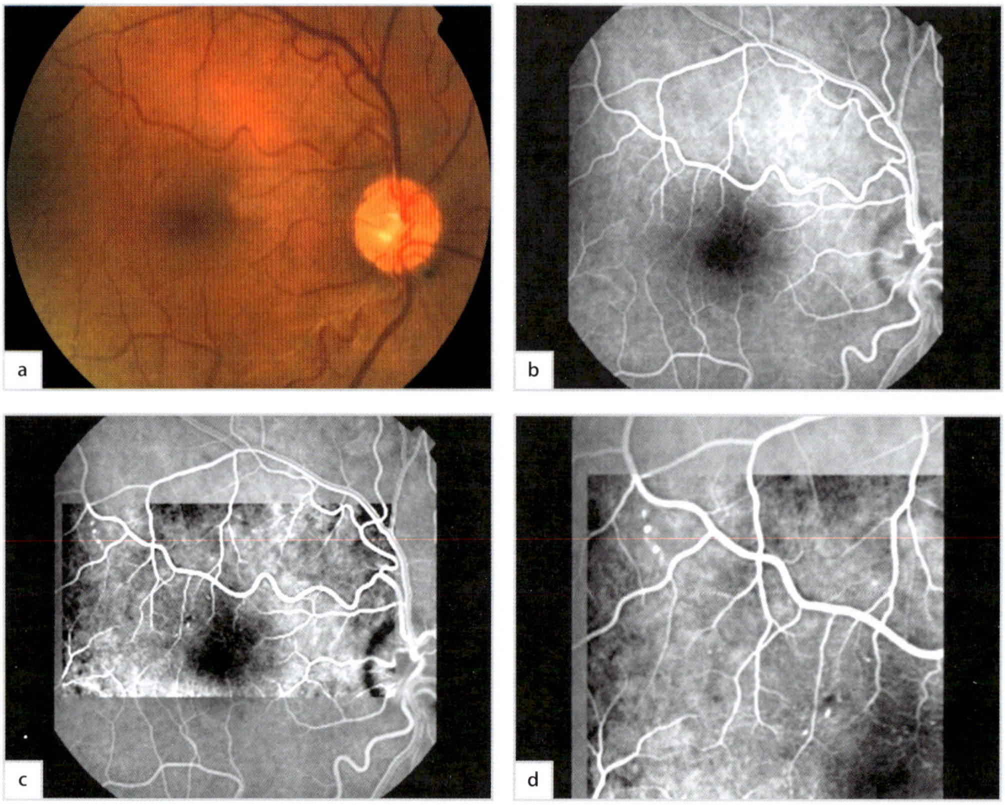

Figure 14.1 Minimal nonproliferative diabetic retinopathy. (a) The right eye shows only a few microaneurysms in the upper temporal area of posterior pole, otherwise the entire fundus is normal. (b) The early transit phase of the fluorescein angiogram shows only a few microaneurysms in the upper temporal part of the posterior pole. (c) The same angiogram has been enhanced to show the microaneurysms more clearly. (d) The enhanced zoomed view of the same region clearly shows the microaneurysms.

Mild nonproliferative diabetic retinopathy

As the retinopathy progresses to the mild stage, the microaneurysms start leaking and lipid exudate is deposited in the deeper layers of the retina around the microaneurysms. This exudation from leaking vessels and microaneurysms contributes to early retinal thickening and edema. The fluorescein angiogram shows hyperfluorescent dots with late leakage (**Figure 14.2**).

Moderate nonproliferative diabetic retinopathy

In the moderate stage of nonproliferative diabetic retinopathy, increasing numbers of microaneurysms, hemorrhages, and lipid exudate are seen with cotton wool spots and retinal edema. Fluorescein angiography shows masking of the background fluorescence due to hemorrhages and cotton wool spots, which appear as gray featureless areas. The late phase shows hyperfluorescence and leakage from microaneurysms and dilated capillaries (**Figure 14.3**).

Severe nonproliferative diabetic retinopathy/preproliferative retinopathy

As the diabetic retinopathy progresses involving the precapillary arterioles and larger retinal arterioles, severe changes characteristic of preproliferative retinopathy begin to develop. These include multiple cotton wool spots, widespread ischemia, dark blot hemorrhages, venous beading and loops, and irregular dilated capillaries commonly defined as intraretinal microvascular abnormalities (IRMA). Fluorescein angiography shows areas of capillary closure related to the cotton wool spots and staining during the late phase. The IRMAs show increasing fluorescence in the arteriovenous phase with late leakage. Hemorrhages mask fluorescence, whereas venous changes are highlighted with late staining of the diseased vessel walls. The areas of retinal edema show some hyperfluorescence due to late leakage of the dye (**Figure 14.4**).

PROLIFERATIVE DIABETIC RETINOPATHY

This is characterized by the development of new blood vessels in response to the production of cytokines such as VEGFs from the ischemic areas. The new vessel growth is often accompanied by fibrous tissue proliferation (Kohner & Dollery 1971).

The new vessels arising from the optic disc are named new vessels on the disc and from elsewhere on the retina as new vessels elsewhere (NVE). Initially, the new vessels are flat on the disc or retina but later break through the internal limiting membrane and grow into the vitreous. When the vitreous fibrous proliferation contracts, the fragile new vessels bleed leading to subhyaloid or vitreous hemorrhages.

These new vessels lack tight endothelial junctions, hence they leak profusely on fluorescein angiography. Initially the vascular pattern grows in a rete or fan-shaped pattern. Long-standing new vessels mature to develop tight endothelial junctions and become competent. This is frequently seen in persisted new vessels following effective panretinal laser photocoagulation. Sometimes the only factor distinguishing between IRMA and early new vessels is the extent and rapidity of leakage of the dye. There are large areas of capillary

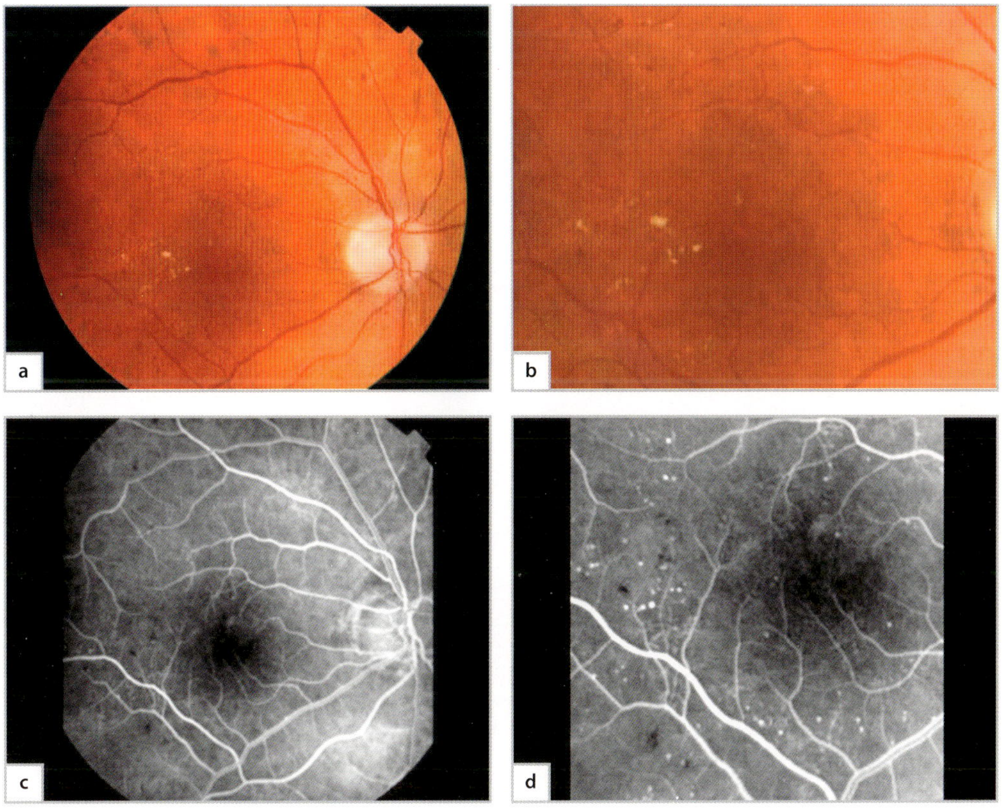

Figure 14.2 Mild nonproliferative diabetic retinopathy. (a) The right eye shows a few microaneurysms and minimal lipid exudate on the temporal side of the fundus. The rest of the fundus is normal. (b) The same affected area has been enlarged to show the background changes well. (c) The early transit phase of the fluorescein angiogram shows the microaneurysms, mainly at the lateral half of the fundus. (d) The same angiogram has been enhanced and zoomed to show the vascular changes well.

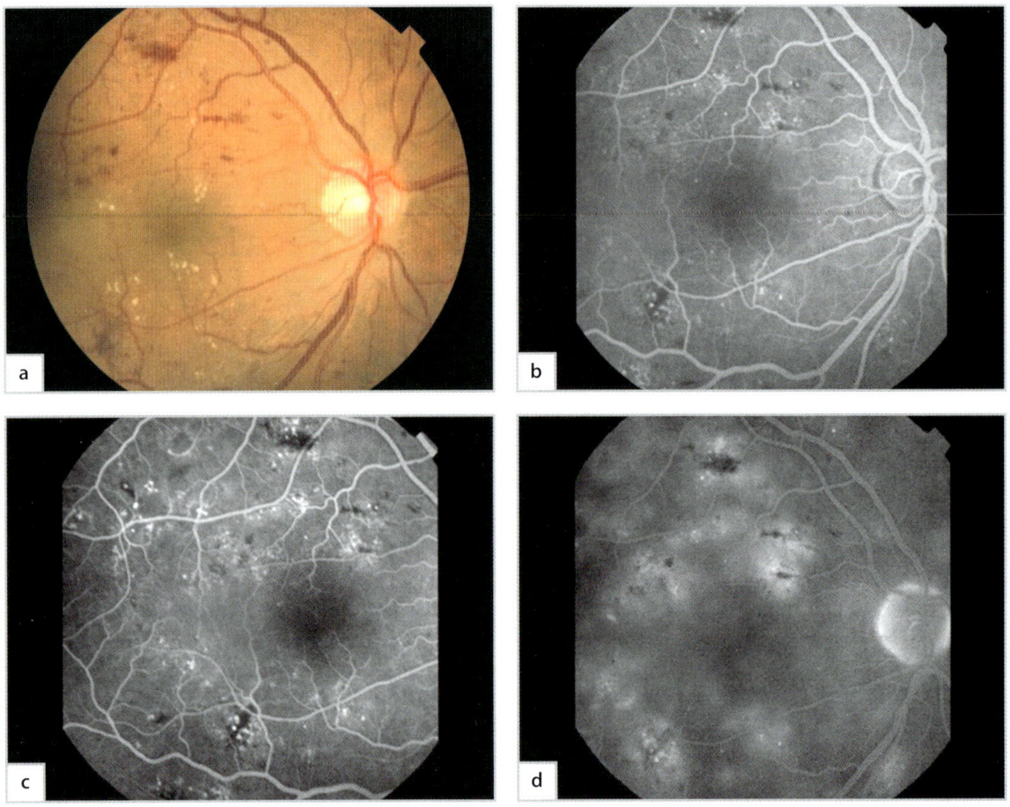

Figure 14.3 Moderate nonproliferative diabetic retinopathy. (a) The right eye shows multiple red dots and several superficial deep retinal hemorrhages in the posterior pole. Some lipid exudates around the macular area. The veins are slightly congested. (b) The arteriovenous phase of the fluorescein angiogram shows the microaneurysms are scattered in the posterior pole. The retinal hemorrhages mask the background fluorescence. The vein may appear minimally congested. (c) The enhanced view of the posterior pole shows all the microaneurysms in the posterior pole. The hemorrhages mask background fluorescence. There is no evidence of any capillary closure. The macula is normal. (d) The late phase shows multiple areas of leaking in the posterior pole. All the leakage sites correspond to the microvascular changes seen in the previous frame. There is no leak from the disc or macula.

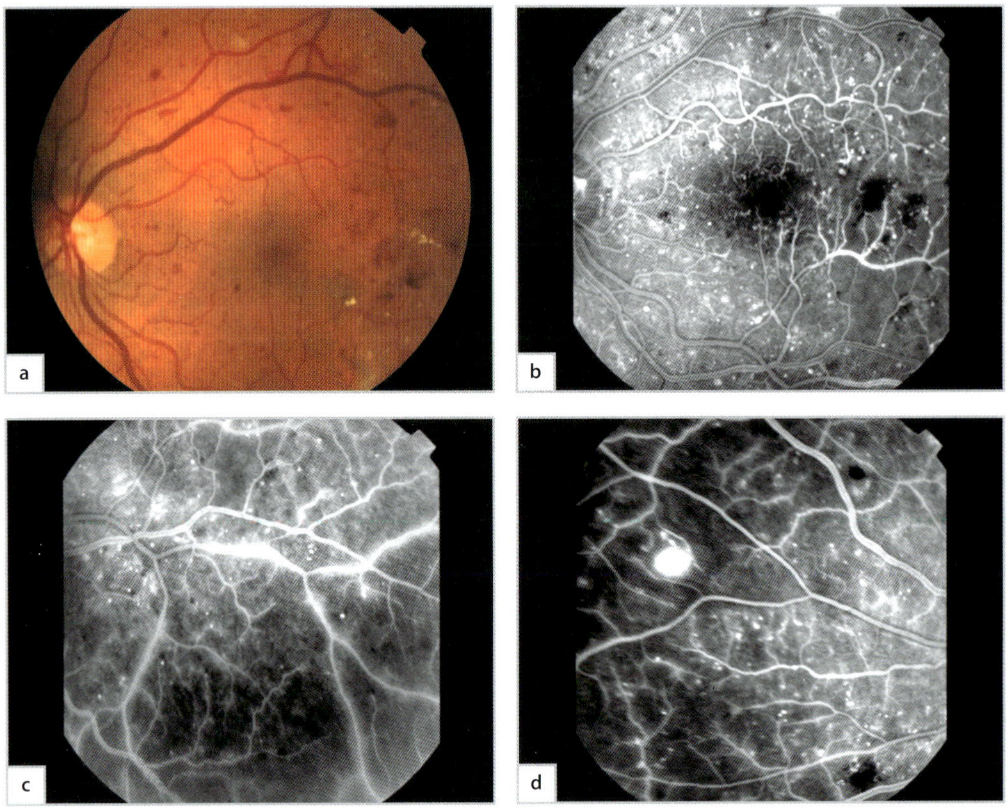

Figure 14.4 Severe nonproliferative diabetic retinopathy. (a) The left eye shows lots of red dots due to microaneurysms associated with retinal hemorrhages, lipid exudate, and small areas of cotton wool spots. (b) The late transit phase of the fluorescein angiogram of the posterior pole shows multiple areas of microvascular changes with microaneurysms, capillary dilatation, and small areas of capillary closure. The lower temporal area of the retina shows retrograde filing of the retinal arteriole adjacent to the capillary closure area. The retinal hemorrhages mask the background fluorescence. (c) The venous phase of the temporal midperipheral area of the fundus shows large areas of capillary closures, dilatation, and irregularity of retinal veins. (d) The late transit phase of the nasal aspect of the fundus shows marked capillary closure and vascular abnormalities. There is one large hyperfluorescent round lesion in the midperiphery, which may be a large microaneurysm or may even be an early new vessel.

nonperfusion next to the new vessels (**Figures 14.5 and 14.6**). In some young diabetes patients, the NVE develops in the perimacular area as clusters of coiled up aneurysmal blood vessels with fibrous proliferation along the vascular arcades causing subhyaloid hemorrhages, which if left untreated progress to a central tabletop retinal detachment.

In advanced diabetic eye disease, persistent and recurrent vitreous hemorrhage, traction retinal detachments, and neovascular glaucoma may occur without specific imaging or angiographic characteristics (**Figure 14.7**). Traction detachments can be detected by OCT or by ultrasound if there are media opacities.

DIABETIC MACULOPATHY OR DME

The classic definition of clinically significant diabetic macular edema (CSME), as given by the ETDRS, is (1) retinal thickening involving or within 500 μm from the center of the macula, (2) hard exudates with thickening of the adjacent retina at or within 500 μm from the center of the macula, and (3) a zone of retinal thickening one disc area or larger, any part of which is within one disc diameter from the center of the macula (ETDRS Report 11).

CSME is the most severe form of DME and leads to moderate visual loss in one out of four persons within 3 years if treated, the risk is reduced by 50%. In the era before OCT, fluorescein angiography was the gold standard for diagnosing and classifying diabetic maculopathy and macular edema. Based on the angiographic findings, diabetic maculopathy was classified as focal, diffuse, ischemic, and mixed types. This classification still holds good in most clinical settings. However, OCT classification is based on the optical reflectivity and three-dimensional images of the central retina. It is now widely used as it provides an objective and quantitative assessment of macular edema that is superior to any other modality.

Fluorescein angiographic findings in diabetic maculopathy

Focal maculopathy

A mixture of microaneurysms and dot hemorrhages with or without hard exudates and retinal edema shows hyperfluorescence and late leakage of the dye. Areas of retinal edema are seen as collections of dye in the late phase (**Figure 14.8**).

Diffuse maculopathy

Fluorescein angiography shows initial masking of the background fluorescence due to retinal edema. The microaneurysms then start showing hyperfluorescence and leakage. There is also leakage from the affected capillary bed in the late phase. The leaking dye collects in a daisy flower petal pattern in the macula generally referred to as cystoid macular edema (CME), related to the collection of edema fluid in the Henle's outer plexiform layer (**Figure 14.9**). The lipid hard exudates are arranged around a bunch of leaking microaneurysms, forming the so-called circinate retinopathy. The DME shows two distinct patterns of dye pooling in the late stage, a petalloid pattern in fovea, and a honeycomb pattern in perifoveal area (Otani & Kishi 2007). Some eyes undergoing panretinal photocoagulation for proliferative diabetic retinopathy may show a worsening of the DME, which is usually of the diffuse type.

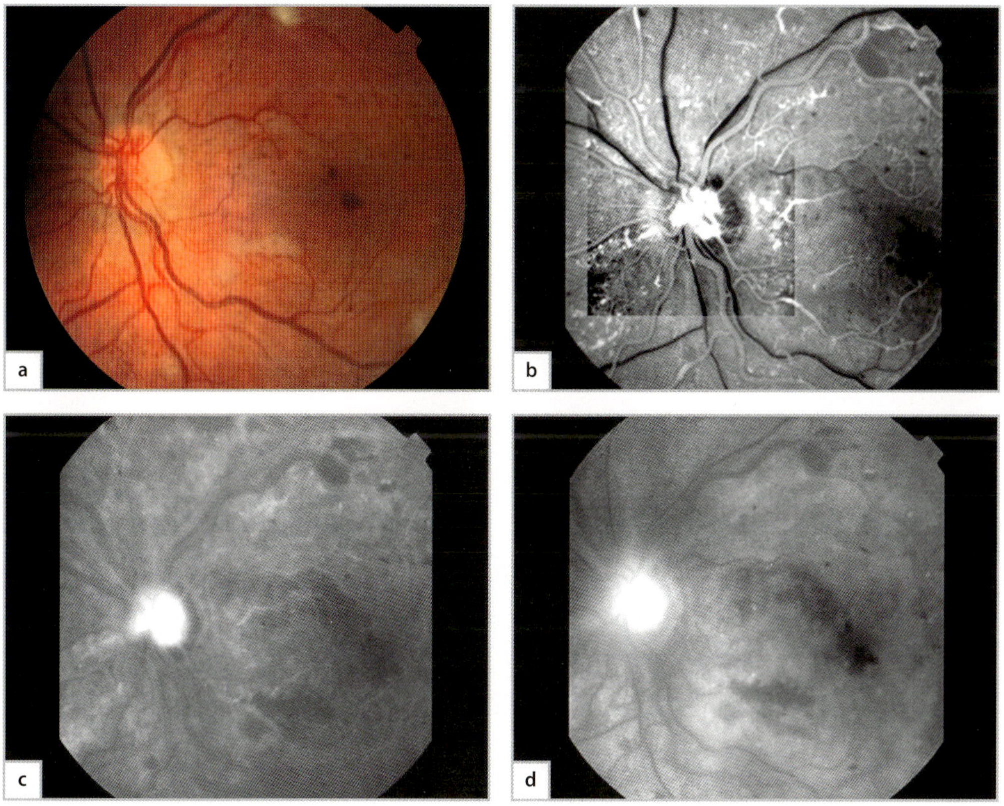

Figure 14.5 Proliferative diabetic retinopathy neovascularization of optic disc. (a) The left eye shows a network of new vessels on the optic disc surface. There are several areas of cotton wool spots scattered in the posterior pole. Generally, there are microaneurysms, capillary dilatation tortuosity, and intraretinal hemorrhages, which dominate the posterior pole. (b) The arterial phase of the fluorescein angiogram shows a network of hyperfluorescence from the optic disc and multiple microvascular angiopathy with capillary closure. (c) The late transit phase shows a moderate increase in hyperfluorescence from the optic disc due to leak from the new vessels. The background appears featureless and shows staining. The dark areas represent capillary closure and correspond to the cotton wool spots. (d) The late phase shows intense hyperfluorescence from the optic disc due to leakage from the new vessels. The background shows some late staining and minimal leak.

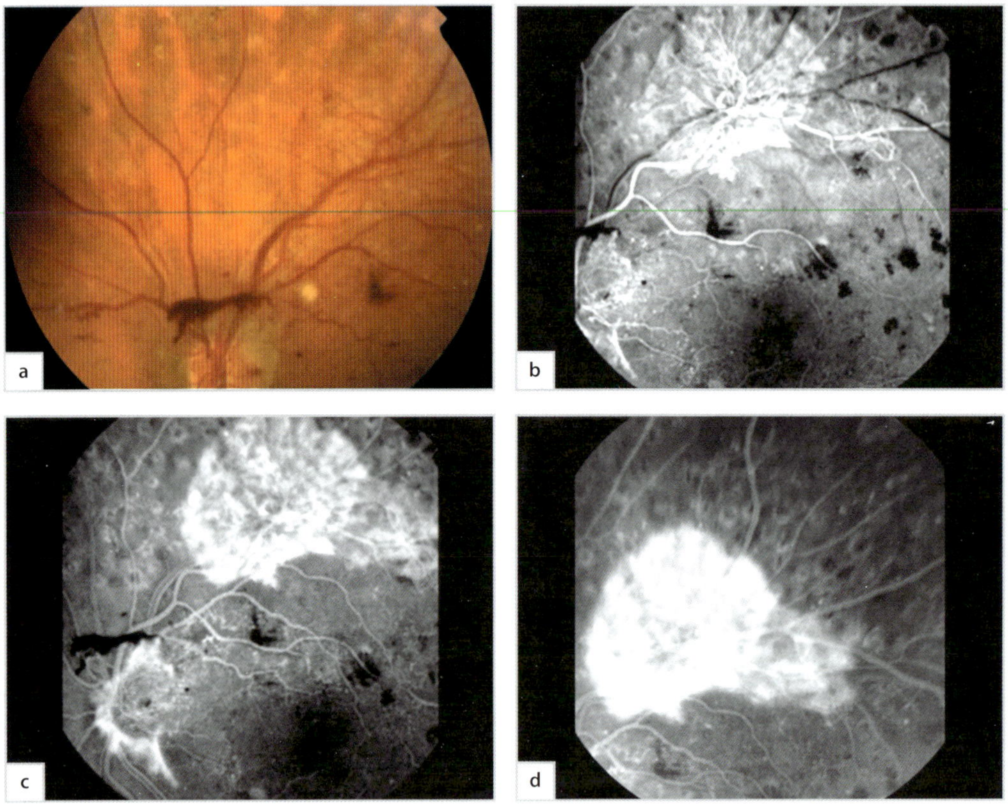

Figure 14.6 Proliferative diabetic retinopathy neovascularization elsewhere and the optic disc. (a) The left eye shows a fine network of new vessels on the surface of the optic disc associated with hemorrhages on the upper part of disc area. There is also a separate area of neovascularization along the superior temporal vessels, approximately one and a half disc diameter, upper temporal to the optic disc margin. There are several areas of retinal hemorrhages and a few cotton wool spots. (b) The early transit phase of the fluorescein angiogram centered at the neovascular complex shows a network of lacy hyperfluorescence architecture of new vessels. The lateral edge of the optic disc also shows a network of new vessels. The dark hypofluorescence areas are due to masking from the retinal hemorrhages. (c) The late arteriovenous phase of the peripheral and optic disc neovascular zone shows increasing hyperfluorescence due to leakage of dye. The hemorrhages continue to mask. (d) The late transit phase centered at the peripheral neovascular complex shows intense leakage of dye.

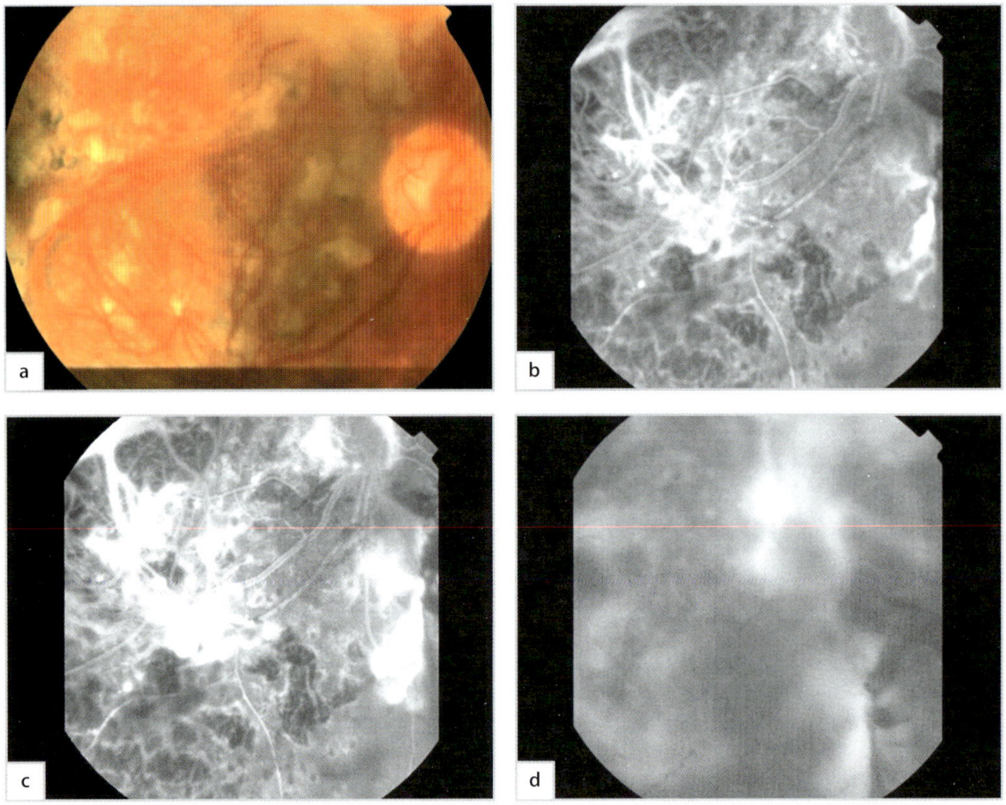

Figure 14.7 Advanced diabetic eye disease. (a) The right eye shows extensive neovascularization of the optic disc. There is widespread fibrovascular scaring of the retina. There are areas of traction retinal detachment at the superior temporal area. Some of the pigment changes seen are the result of previous laser photocoagulation marks. (b) The mid transit phase of the fluorescein angiogram shows gross distortion of vascular structures, particularly at the inferior temporal quadrant. (c) The late transit phase shows increasing hyperfluorescence due to leakage of dye. (d) The late phase shows massive leakage of dye.

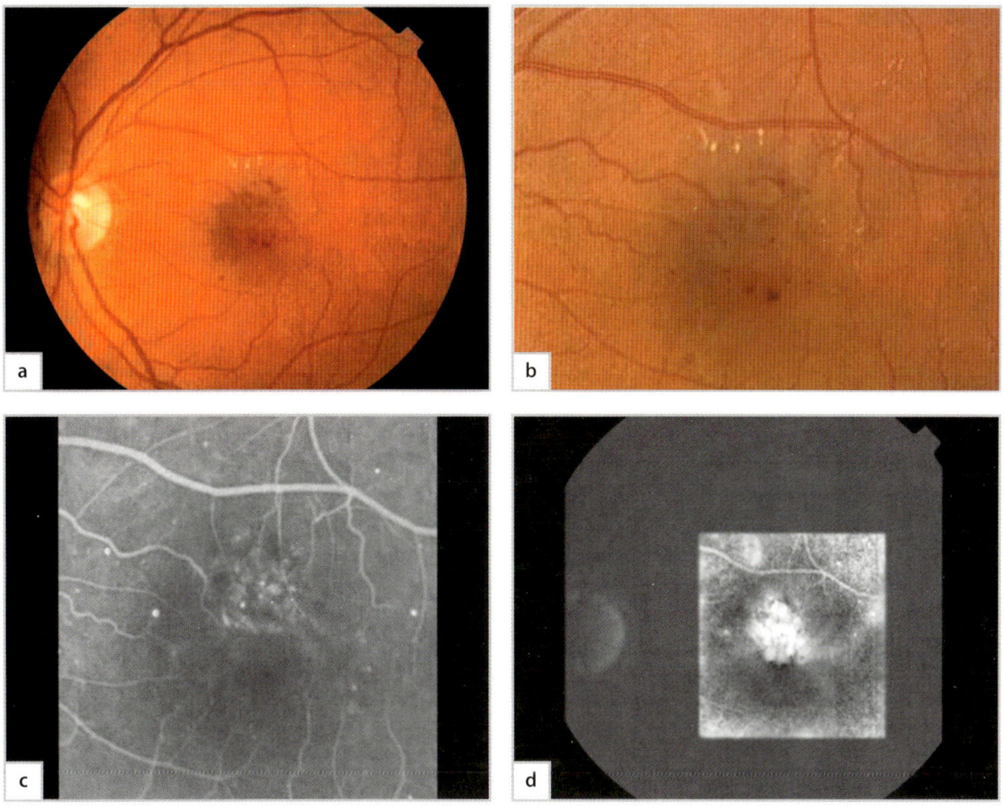

Figure 14.8 Focal diabetic maculopathy. (a) The left eye shows a localized area of microaneurysms and microvascular changes, just above the macular area. Note a few hemorrhages are on the macula itself. (b) The enlarged view of the macular area shows the microvascular changes affecting the macula and its upper part quite clearly associated with slight macular edema. (c) The mid transit fluorescein angiogram of the macular area shows the group of microaneurysms, just above the macula with a few odd ones elsewhere. (d) The late phase shows a leakage of dye arising from the microvascular changes above the macular area and is spreading into the macula in a fingerlike projection, an indication of early cystoid macular edema. The edema is localized to the upper part of the macula only.

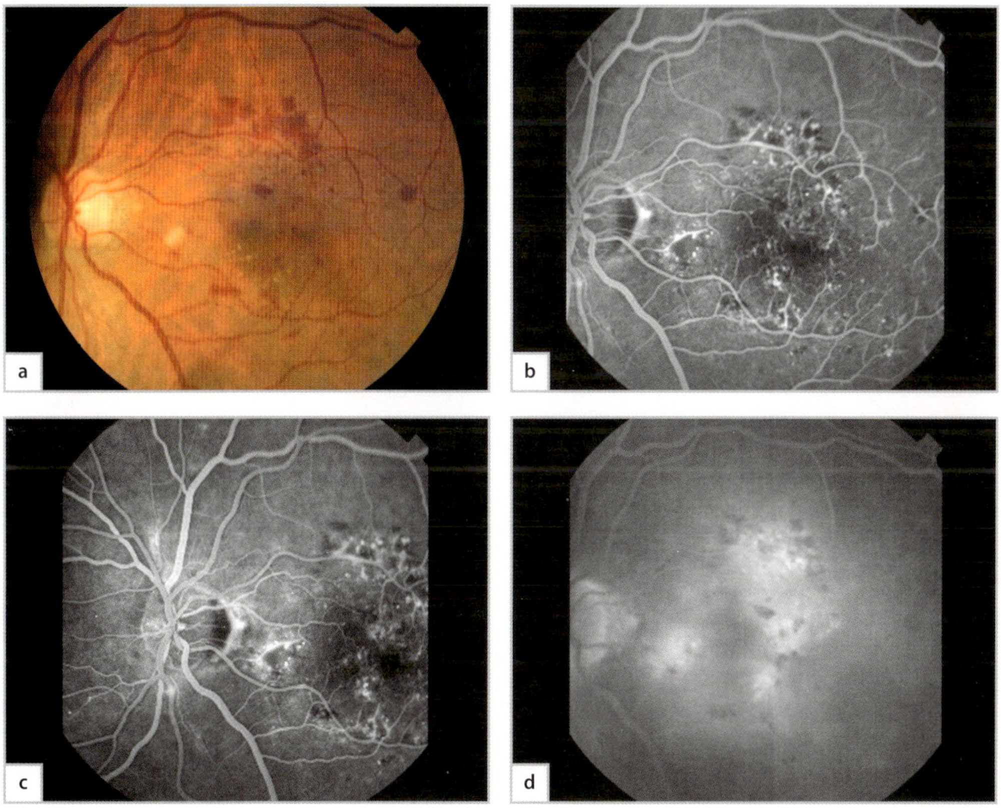

Figure 14.9 Diffuse diabetic maculopathy. (a) The left eye shows scattered areas of microaneurysms and retinal hemorrhages, affecting the macular area. There is minimal macular edema and a cotton wool spot inferiorly. (b) The arteriovenous phase of the fluorescein angiogram shows capillary dilatation, closure, and microaneurysm, affecting the entire macular area. (c) The late transit phase shows the commencement of the leak from the vascular abnormalities from the macular area. The rest of the fundus appears near normal. (d) The late phase shows multiple sites of hyperfluorescence due to leakage of dye. All the leaking areas seem to spread toward the macula forming a petalloid appearance due to early cystoid macula edema.

Ischemic maculopathy

Diabetic retinopathy with capillary closure and reduced perfusion of the retina within the macular area is called diabetic macular ischemia (DMI). Involvement of the perifoveal arcade does not exhibit much edema, but may show a few hemorrhages. Visual loss is profound and does not correlate with the extent of changes seen clinically. The perifoveal inter-capillary area and the foveal avascular zone (FAZ) increase in size as the diabetic retinopathy progresses. The extent of DMI is related to the severity and duration of hyperglycemia. Macular nonperfusion occurs earlier in type 2 than in type 1 diabetes, possibly due to coexistent hypertension in type 2 diabetes.

Fluorescein angiography is the best modality to demonstrate ischemic maculopathy, where areas of capillary closure are seen as hypofluorescent. The perifoveal arcade is distorted or broken with an increase in FAZ size. In the late phase, some leakage of the dye may be seen surrounding the hypofluorescent areas (**Figure 14.10**). The arterioles appear narrowed and show pruning of the perpendicular side branches. The normal average longest diameter of the FAZ is 0.65 mm with a range of 0.12–1.2 mm, and the mean diameter as measured by fluorescein angiography ranges from 0.74 to 1.02 mm with an average of 0.94 mm. In diabetic eyes, this is reduced to 0.53–0.73 mm.

Grading of DMI can be done by FFA but it lacks uniformity and is limited by the presence of media opacities. The ETDRS grading of macular ischemia is based on the degree of capillary loss, FAZ size, capillary dilatation, and arteriolar abnormalities and retinal pigment epithelial (RPE) defects (ETDRS Report 11). The ETDRS standard photo 2 is used to quantify the DMI. The central 2F field is subdivided into 10 subfields and the size of the normal FAZ is 500–600 μm. The margins of the FAZ correspond roughly to the dashed circle of the grid (300 μm).

Mixed maculopathy

In a considerable number of diabetic patients' eyes, features of both exudative and ischemic maculopathy may be seen concurrently and the fluorescein findings show features of both types.

Ocular coherence tomogram and DME

OCT is playing an increasing role in diagnosis and management of DME in spite of substantial disagreement on the OCT and the ETDRS definitions of CSME (Danis & Hubbard 2011). The OCT measures the macular edema, compact retinal thickening, intraretinal cystic changes, and subretinal fluid. It detects hard exudates in its early stage even before their clinical appearance as hyper-reflective dots. The presence of serous detachments, vitreomacular traction, and thickness of the photoreceptor outer segments (POS) cannot be detected clinically and are demonstrated clearly by the OCT (Alasil et al. 2010). The high-resolution B-scan OCT picks up early changes in the retinal morphology even in the absence of visual loss or other clinical signs. The OCT is also invaluable in monitoring the progress and response to treatment with both laser photocoagulation and anti-VEGF agents and has also been used for the screening of diabetic retinopathy (Bernardes et al. 2011). Currently, the spectral domain OCT scanner (SD-OCT) is the best type available for clinical use. The OCT classification of DME shows five distinct patterns (Kim et al. 2006):

1. Diffuse sponge-like retinal thickening is seen as increased retinal thickness ≥ 200 μm with reduced intraretinal reflectivity and expanded areas of lower reflectivity, especially in the outer retinal layers ≥ 200 μm in width. The outer retina is the predominant location of fluid in DME. Well-demarcated hyper-reflective dots or foci may be seen in the walls of intraretinal microaneurysms and scattered throughout all retinal layers forming confluent plaques

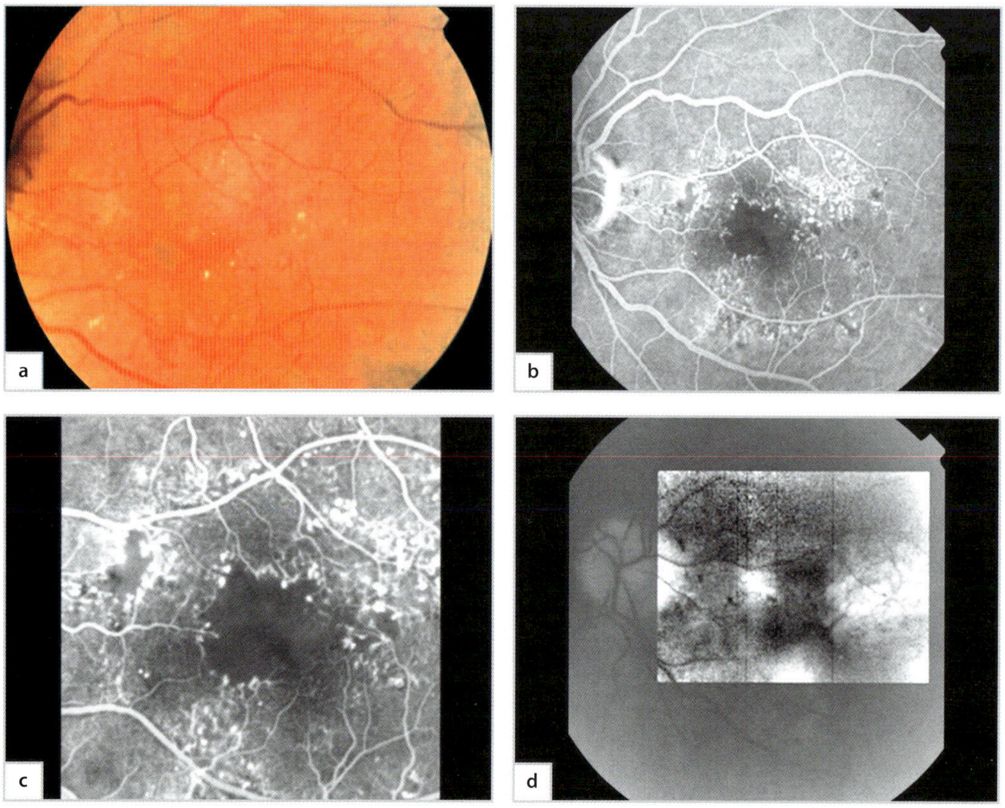

Figure 14.10 Ischemic diabetic maculopathy. (a) The left eye shows only a few red dots, possible microaneurysms associated with minimal degree of lipid exudate. (b) The arteriovenous phase of the fluorescein angiogram shows wide scattering of the microaneurysms, surrounding the macular area. Note that the perifoveal arcade is hugely distorted due to capillary loss. (c) The enlarged view of the macular area shows the capillary dilatation, tortuosity, and microaneurysms, surrounding the macular area with several areas of extended capillary loss. The perifoveal arcade is irregular and has lost its normal pattern due to capillary closure of the perifoveal arcade, a sign of severe ischemia of the fovea. (d) The late phase shows some leakage of dye from the lateral and medial aspect of the macula. However, the leakage is only moderate due to ischemia.

in the outer plexiform layer, which correspond to the areas of hard exudates (**Figures 14.11a** and **b** and **14.12**) (Bolz et al. 2009). These dots may be seen in the absence of clinically apparent hard exudates (and may represent extravasated lipoproteins, an early subclinical barrier breakdown sign in DME) (Ota et al. 2010). Eyes with moderate macular thickening of 300–400 μm) benefit most from laser treatment (Eastbrook et al. 2007)

2. CME is characterized by round or oval areas of low reflectivity with highly reflective septae, separating the cystic cavities located within the intraretinal cystic spaces (**Figure 14.13**). These are usually present in the outer nuclear and outer plexiform layers. There is no correlation between cystic spaces and visual acuity. Initially, these spaces are discrete and uniform in size but later coalesce to form a dome-shaped macular elevation
3. Serous retinal detachment is defined as an accumulation of subretinal fluid that appears dark beneath a highly reflective detached retinal elevation resembling a dome (**Figure 14.14**). The highly reflective posterior border of detached retina differentiates subretinal from intraretinal fluid. Detection of subretinal fluid (SRF) is as important as these eyes are unresponsive to a grid laser to attain flattening with anti-VEGF prior to laser photocoagulation. The height of serous retinal detachment does not correlate with retinal thickening or severity of DME, but is associated with microalbuminuria or overt nephropathy (Gaucher et al. 2008)
4. Taut posterior hyaloid membrane is defined as a highly reflective signal arising from the inner retinal surface and extending toward the optic nerve and toward peripheral retina (**Figure 14.15a–c**). This represents the thickened posterior hyaloid and may be seen in about 4% of eyes with DME. This entity is diagnosed only by OCT and does not respond to conventional laser or antiVEGF therapy but is best treated with vitrectomy and peeling of the membrane (Thomas et al. 2005)
5. Traction macular detachment at the fovea is defined as a peak-shaped detachment of the retina in the macular area, arising as a result of the pull or traction exerted by the posterior hyaloid interface or epiretinal membranes. This may be responsible for persistent DME after focal laser treatment (**Figure 14.16a–d**)

The OCT is a modest predictor of visual acuity in patients with DME, and POS is a key predictor of the visual function and visual acuity. Eyes where OCT demonstrates higher reflectivity of the inner retinal layers achieve better visual acuity, and conversely lower optical reflectivity represents atrophy and is a predictor of poor visual acuity. This may help in predicting the response to intravitreal therapies and help in preoperative counseling of patients.

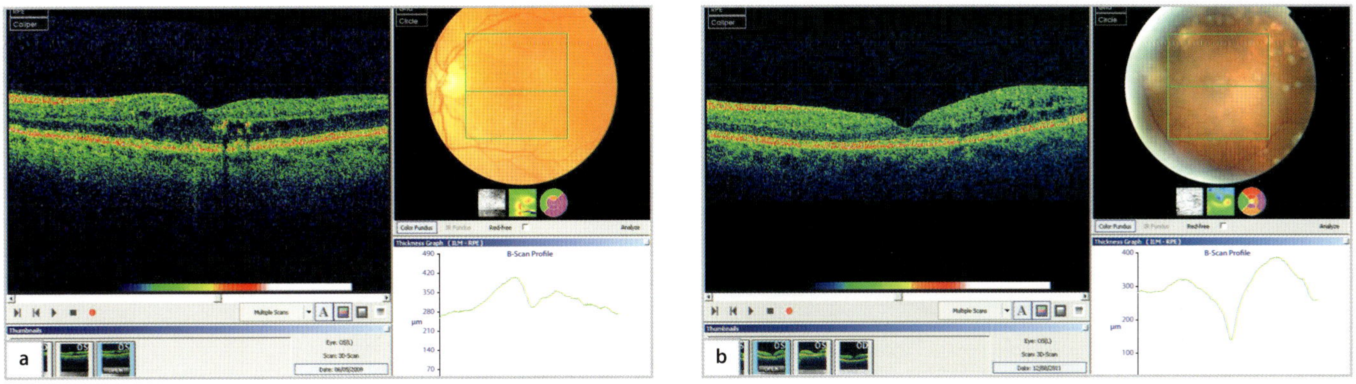

Figure 14.11 Spongiform diabetic macular edema. (a) Ocular coherence tomogram of the left macula shows fluid thickening of the outer retinal layers in the foveal area, causing reduction in optical backscatter. (b) Ocular coherence tomogram of the left macula shows fluid accumulation in the outer retinal layers, temporal to the fovea resulting in spongiform macular edema.

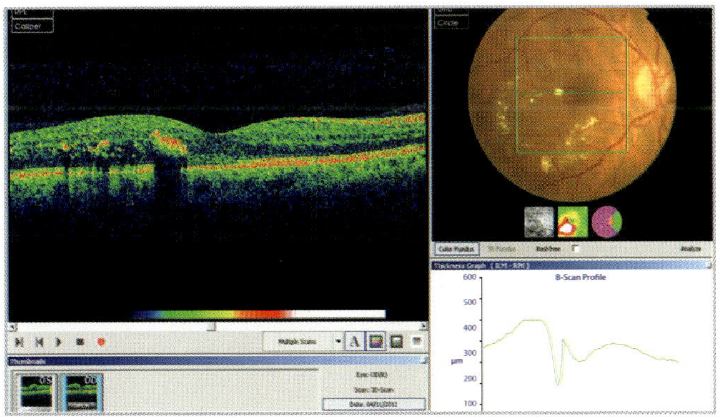

Figure 14.12 Diabetic macular edema with hard exudate. Ocular coherence tomogram of the right macula shows hyper-reflective dots in the outer retinal layers, corresponding to the hard exudates.

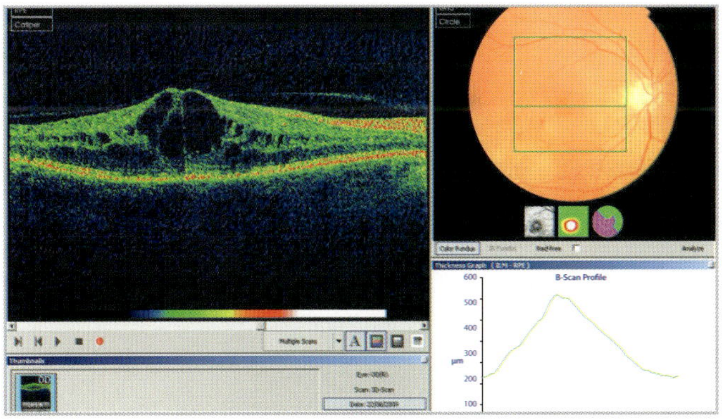

Figure 14.13 Cystoid macular edema. Ocular coherence tomogram of the right eye shows macular thickening with several large cystoid spaces with intervening septae separating them. The vitreous is still attached at the fovea, although it is separated on either side of it.

The OCT can detect ischemic changes, especially in the early stages. In diabetic eyes, the pericentral retinal thickness is reduced due to ischemic neurosensory tissue loss, even before the retinopathy is detected clinically. Retinal nerve fiber layer is significantly decreased in preproliferative retinopathy. In the absence of edema, the ischemic areas in the retina appear thinner. Coexisting macular edema makes OCT interpretation complicated. Epiretinal membranes and DMEO cause retinal thickening and formation of cystic changes, masking underlying ischemia that cannot be detected by the OCT. The other consequence from this phenomenon is underlying distortion between visual acuity and macular thickness due to ischemia.

There is some correlation between the findings on fluorescein angiography and OCT in DME. The severity of dye leakage compares positively with the severity of outer retinal edema (Brar et al. 2010).

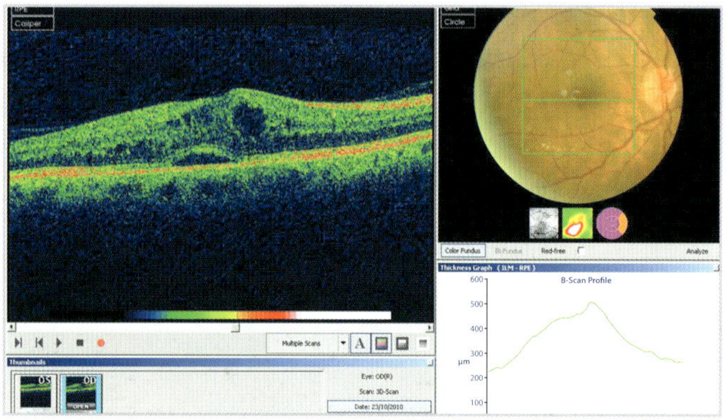

Figure 14.14 Cystoid macular edema with serous retinal detachment. Ocular coherence tomogram of the right eye shows cystoid spaces over an area of hyporeflectivity due to a serous detachment of the macula.

Cystic changes in the outer and inner retina are also correlated with severity of fluorescein leakage. Large foveal cysts in the outer nuclear layer and outer plexiform layers on SD-OCT correspond to cystoid leakage patterns in fluorescein angiography. A honeycomb pattern of leakage on angiography matches to the swelling and cystic spaces in the inner nuclear layers of the retina. Diffuse patterns of hyperfluorescence did not correlate with the changes on high-definition OCT (HD-OCT). The loss of inner retinal layers specifically correlates with capillary nonperfusion and severe ischemia, and therefore is a poor prognostic factor (Bolz et al. 2009). Although both HD-OCT and fluorescein angiography are highly sensitive techniques and correlate well in the detection of DME, there is a small chance that when performed alone, they might miss existing subtle DME.

MICROPERIMETRY

Perimetry can provide useful information on functional visual loss beyond visual acuity. There is decrease in retinal sensitivity in diabetic eyes even before diabetic retinopathy is detected clinically, thus it may be a predictor of development of diabetic retinopathy (Vujosevic et al. 2006). Short-wave automated perimetry (SWAP) is considered to be more sensitive than standard automated perimetry (SAP) as it isolates the blue-yellow neural pathway. There is a good correlation between areas of ischemia on FFA to areas of decreased retinal sensitivity on SWAP. The SWAP can detect visual field defects, which worsen with progression of diabetic retinopathy and probably reflect ischemia rather than edema.

With the introduction of fundus-related perimetry, known as microperimetry, macular sensitivity can be linked with the precise location of diabetic change. Microperimetry demonstrates loss of retinal sensitivity in ischemic areas and decreased sensitivity at the borders of ischemia. Therefore, microperimetry is useful in evaluating the sites

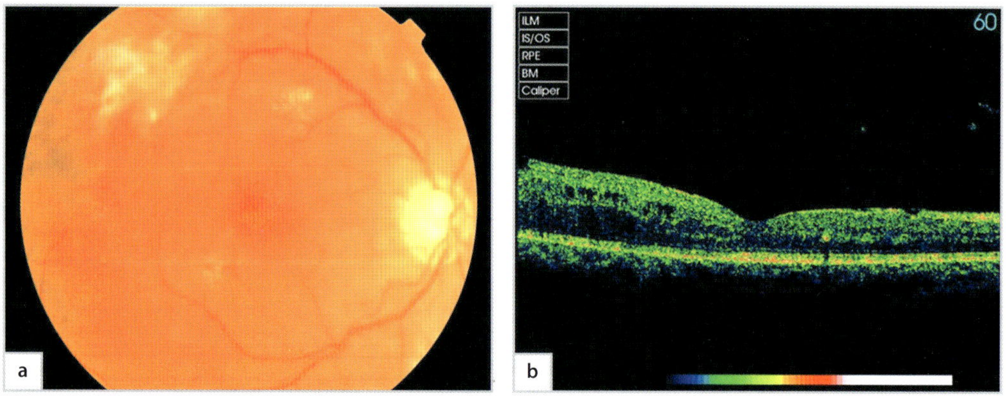

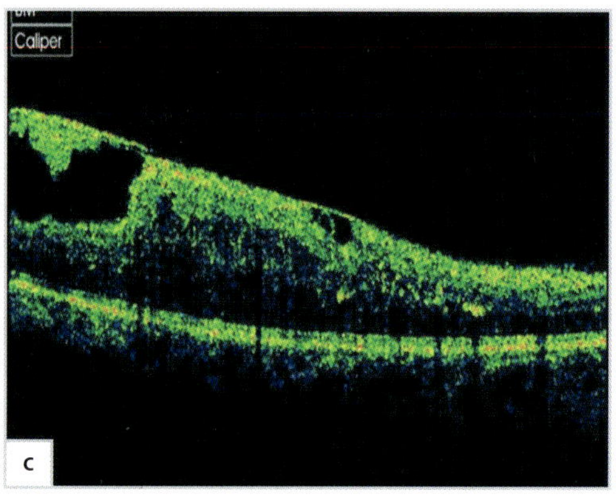

Figure 14.15 Taut thickened posterior hyaloid face. (a) The right eye shows macular edema associated with a taut and thickened posterior hyaloid face. (b) Ocular coherence tomogram of the right eye shows increased retinal thickening and a taut posterior hyaloid membrane. (c) The ocular coherence tomogram of the temporal periphery of the fundus nearer to the epiretinal membrane shows typical thickening due to a taut hyaloid face.

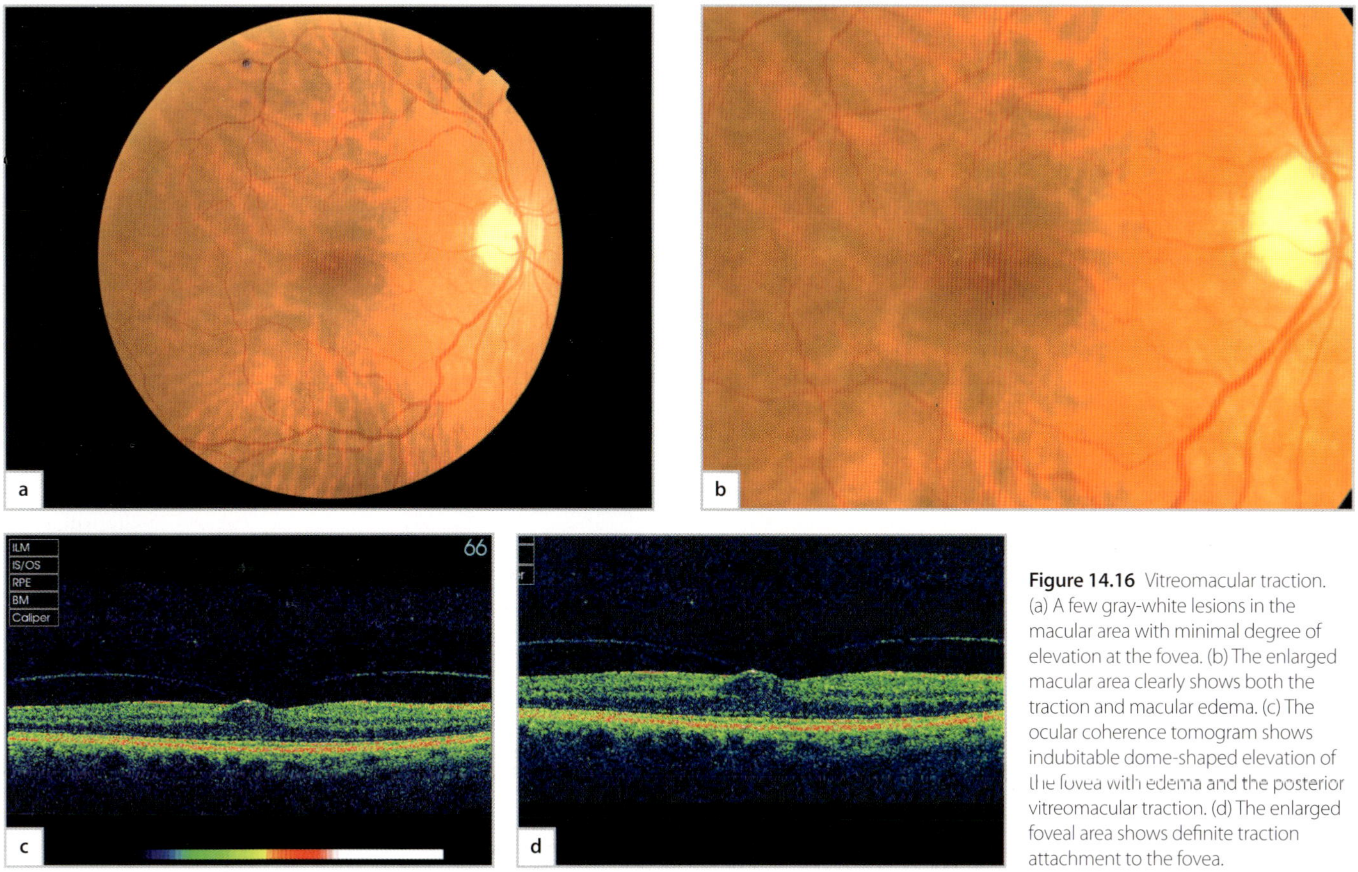

Figure 14.16 Vitreomacular traction. (a) A few gray-white lesions in the macular area with minimal degree of elevation at the fovea. (b) The enlarged macular area clearly shows both the traction and macular edema. (c) The ocular coherence tomogram shows indubitable dome-shaped elevation of the fovea with edema and the posterior vitreomacular traction. (d) The enlarged foveal area shows definite traction attachment to the fovea.

of relative and absolute scotoma and fixation characteristics. These parameters have been useful in quantifying and predicting functional impact of macular edema and other disorders. Macular sensitivity and the fixation pattern in DME can be quantified by using the automatic technique of microperimetry related to macular thickness determined by OCT. Macular edema can be better outlined by measuring macular sensitivity using microperimetry then using OCT and visual acuity as measures of macular sensitivity. Therefore, microperimetry is valuable in predicting the outcome in DME. Microperimetry is also of great help in treating CSME with the less aggressive subthreshold micropulse diode laser (MPDL) as it preserves the retinal sensitivity.

FUNDUS AUTOFLUORESCENCE

Fundus autofluorescence (FAF) has been used in the recent years as an imaging technique to evaluate macular disorders. FAF is thought to derive from lipofuscin in RPE cells, reflecting some aspect of RPE function and integrity. In the macular area, the FAF signal is reduced at the fovea because of its absorption by the luteal pigment, whereas the signal is relatively increased in the parafoveal area, although it is still reduced when compared with the diffuse background signal in the more peripheral retinal areas. FAF showed 81% sensitivity and 69% specificity in detecting CME, offering a rapid and noninvasive technique in the study of this entity. All cases of CME of different cause produce similar changes (Vujosevic et al. 2010). Three different increased patterns of FAF are seen in patients with cystoid DME that relates positively with fluorescein angiography and OCT findings; these are single cyst increased, multicystic increased, and combined single and multicystic increased FAF. The FAF parameters link to both structural and functional parameters more commonly in DME. The presence of increased FAF was associated with functional and structural impairment of the macula. This group of eyes with increased FAF pattern also has poorer macular sensitivity than the normal FAF group. Therefore, the DME with increased FAF pattern is functionally more severe than DME with a normal FAF pattern.

There is a significant link between the presence of increased FAF areas and decreased retinal sensitivity, regardless of visual acuity. There are two hypotheses about the increased FAF areas observed in DME. The first is due to accumulation of oxidative metabolic products induced by activated microglia. The second is related to the mechanical effect of CME: cysts are mostly present in the outer plexiform and inner nuclear layers, where there is a maximum accumulation of luteal pigment, and cysts may displace luteal pigment preventing the normal blockage of foveal FAF signal at the level of each of them, therefore increased FAF may be a pseudo-autofluorescence due to a window defect. FAF is used in conjunction with microperimetry in managing eyes that receive MPDL for treatment of DME.

ULTRASOUND

B-scan ultrasonography is of great use when examining eyes with proliferative retinopathy, especially in the presence of opaque media, and can be invaluable to the vitreoretinal surgeon when planning surgery in these eyes. Vitreous hemorrhage, epiretinal membranes, posterior vitreous detachments, and retinal detachments can be clearly demonstrated by the use of B-scan ultrasound (Mcleod & Restori 1979).

Hemorrhage within the vitreous cavity gives rise to scattered pointlike echoes of varying amplitudes. Arrangement of such echoes in intragel membranes is sometimes observed during sedimentation of hemorrhage within fluid vitreous producing a flat sheet (fluid-level) of very high amplitude echoes. If a sheet of high amplitude echoes, lower in amplitude than sediment blood but showing more internal structure, is detected on the retinal surface the echoes are considered to arise from epiretinal membranes.

Posterior vitreous detachment is indicated by the presence of pointlike echoes confined to the gel compartment or retrohyaloid space. The distinction between these compartments is often emphasized during dynamic studies, the detached gel moving as a corporate body within the fluid retrohyaloid space. Posterior vitreous detachment is indicated by the presence of echoes from the posterior hyaloid interface. If the gel is mobile and contains opacity, echoes along this interface are considered to arise from blood products in the cortical gel. A gradual compaction of such intragel echoes within the posterior hyaloid interface is characteristic of ochre membrane formation. If a fine sheet of high-amplitude echoes is seen arising from the posterior hyaloid interface with a rigid gel boundary, the posterior hyaloid membrane is considered to be fibrocellular in nature. However, if a thicker sheet of high-amplitude echoes is seen arising from the rigid gel boundary, the posterior hyaloid membrane is considered to be fibrovascular in nature. Occasionally, several different types of membrane are found in the same eye. Posterior vitreous detachment can be complete or incomplete. If incomplete, there might only be a single vitreoretinal adhesion, which is often stalk like.

Multiple vitreoretinal adhesions are also demonstrable, especially by consecutive serial scanning of various levels within the eye. Retinal detachment is demonstrated by membrane-like echoes of high amplitude, which tether at the ora serrate and, if total, at the optic nerve head. Some retinal detachments show undulating movements on dynamic testing, but movement of the retina is usually restricted or absent. Occasionally, a fibrotic posterior hyaloid membrane tethering at the optic nerve head can mimic a total retinal detachment in topography and in echo amplitude. Ultrasound is not of much benefit in detecting nonproliferative diabetic retinopathy or macular edema.

ELECTROPHYSIOLOGY

This is not routinely used in the diagnosis of diabetic retinopathy, although it can provide an objective measurement of clinical and fluorescein angiographic findings of diabetic retinopathy. There is a good corelation between the progressive retinal dysfunction seen on electroretinogram (ERG) and the progression of diabetic microangiopathy. Multifocal ERG, which is used to study macular dysfunction, does not localize well to the areas of pathology, possibly due to the presence of underlying macular ischemia. Foveal cone ERG parameters are seen to be abnormal in diabetic retinopathy and the severity corelates with the degree of retinal thickness. Electrophysiology does not allow any distinction between DME and DMI.

IMAGING FOR DIABETIC RETINOPATHY SCREENING

Currently, diabetic retinopathy screening is mainly done by digital fundus photography, which is then graded and screened by trained experts. To increase the efficiency of diabetic retinopathy screening and to be able to deal with the anticipated rapid rise in the number of people with diabetes, private and public health authorities may consider alternative methods of screening for diabetic retinopathy.

The adoption of digital camera technology with automated detection systems, such as Eye Check and Challenge 2009, may fulfill the current and future needs of diabetic retinopathy screening. Both these systems detect early changes of diabetic retinopathy, such as microaneurysms and hemorrhages. It would be right to anticipate that automated systems based on algorithms will allow cost-effective early detection and diagnosis of diabetic retinopathy in a large population with diabetes and enable triage of patients who need further investigations (Abramoff et al. 2010). Screening systems are unable to detect early ischemic changes.

OCT has also been used to perform screening for diabetic retinopathy in the community, with varying success. In summary, retinal imaging for diabetic retinopathy encompasses a wide variety of modalities, which help us to understand its pathology and presentation, to diagnose and prognosticate the disease and manage it effectively. These techniques are in the process of being refined even further to be able to detect a wider aspect of retinal vascular and photoreceptor dysfunction at a cellular level and during the early stages before the disease becomes clinically apparent.

REFERENCES

Abramoff MD, Reinhardt JM, Russel SR, et al. Automated early detection of diabetic retinopathy. *Ophthalmology* 2010; **117**:1147–1154.

Alasil T, Keane PA, Updike JF, et al. Relationship between optical coherence tomography retinal parameters and visual acuity in diabetic macular edema. *Ophthalmology* 2010; **117**:2379–2386.

Ashton N. Vascular changes in diabetes with particular reference to the retinal vessels: preliminary report. *Br J Ophthalmol* 1949; **33**:407–420.

Ashton N. Arteriolar involvement in diabetic retinopathy. *Br J Ophthalmol* 1953; **37**:282–292.

Baskin DE. Optical coherence tomography in diabetic macular oedema. *Curr Opin Ophthalmol* 2010; **21**:172–177.

Bernardes R, Serranho P, Lobo C. Digital ocular fundus imaging: a review. *Ophthalmologica* 2011; **226**:161–181.

Bolz M, Ritter M, Schneider M, et al. A systematic correlation of angiography and high-resolution optical coherence tomography in diabetic macular oedema. *Ophthalmology* 2009; **116**:66–72.

Bolz M, Schmidt-Erfurth U, Deak G, et al. Ocular coherence tomographic hyperreflective foci: a morphologic sign of lipid extravasation in Diabetic macular oedema. *Ophthalmology* 2009; **116**:914–920.

Brar M, Yuson R, Kozak I, et al. Correlation between morphologic features on spectral domain optical coherence tomography and angiographic leakage patterns in macular edema. *Retina* 2010; **30**:383–389.

Early Treatment of Diabetic Retinopathy Research Group. Classification of diabetic retinopathy from fluorescein angiograms. ETDRS report number 11. Early Treatment Diabetic Retinopathy Study Research Group. *Ophthalmology* 1991; **98**:807–822.

Cogan D, Toussant D, Kubawara T. Retinal vascular patterns. IV Diabetic retinopathy. *Arch Ophthalmol* 1961; **66**:366–378.

Danis RP, Hubbard LD. Imaging of diabetic retinopathy and diabetic macular edema. *Curr Diab Rep* 2011; **11**:236–243.

Danis RP, Scott IU, Qin H, et al. Diabetic retinopathy Clinical research network. Association of fluorescein angiographic features with visual acuity and with optical coherence tomographic and stereoscopic colour fundus photographic features of diabetic macular edema in a randomized clinical trial. *Retina* 2010; **30**:1627–1637.

Early Treatment of Diabetic Retinopathy Study Research Group. Photocoagulation for diabetic macular oedema. ETDRS report number 4. *Invest Ophthalmol Clin* 1987; **27**:265–272.

Early Treatment of Diabetic Retinopathy Study Research Group. The ETDRS Study: design and baseline patient characteristics. ETDRS report number 7. *Ophthalmology* 1991; **98**:741–756.

Eastbrook EJ, Madusudana KC, Hannan SR, Newsom RS. Can optical coherence tomography predict the outcome of laser photocoagulation for diabetic macular edema. *Ophthalmic Surg Lasers Imaging* 2007; **38**:478–483.

Gaucher D, Sebah C, Erginay A, et al. Optical coherence tomography features during the evolution of serous retinal detachment in patients with diabetic macular edema. *Am J Ophthalmol* 2008; **145**:289–296.

Ghazi NJ, Ciralsky JB, Shah SM, et al. Optical coherence tomography findings in persistent diabetic macular edema: the vitreomacular interface. *Am J Ophthalmol* 2007; **144**:747–754.

Kim BY, Smith SD, Kaiser PK. Optical coherence tomographic patterns of diabetic macular edema. *Am J Ophthalmol* 2006; **142**:405–412.

Kohner EM 1969. Cottonwool spots in diabetic retinopathy. Proceedings of the Royal Society of Medicine,62(12),1269–1271

Kohner EM, Dollery CT. Fluorescein angiography of the fundus in diabetic retinopathy. *Br Med Bull* 1970; **26**:166–170.

McLeod D, Restori M. Ultrasonic examination in diabetic Eye disease. *Br J Ophthalmol* 1979; **63**:533–538.

Norton EW, Gutman F. Diabetic retinopathy studied by fluorescein angiography. *Trans Am Ophthalmol Soc* 1965; **63**:108–128.

Ota M, Nishijima K. Sakamoto A, et al. Optical coherence tomographic evaluation of foveal hard exudates in patients with diabetic maculopathy accompanying macular detachment. *Ophthalmology* 2010; **117**:1996–2002.

Otani T, Kishi S. Correlation between optical coherence tomography and fluorescein angiography findings in diabetic macular edema. *Ophthalmology* 2007; **114**:104–107.

Scott JD, Dollery CT, Hill DW, et al. Fluorescein studies of the retinal circulation in diabetics. *Br J Ophthalmol* 1963; **47**:588–589.

Thomas D, Bunce C, Moorman C, Laidlaw AH. Frequency and association of a taut thickened posterior hyaloid, partial vitreomacular separation and subretinal fluid in patients with diabetic macular oedema. *Retina* 2005; **25**:883–888.

Vujosevic S, Bottega E, Casciano M, et al. Microperimetry and fundus autofluorescence in diabetic macular edema: subthreshold micropulse diode laser versus modified early treatment diabetic retinopathy study laser photocoagulation. *Retina* 2010; **30**:908–916.

Vujosevic S, Madena E, Pilotto E, et al. Diabetic macular edema: correlation between microperimetry and ocular coherence tomography findings. *IOVS* 2006; **47**:3044–3051.

Yamana Y, Ohnishi Y, Taniguchi Y, Ikeda M. Early signs of diabetic retinopathy by fluorescein angiography. *Jpn J Ophthalmol* 1983; **27**:218–227.

Chapter 15 Imaging of the optic disc and retinal nerve fiber layer in glaucoma

John Mark S. de Leon, Shamira Perera, Tin Aung

INTRODUCTION

Accurate evaluation of the optic nerve head (ONH) and retinal nerve fiber layer (RNFL) are an essential part of the management of patients with suspected glaucoma and patients with established glaucoma. Even though the mainstay of clinical practice is still careful stereoscopic optic disc evaluation, several new imaging devices provide excellent adjuncts to the diagnosis and follow-up of glaucoma. These offer considerable advantages over previous methods (drawings and photographs) for recording and monitoring the appearance of the ONH and the RNFL. However, the printed outputs of these devices merely provide valuable measurement information that should be integrated with and taken in the context of other clinical findings and not used in isolation to make management decisions in glaucoma.

The ONH and RNFL are biological structures and therefore exhibit wide variation within the normal population. Imaging devices often have an integrated database of measurements from normal eyes, and the structural measurements of the patient's ONH/RNFL are statistically compared with the database and abnormalities flagged up. It should be noted that these are not diagnostic but should be considered only as levels of probability as belonging to normal measurements within the database. Responsibility rests with the operator to key the proper demographic data into the device (e.g. date of birth and ethnicity) for the context of the scan. Conditions other than glaucoma, such as tilted discs, high refractive errors, small or large optic discs, disc hemorrhages, and atypical retardation patterns (ARPs), and inaccurate reference planes may cause measurements to fall outside the normal range. Because of the good reproducibility, accuracy, and precision of measuring discrete structural parameters, the greatest potential of these ONH/RNFL imaging devices lies in their ability to detect subtle changes that are difficult to detect clinically and difficult to follow faithfully over time.

All the available technologies have a proven ability to discriminate well between healthy and glaucomatous nerves (Lin et al. 2007). Studies comparing the different imaging technologies have concluded that they all perform similarly well in diagnosing early glaucoma. However, all are relatively expensive and their technological improvements are constantly in flux to address increasingly exacting clinical demands, while they seek to retain some backward compatibility with previous versions.

In this chapter, the ONH and RNFL that are diseased due to glaucoma shall be illustrated with printouts from the various types of imaging devices [confocal scanning laser ophthalmoscopy (CSLO), scanning laser polarimetry (SLP), and optical coherence tomography (OCT)]. Illustrated actual clinical cases shall be presented to emphasize the utility of these devices and highlight the more important parameters. Common printout assessment pitfalls shall also be illustrated and emphasized for each of the different imaging devices.

CONFOCAL SCANNING LASER OPHTHALMOSCOPY

The Heidelberg Retina Tomograph (HRT; Heidelberg Engineering, Dossenheim, Germany), a CSLO, uses confocal optics (including a 675 nm diode laser) to create a three-dimensional topographic map of the ONH using 16–64 planes (384 × 384 pixels) up to a scan depth of 4 mm (from anterior retinal surface to the lamina cribrosa) so that the ONH's structural parameters can be compared with a normal database and can be evaluated and monitored through time. The HRT-2, compared with the initial version (HRT-1), possesses additional automated features such as serial scans, scan averaging, fine focus, and scan depth. Both devices require the operator to outline the disc border at the scleral rim, but the latest version (HRT-3) has an operator-independent disc delineation system. In addition, the new HRT-3 software has a higher analytic accuracy, larger normative, and ethnic-specific database that adjusts to age-related ONH changes and optic disc size (Zangwill et al. 2007). The new scaling and alignment algorithm improves HRT-3's ability to measure stereometric parameters such as area and volume-based measurements, height variation contour, and RNFL cross-sectional area, and also improves the progression analyses (Ferreras et al. 2008). ONH parameters are then quantified as they relate to the reference plane (defined as that plane 50 μm below the neuroretinal rim as measured along the contour line at the inferior papillomacular bundle) (Lin et al. 2007). The neuroretinal rim is considered above and the cup below this arbitrary reference plane.

HRT-3 image quality is acceptable if the topographic standard deviation (**Figure 15.1**) is < 40 μm, but better quality images are obtained with values < 20 μm. Standard deviation alone, however, does not assure a good quality image and the clinician must further examine the HRT image for artifacts. A good quality HRT image has a well-centered optic disc, even illumination, minimal movement, good focus, and no doubling of vessels. A reflectance image **Figure 15.1** of the ONH is created in which darker colors represent elevated structures, and lighter colors represent depressed structures.

When assessing the HRT-3 printout to identify whether the ONH stereometric parameters fall outside the normal range, it is important to focus on only a few quantitative parameters because of the overwhelming amount of data. Of these parameters, the rim area and cup shape measure **Figure 15.1** are the most useful parameters that aid in discrimination between normal and glaucomatous eyes (Wollstein et al. 1998).

The Moorfield's regression analysis (MRA) (**Figure 15.1**) is the most commonly used glaucoma detection algorithm for measuring neural rim area in a number of sectors around the optic disc and compares these with predicted values adjusted for disc area and age. The MRA (seen as red and green histograms in the HRT-1 and -2) (**Figure 15.1**) classifies the ONH's specific six sectors (also seen on the reflectance map) as 'normal' (a green check mark), 'borderline' (a yellow exclamation mark), or 'outside normal limits' (a red cross based on the ratio of rim area to disc area based on a normative database). This regression analysis compensates for age and identifies glaucomatous eyes with a relatively high level of sensitivity and specificity (clinic-based studies) (Wollstein et al. 2000, Miglior et al. 2003, De Leon-Ortega et al. 2007), and thus makes it attractive for glaucoma screening, but only within certain limits of disc area and age.

Very large and very small ONHs can also confuse the MRA (Coops et al. 2006, Zangwill et al. 2007), and results in these cases must be interpreted with caution. The first stereometric parameter that the HRT provides is the disc area (mm^2) measurement, which is very useful in identifying small discs or further assessing asymmetric discs (**Figure 15.2**). Small discs tend to be overlooked in glaucoma screening because they usually have small cups, and glaucoma may be underdiagnosed. In this case the HRT and OCT show that these small and asymmetric discs have thinning of the neuroretinal rim and confirm glaucomatous optic neuropathy.

Big discs (**Figure 15.3**) also have a tendency to have big cups, and the HRT will give information about the exact size of the disc and the status of the rim, and in this case the HRT (normal rim parameters) confirms the impression that we are dealing with a case of physiological cupping. In contrast (**Figure 15.4**), a large disc may appear glaucomatous clinically and be flagged by the HRT as abnormal but may have a normal visual field exam and in fact have reassuringly normal RNFL with an OCT.

The Glaucoma Probability Score (GPS) is a newer classifier that is similar to the MRA but does not require drawing a contour line on the disc. It is based on a three-dimensional geometric model with three parameters to characterize the ONH (cup size, cup depth, and rim steepness) and two parameters to characterize the RNFL (horizontal RNFL curvature and vertical RNFL curvature). Through vector machine analysis and compared with a normative database, it gives the probability of the disc being glaucomatous. The results are displayed on the printout as 'within normal limits,' 'borderline,' or 'outside normal limits,' both globally and for all six sectors. The GPS

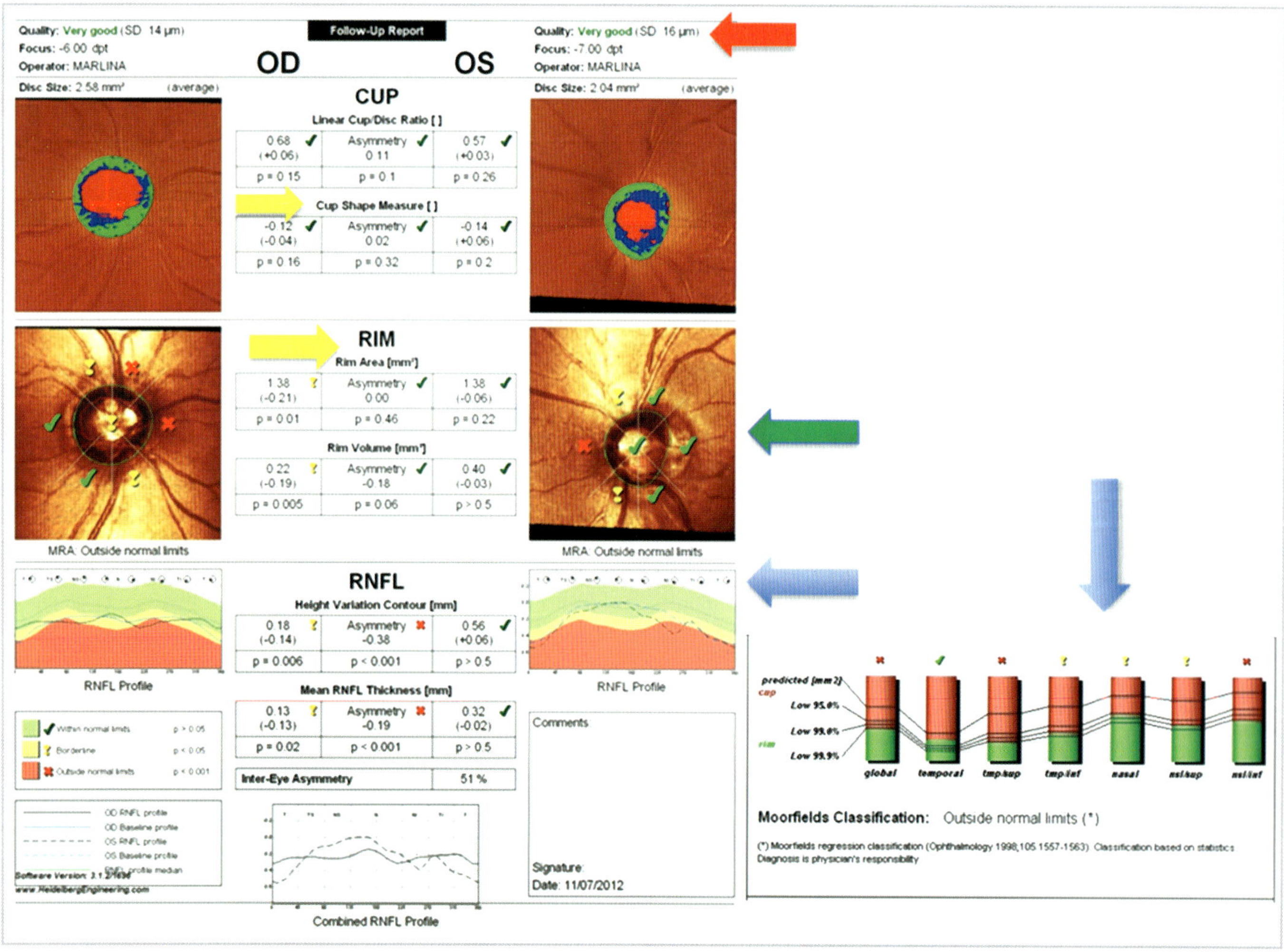

Figure 15.1 The Heidelberg Retina Tomograph 3 printout shows the parameters of the Moorfield's regression analysis (MRA): red arrow—image quality; green arrow—reflectance image; yellow arrows—cup-shaped measure and rim area; blue arrows—MRA.

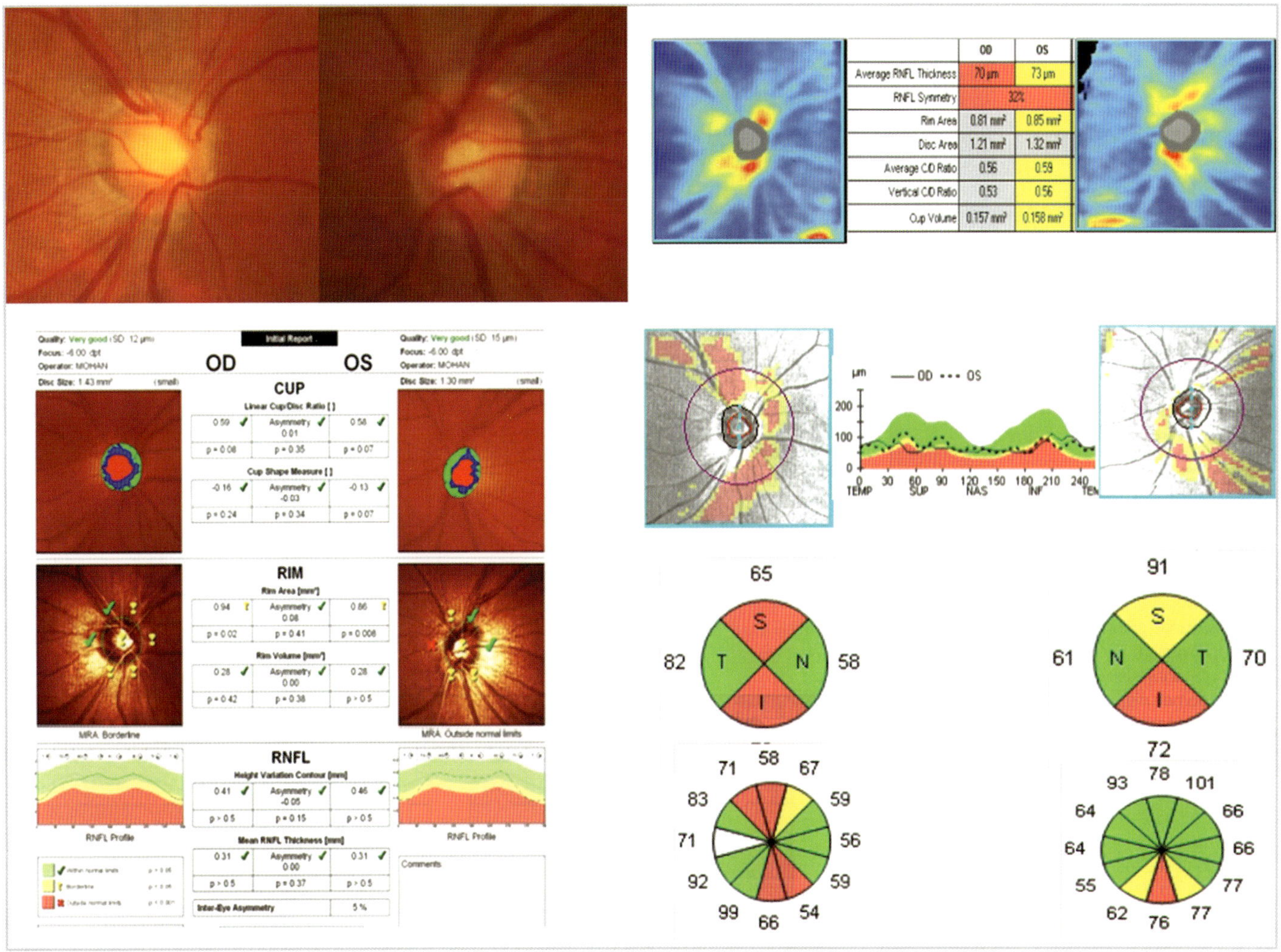

Figure 15.2 Small discs with glaucoma. Heidelberg Retina Tomograph and optical coherence tomography show that these small and asymmetric discs have thinning of the neuroretinal rim and confirm glaucomatous optic neuropathy.

must be viewed from the computer screen because it is not featured in any of the HRT printouts. The GPS and the MRA have similar ability to discriminate between normal and glaucomatous discs.

A test–retest study (Strouthidis et al. 2005) has identified the HRT's rim area as the most repeatable and reliable stereometric parameter, and therefore a good parameter for identifying subtle changes through time (**Figure 15.5**). The HRT-3 software features two algorithms to determine progression—trend analysis and topographical change analysis (TCA). Trend analysis represents progression of a selected parameter (e.g. rim area) over time through a graph from baseline; however, interpretation is empirical and one cannot generate a rate of change. Progression by TCA is determined by statistically estimating the probability that change in height at a pixel is by chance. Progression by TCA is defined as a cluster of 20 or more significantly depressed superpixels within the ONH margin.

SCANNING LASER POLARIMETRY

The RNFL is made of ordered parallel axon bundles containing microtubules, cylindrical intracellular organelles with diameters shorter than the wavelength of light. SLP, which was designed to measure the RNFL thickness, is a CSLO with an integrated polarimeter that measures the amount of retardation (phase shift) of a polarized, near-infrared laser beam as it passes through the RNFL structures. This is the source of birefringence and different patterns of RNFL birefringence are detected when the RNFL is atrophic and thinned in comparison with a healthy thick RNFL. The greater the number of microtubules, the larger the amount of retardation measured by SLP, thus indicating the presence of more nerve fibers.

The fifth-generation GD× VCC (Carl Zeiss Meditec, Inc., Dublin, California, USA) uses a diode laser to generate a retardation map (**Figure 15.6**) produced through the different birefringence patterns. The cornea and, to a lesser extent, the lens also produce significant birefringence, and early attempts at compensating for this error included the fixed corneal compensator (FCC). Because of wide interindividual variability in the axis and magnitude of corneal birefringence, deviation from the preset FCC settings led to incomplete neutralization of corneal birefringence and hence errors in RNFL measurements. The variable corneal compensator (VCC) uses the macula as an internal polarimeter and is better able to compensate for variable anterior segment birefringence (assuming a normal macula for birefringence correction). Another source of error in RNFL mea-

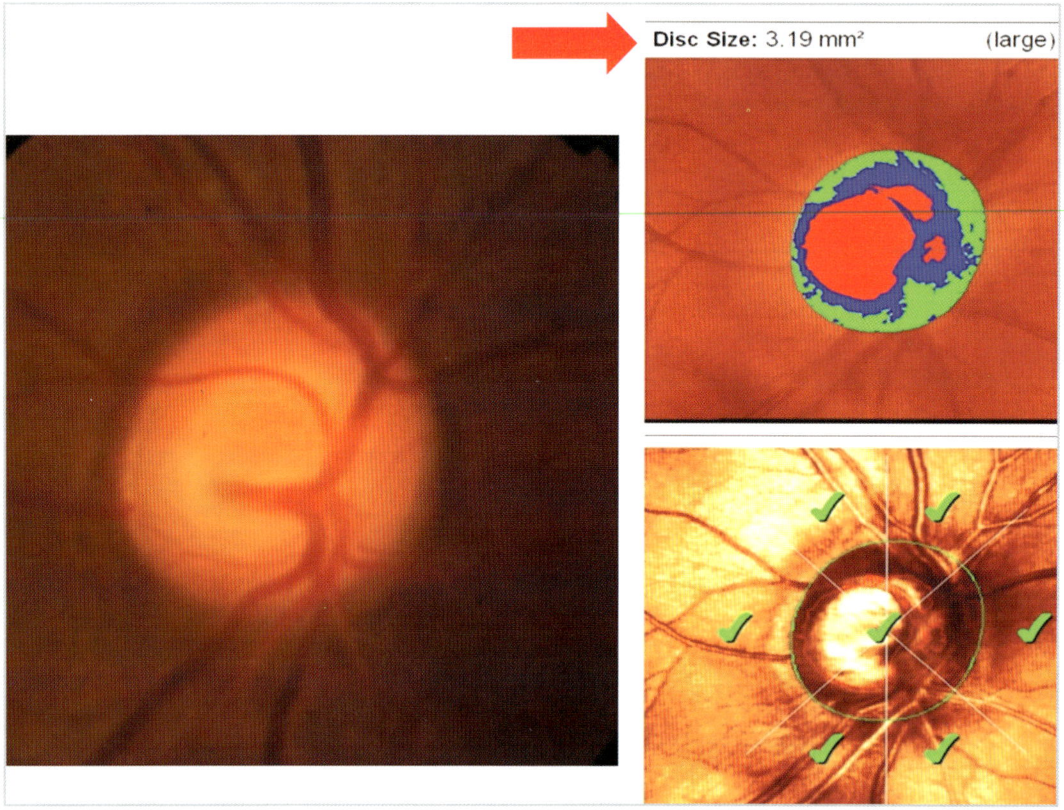

Figure 15.3 Physiological cupping of optic disc in glaucoma.

surement by the GD× is an artifact associated with ARPs. ARPs are due to light scattering and may be seen in glaucomatous eyes and are more frequently observed in older and highly myopic patients (Mai et al. 2007, Lemij & Reus 2008). In order to minimize the ARP, a new algorithm known as enhanced corneal compensation (ECC) has been developed. The new ECC algorithm increases the ability of GD× to discriminate between healthy and glaucomatous patients, especially in those cases with high ARPs and moderate-to-high myopia (Bowd et al. 2007, Lemij & Reus 2008).

When using the GD×, it is preferable that the patient's eyes are not dilated; the room lights can be left on. A near-infrared laser (785 nm wavelength) scans the fundus twice, first to determine anterior segment birefringence and second to image the retina with adjusted compensation. The GD× VCC automatically generates a quality (Q) score between 1 and 10 (**Figure 15.6**) based on several factors (fixation, refraction, and ocular alignment); a score of ≥ 8 is considered acceptable. A high-quality GD× scan has a sharply focused reflectivity image and a 3.2 mm diameter ellipse well-centered on the ONH to generate an RNFL analysis (**Figure 15.6**). Below this is a retardation image shown as a heat map of RNFL thickness with the hotter colors representing greater retardation (and therefore thicker RNFL) values so a normal image will appear as a red upright bow tie pattern (**Figure 15.6**)—bright yellow and red (thicker RNFL) are seen in the superior and inferior arcuate areas following the anatomy of the RNFL bundles, while green and blue (thinner RNFL) are seen in the nasal and temporal sectors. Below this is the statistical deviation map that highlights pixels with retardation values falling below those seen in the normative database. The color of the pixel indicates the level of probability of deviation from the normal database. The temporal-superior-nasal-inferior-temporal (TSNIT) graphs (RNFL profile plots) at the bottom of the printout display the RNFL thickness values around the measurement annulus in relation to the normal range of thickness values. The green- and purple-shaded areas indicate the normal range of thickness values for the left and right eyes, respectively. In between these two graphs with shaded areas is the TSNIT symmetry graph with the right and left eye plots superimposed on each other. Retardation parameters generated automatically by the software are displayed in the top central panel and include values for TSNIT average, superior average, inferior average, TSNIT standard deviation, inter-eye symmetry, and Nerve Fiber Index (NFI). These are also color coded to indicate statistical deviation from the normative database values. Inter-eye symmetry values near 1.0 represent good symmetry and near 0 represent poor symmetry.

Studies (Bowd et al. 2007, Mai et al. 2007) have demonstrated good correlation between GD× measurements and RNFL thickness. Though, better correlations were described for the inferior and superior quadrants, with underestimates in the nasal and temporal sectors (Lemij & Reus 2008). Nevertheless, studies have consistently demonstrated the utility of the GD× to discriminate between healthy and glaucomatous eyes (Bowd et al. 2007, Lemij & Reus 2008). The most discriminating parameter (high specificity and sensitivity) of the GD× to identify glaucoma is the NFI, a support vector machine-derived parameter that represents the overall integrity of the RNFL. The higher the NFI, the more likely the scan comes from a glaucomatous eye. NFI values > 50 are used as cutoff for $p < 1\%$ level and > 30 is used for $p < 5\%$ level. A consensus regarding the definition of an abnormal GD× scan has not been established, but a scan may be considered as abnormal if the TSNIT parameters are outside 95% normal limits and may suggest RNFL atrophy and need for clinical correlation.

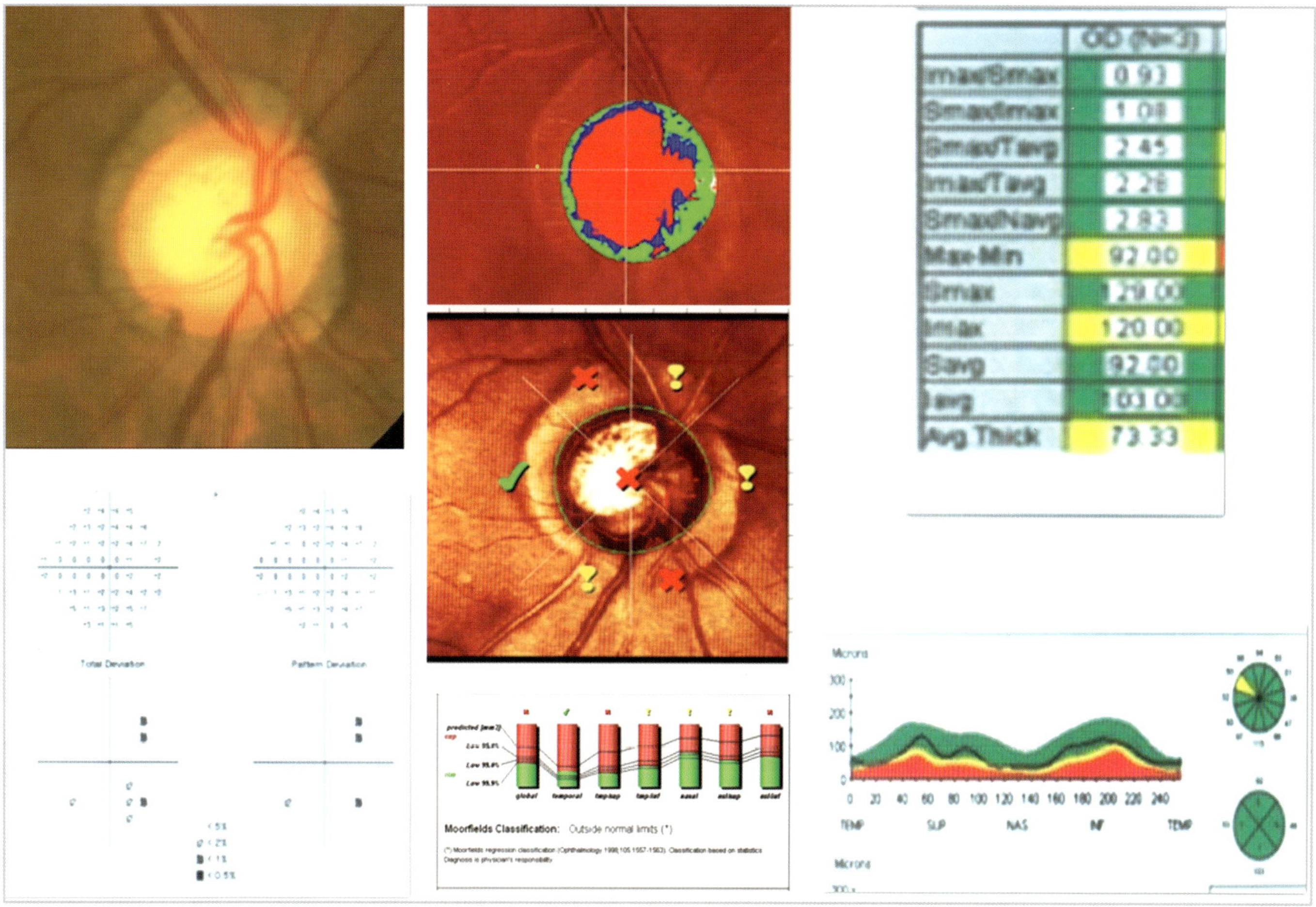

Figure 15.4 Large normal disc flagged as abnormal by the Heidelberg Retina Tomograph may appear glaucomatous, but may have a normal visual field; reassuringly, the retinal nerve fiber layer is normal with an optical coherence tomography.

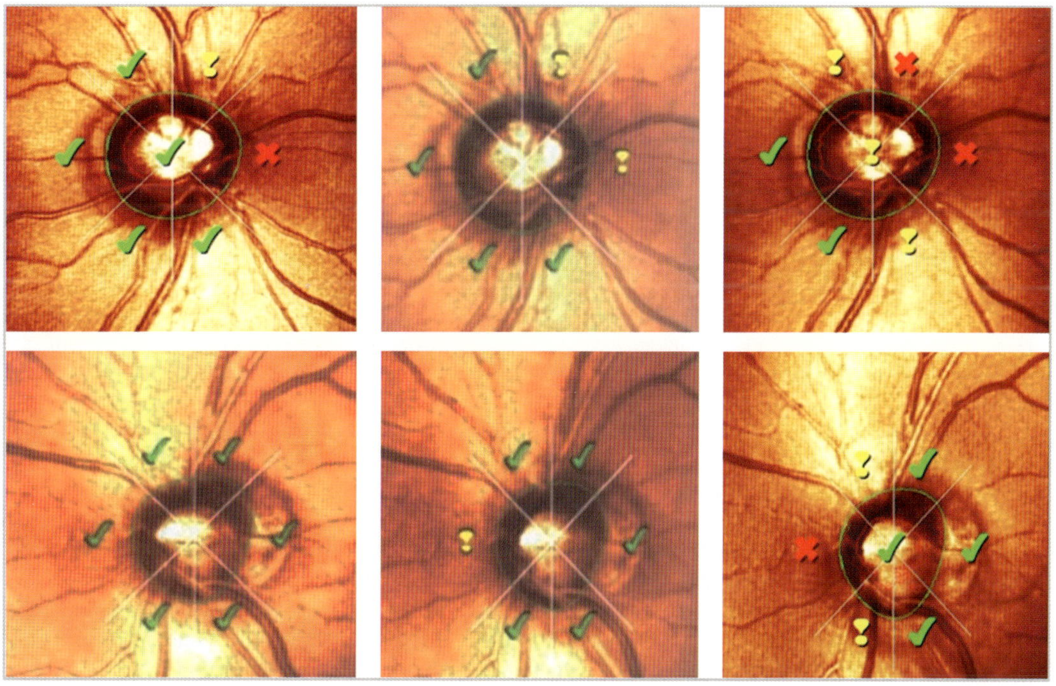

Figure 15.5 A series of Heidelberg Retina Tomograph printouts that highlight bilateral progression of juvenile open angle glaucoma.

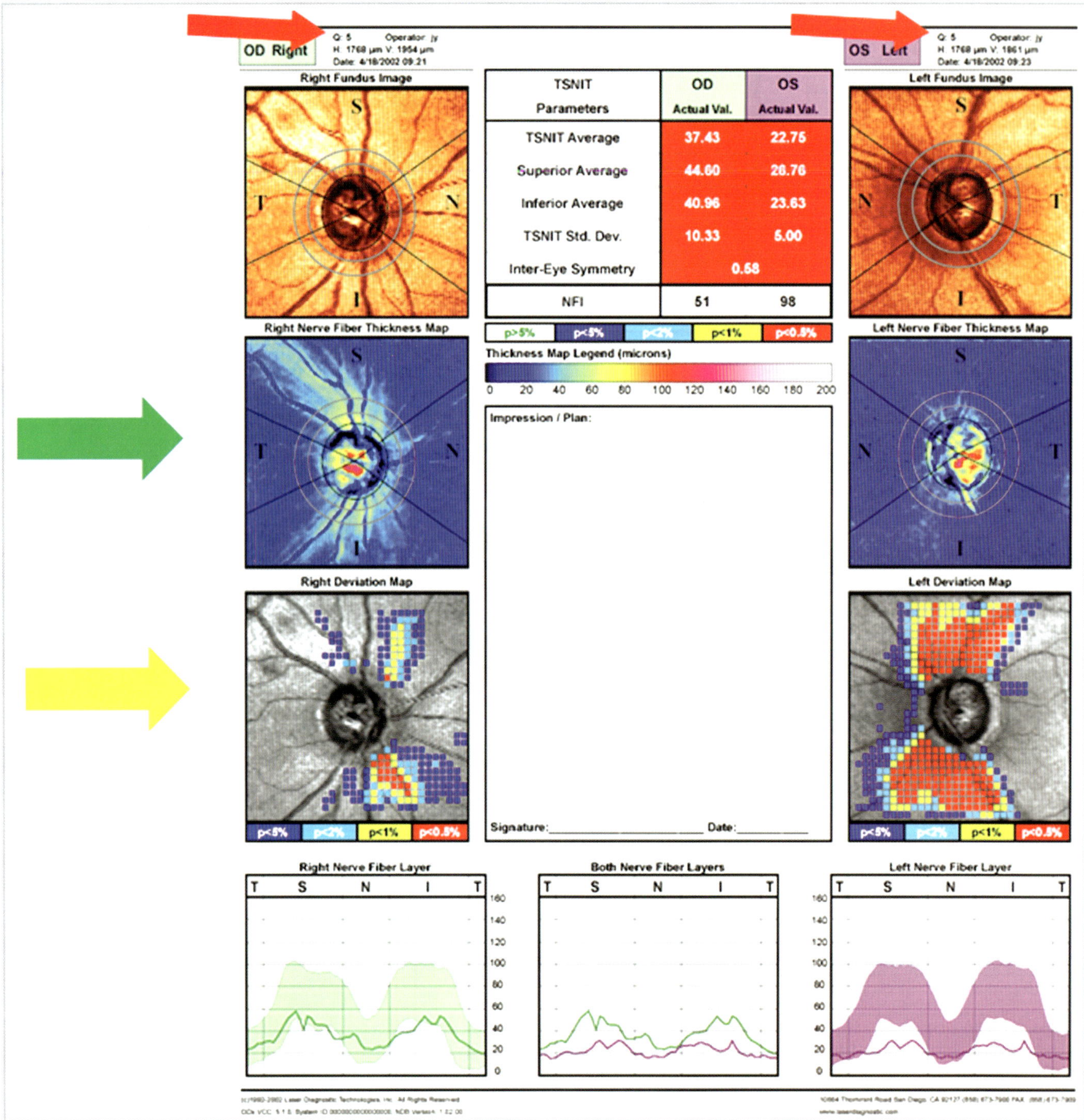

Figure 15.6 GDx VCC print-out: red arrows—image quality (Q) score; Green arrow—RNFL thickness map (yellow, orange, red = thick RNFL; blue, green = thin RNFL); yellow arrow—RNFL deviation map reveals color-coded location and severity of RNFL loss (warm colors = more severe loss; blue colors = less severe loss)

Even in red-free light, it is very difficult to detect discrete RNFL defects clinically or on a photograph, and the GD× detects these defects more readily (**Figure 15.7**). The progression analysis software of the GD× VCC assesses serial images and flags progression if there is detection of change of three consecutive follow-up images compared with an average of two high-quality baseline scans, a manner similar to the Guided Progression Analysis of the Humphrey Field Analyzer (Carl Zeiss Meditec, Inc., Dublin, California, USA). Studies are still needed to validate this progression strategy.

OPTICAL COHERENCE TOMOGRAPHY

OCT is an imaging technology that can image and measure glaucomatous RNFL thinning and allow in vivo noninvasive quantitative evaluation of RNFL thickness. Its principle is analogous to that of ultrasonography, but it uses light instead of sound to acquire high-resolution images of ocular structures. The dimensions of the different

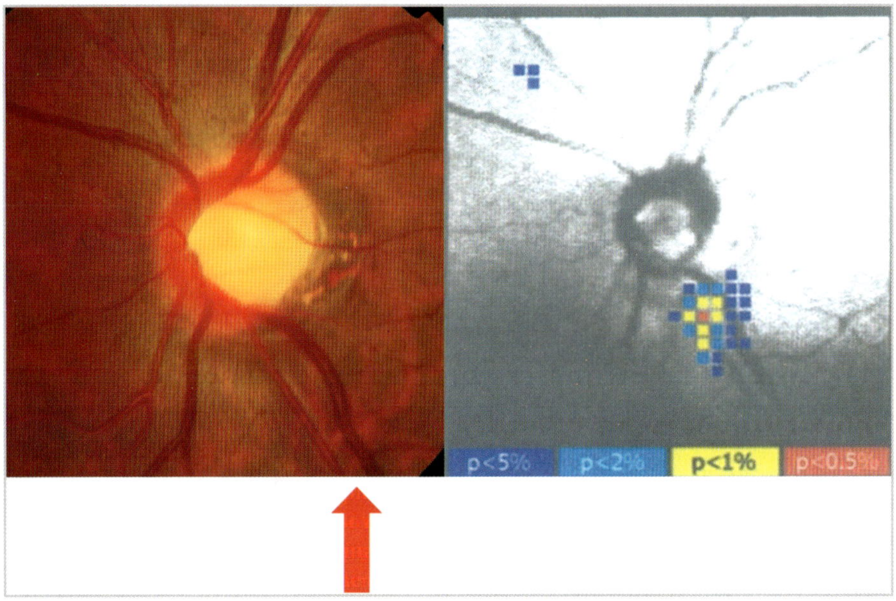

Figure 15.7 It is difficult to detect discrete retinal nerve fiber layer (RNFL) defects clinically using a red–free photograph. However, GDx VCC is better positioned to detect RNFL defects.

ocular structures can be determined by measuring the time it takes for light to be reflected from the different structures. RNFL thickness is determined by measuring the difference in delay of backscattered light from the RNFL inside the imaged tissue. Algorithms pinpoint the RNFL by detecting the anterior edge of the retinal pigment epithelium and determining the photoreceptor layer position that determines the posterior boundary of the RNFL. Each scan of the RNFL is a 360° thickness measurement around the ONH at a fixed distance (usually a diameter of 3.4 mm) to produce almost histologic-like cross-sectional images. The algorithm to detect ONH/RNFL boundaries remains imperfect, especially in cases in which the RNFL reflectance is low, such as in severe glaucoma. A good quality OCT image is well-centered and focused on the ONH. A signal score of 6 is considered just acceptable.

A time domain OCT (TD-OCT) system (Stratus OCT 3, Carl Zeiss Meditec, Inc., Dublin, California, USA) can provide 8–10 μm axial resolution and 512 axial scans in 1.3 seconds using a diode laser to generate a near-infrared (820 nm) light beam that is directed into the eye via a conventional slit-lamp biomicroscope and focused on the retina using a 78-diopter condensing lens. The limitations of the relatively slow standard TD-OCT are partially due to the subject eye motion and inferior resolution. Using best RNFL thickness parameters, TD-OCT has reported sensitivities and specificities for glaucoma diagnosis ranging from 66% to 100%.

For the Stratus OCT (**Figure 15.8**), there are many good reproducibility studies of RNFL thickness (Schuman et al. 1996, Budenz et al. 2007). Several studies have confirmed that RNFL thickness is useful to distinguish mild-to-moderate glaucoma patients from healthy subjects (Medeiros et al. 2005, Wollstein et al. 2005). ONH parameters appear to be less useful and reproducible than RNFL thickness in detecting glaucoma, and they are limited by the lack of morphometric data. Age, ethnicity, axial length, and refractive error (myopia) are known to affect the RNFL thickness measurements. The Stratus OCT overall, inferior quadrant, and superior quadrant RNFL parameters are the most important ones for glaucoma clinical assessment. Movement artifacts, media opacity, high myopia, and severe glaucoma can limit OCT scan measurements and reproducibility (Chang & Budenz 2008).

The Stratus TD-OCT delineates early-to-moderate inferior RNFL loss (also documented with the HRT-3), which correlates well with the visual field loss (**Figure 15.9**). The next-generation Cirrus OCT (Carl Zeiss Meditec, Inc., Inc., Dublin, California, USA) is a spectral domain OCT (SD-OCT) with better resolution and a much faster scan rate. While the TD-OCT collects 400 axial measurements per second with an axial resolution of around 10 μm, the scan rate of SD-OCT is at least 20,000 axial measurements per second with an axial resolution of 5 μm. This serves to reduce motion artifacts, and allows higher resolution three-dimensional imaging. A data cube centered on the ONH is created, made up of 200 B-scans with 200 A-scans per B-scan, generating more than 40 million data points. The high-density three-dimensional data cube is automatically corrected for optic disc tilt and other anatomic anomalies, such as staphylomas. Thus, for myopic and tilted discs, measurements of the optic disc and the rim area correspond to the anatomy in the same plane as the optic disc. The ONH and RNFL analyses generated by the Cirrus high-definition (HD-OCT) provide specific calculations with key parameters displayed in table format (**Figure 15.10**). The color-coded comparison to normative data allows quick determination if it deviates from the age-corrected normal values. The most valuable function of the Cirrus HD-OCT is the evaluation of the RNFL. The RNFL and neuroretinal rim thickness profiles demonstrate symmetry between the two eyes and show the comparison with normative data. The RNFL thickness is also compared with normative data in quadrant and clock hour displays. Quadrants may reveal diffuse thinning, while clock hours may show localized thinning.

The RTVue SD-OCT (Optovue, Inc., Fremont, California, USA) offers the ganglion cell complex (GCC) protocol (**Figure 15.11**) that is designed to measure the inner retinal thickness, including the nerve fiber layer, ganglion cell layer, and the inner plexiform layer, collectively called the GCC. It is believed to be the primary region of affection in glaucoma (Tan et al. 2009). Another SD-OCT, the Spectralis (Heidelberg Engineering, Inc., Dossenheim, Germany), has a faster scan speed of 40,000 A-lines per second and has the advantage of simultaneous real-time imaging with eye-movement tracking with scanners that ensure that the same location of the retina is scanned over time. The Spectralis OCT RNFL thickness printout (**Figure 15.12**) provides the RNFL scan and profile corresponding to a circle of 3.4 mm diameter centered on the optic disc, and the RNFL thickness around

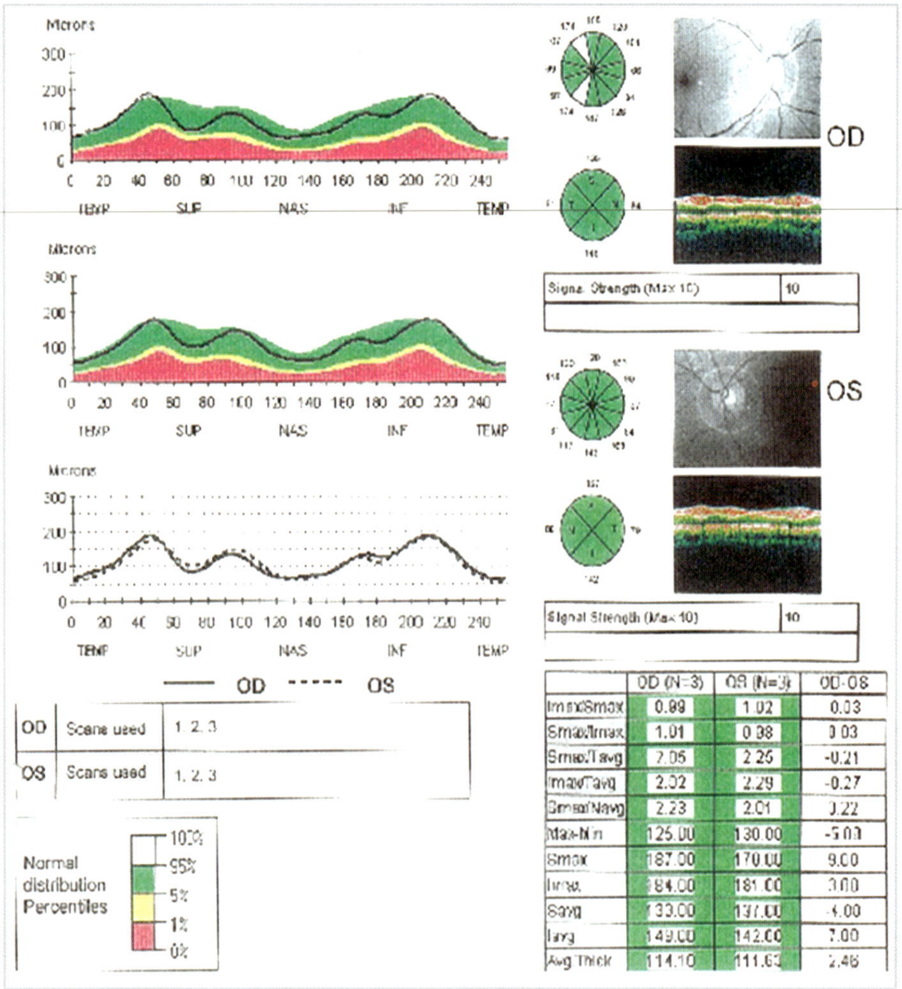

	OD (N=3)	OS (N=3)	OD-OS
Imax/Smax	0.89	1.02	0.03
Smax/Imax	1.01	0.98	0.03
Smax/Tavg	2.05	2.26	-0.21
Imax/Tavg	2.02	2.29	-0.27
Smax/Navg	2.23	2.01	0.22
Max-Min	125.00	130.00	-5.00
Smax	187.00	170.00	9.00
Imax	184.00	181.00	3.00
Savg	133.00	137.00	-4.00
Iavg	149.00	142.00	7.00
Avg Thick	114.10	111.63	2.48

Figure 15.8 The stratus time domain optical coherence tomography printout shows good reproducibility studies of retinal nerve fiber layer thickness.

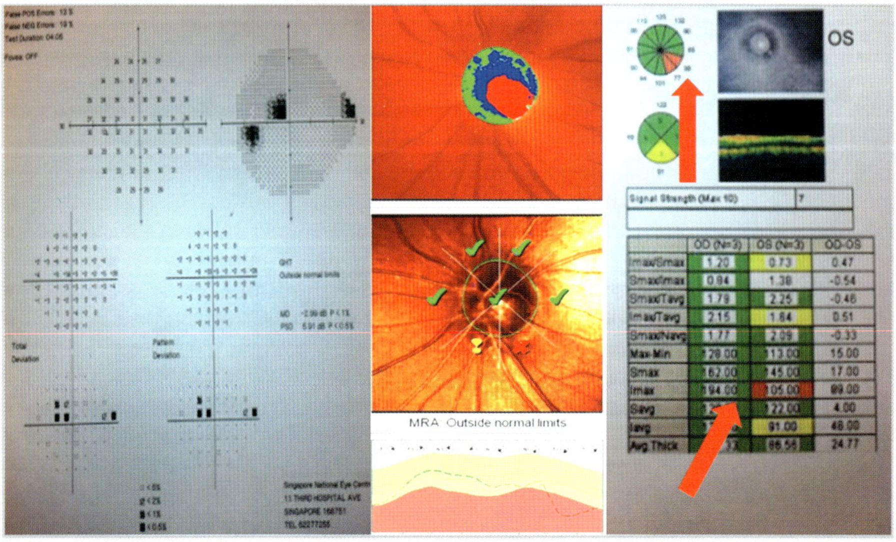

Figure 15.9 Stratus time domain optical coherence tomography delineates early retinal nerve fiber layer loss.

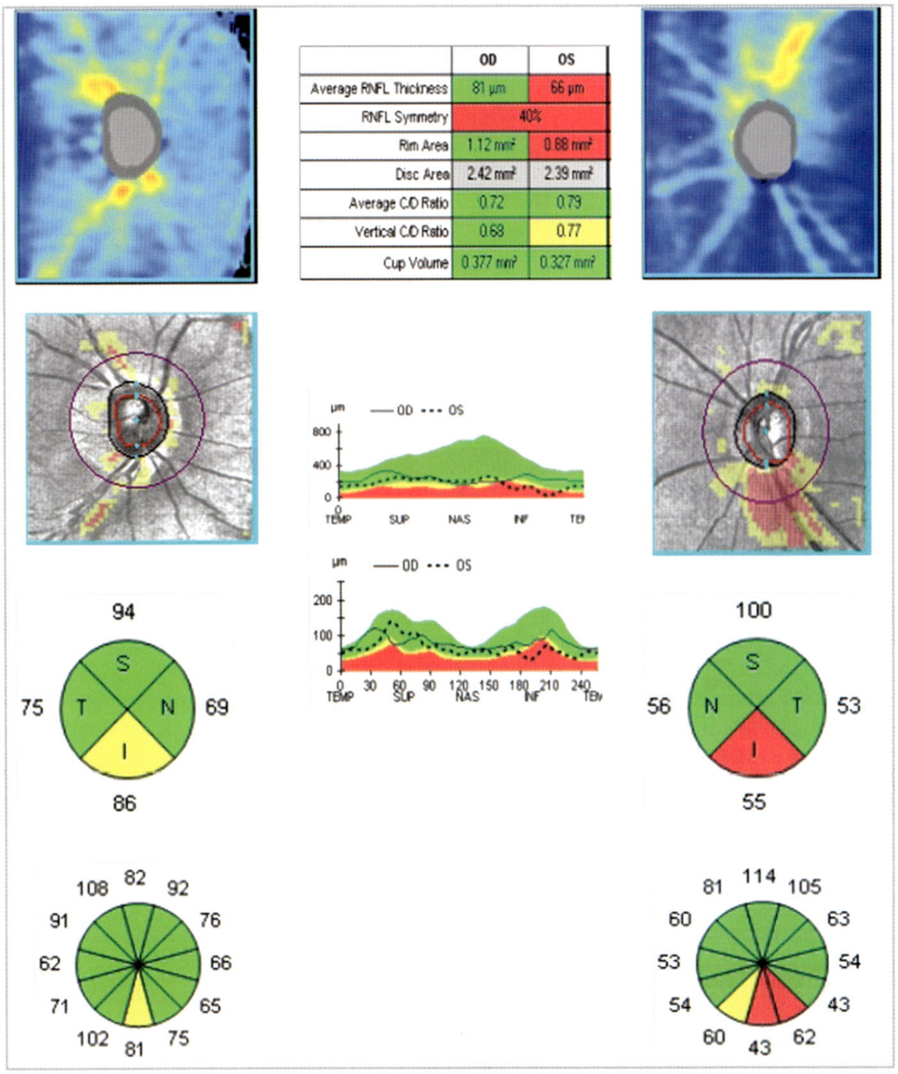

Figure 15.10 Cirrus spectral domain optical coherence tomography printout. The most valuable function of the Cirrus high-definition optical coherence tomography is the evaluation of the retinal nerve fiber layer.

the optic disc is measured in six sectors corresponding to the sectors generated similar to the HRT.

In summary, all types of SD-OCT devices tested show a good glaucoma diagnostic capability and most of the studies consistently show no statistically significant differences in glaucoma diagnostic capability between TD-OCT and the newer SD-OCT. An equivocal optic disc with a normal visual field printout highlights the utility of the SD-OCT (Cirrus) in identifying pre-perimetric glaucoma in **Figure 15.13**. The Cirrus SD-OCT shows focal thinning of the superior neuroretinal rim, thus confirming the diagnosis of pre-perimetric glaucomatous optic neuropathy.

On the SD-OCT printout in **Figure 15.14**, OS emphasizes structural correlation of an inferior RNFL defect with an inferior rim notch on the disc photograph. In **Figure 15.15**, SD-OCT detects structural losses better than a TD-OCT in a case of small optic disc that appears normal because of its small cup. The following image (**Figure 15.16**) exemplifies again the utility of a TD-OCT (Stratus) and SD-OCT (Cirrus) in detecting a structural defect that otherwise could have been missed clinically. The defect is more clearly seen with the SD-OCT (Cirrus).

The images in **Figure 15.17** highlight the fact that different imaging devices cannot be compared with each other and some parameters may be flagged as normal in one device but abnormal in another. A study by Foo et al. (2012) showed that the SD-OCT underestimates ONH rim area and overestimates cup parameters compared with HRT-3. The images in **Figure 15.18** highlight the fact that nonglaucomatous myopic and tilted discs are poorly classified by these ONH/RNFL devices.

SUMMARY: COMPARISON OF THE THREE IMAGING ONH/RNFL IMAGING DEVICES

All these devices have their inherent advantages and disadvantages and all have been proven to discriminate well between normal eyes and glaucoma. Many studies that evaluate and compare the different technologies have concluded that they perform similarly in the diagnosis of early glaucoma, while other studies have demonstrated that one technology may outperform the others in detecting early ONH and RNFL defects. All these devices have high reproducibility good correlation with structural (stereoscopic disc photography) and functional (visual fields) tests.

The OCT may have the strongest correlation with visual field findings and may be able to detect early RNFL changes before defects are seen in perimetry. The OCT, however, does not have a normative morphometric database and statistical analysis for the ONH evaluation. It has a normative database for RNFL thickness evaluation, which is its best performing parameter and is the most reproducible of all measurements. OCTs may not be compatible with previous versions, making it difficult to make a longitudinal evaluation of progression detection.

The HRT-3 has the strength of having a large, normative ethnic-specific database and a statistical analysis program that helps in diagnosis and monitoring. HRT-3 is backward compatible with the previous HRT versions, so longitudinal follow-up of patients with glaucoma is not compromised. The HRT has been demonstrated to correlate well with stereo photographs and automated perimetry (Mai et al. 2007, Zangwill et al. 2007). It is a promising technology in detecting and quantifying glaucoma progression. Unlike the OCT, RNFL thickness is less useful when using the HRT because it is not directly measured by the instrument. However, RNFL thickness values measured from the HRT's reference plane may be prone to error, especially in unusual discs. This plane's position (influenced by the operators drawing of the contour line for HRT-1 and -2) has been shown to be a major factor influencing HRT measurement variability. The introduction of the contour line and reference plane-independent GPS classifier is a significant improvement because it allows user-independent analysis and tends to perform similarly to, or better than, the reference plane-dependent MRA. Other limitations of the HRT include blood vessels that can affect measurements because the machine erroneously considers them as part of the neuroretinal rim, and the stereometric measurements can be influenced by moderate intraocular pressure changes. HRT does not require pupil dilation but image quality with dilation may improve in eyes with cataracts and small pupils.

The SLP-ECC increases its ability to discriminate between healthy and glaucomatous nerves and reduces the effects of ARPs, making it a promising technology to diagnose glaucoma early; however, it does not have a progression analysis program. Corneal pathology, corneal surgery, and macular pathology can lead to inadequate compensation of corneal birefringence and erroneous RNFL thickness assessment. Highly myopic eyes also reveal atypical patterns of birefringence. GD× measurements are affected by various conditions, such as media opacity, ocular surface, macular diseases, and peripapillary atrophy. The VCC device has an artifact from compensating for poor signal-to-noise ratio, which is partially rectified in the ECC version, but upgrading requires new hardware and images taken with older devices cannot be analyzed for change with the newer device. The major strength of the SLP relies on the ability to obtain reproducible measurements of the RNFL thickness without pupil dilation, a reference plane or magnification correction. Analysis of progressive glaucomatous loss is done subjectively by evaluating retardation maps in chronological order, and studies are still ongoing regarding automated statistical progression analysis software for this device.

Since glaucoma is an integrative diagnosis that assesses both structural and functional parameters and a multiple risk factor, these imaging devices have come up with software capabilities that assemble all the data for quick interpretation. The Forum (Carl Zeiss Meditec, Inc., Dublin, California, USA) and Heyex (Heidelberg Eye Explorer Heidelberg Engineering, Dossenheim, Germany) prepare preconfigured clinical displays and combine reports presenting diagnostic data immediately in clinically relevant ways and encourage networking.

In conclusion, imaging devices show promise for enhancing documentation and detection of ONH/RNFL changes for use in the clinical management of glaucoma. Their increasing role as important adjuncts to the gold standard of a careful clinical evaluation of ONH/RNFL stereoscopic photographs is being further recognized. Just like any sophisticated devices nowadays, each imaging instrument is in a constant technological flux with important software improvements anticipated, particularly for progression detection.

Each glaucoma patient will have different circumstances that dictate the frequency of imaging. The patient's category of glaucoma risk could further guide the clinician as to the frequency of imaging. A low-risk ocular hypertension patient may have imaging done less frequently than a patient who has moderate glaucoma with uncontrolled eye pressures. It is important to remember that the imaging quality of the scan and glaucoma severity can influence the diagnostic accuracy of these imaging instruments. Diagnostic accuracy of even the most sophisticated analyses of ONH/RNFL data may be limited if poor quality scans are used, and will be much higher in eyes with advanced glaucoma. It is therefore essential that clinicians understand the strengths and limitations of each instrument and that they interpret the data in the context of the other ocular clinical findings, particularly with a careful intelligent clinical examination of stereoscopic ONH/RNFL photos and assessment of visual function for appropriate glaucoma management decisions.

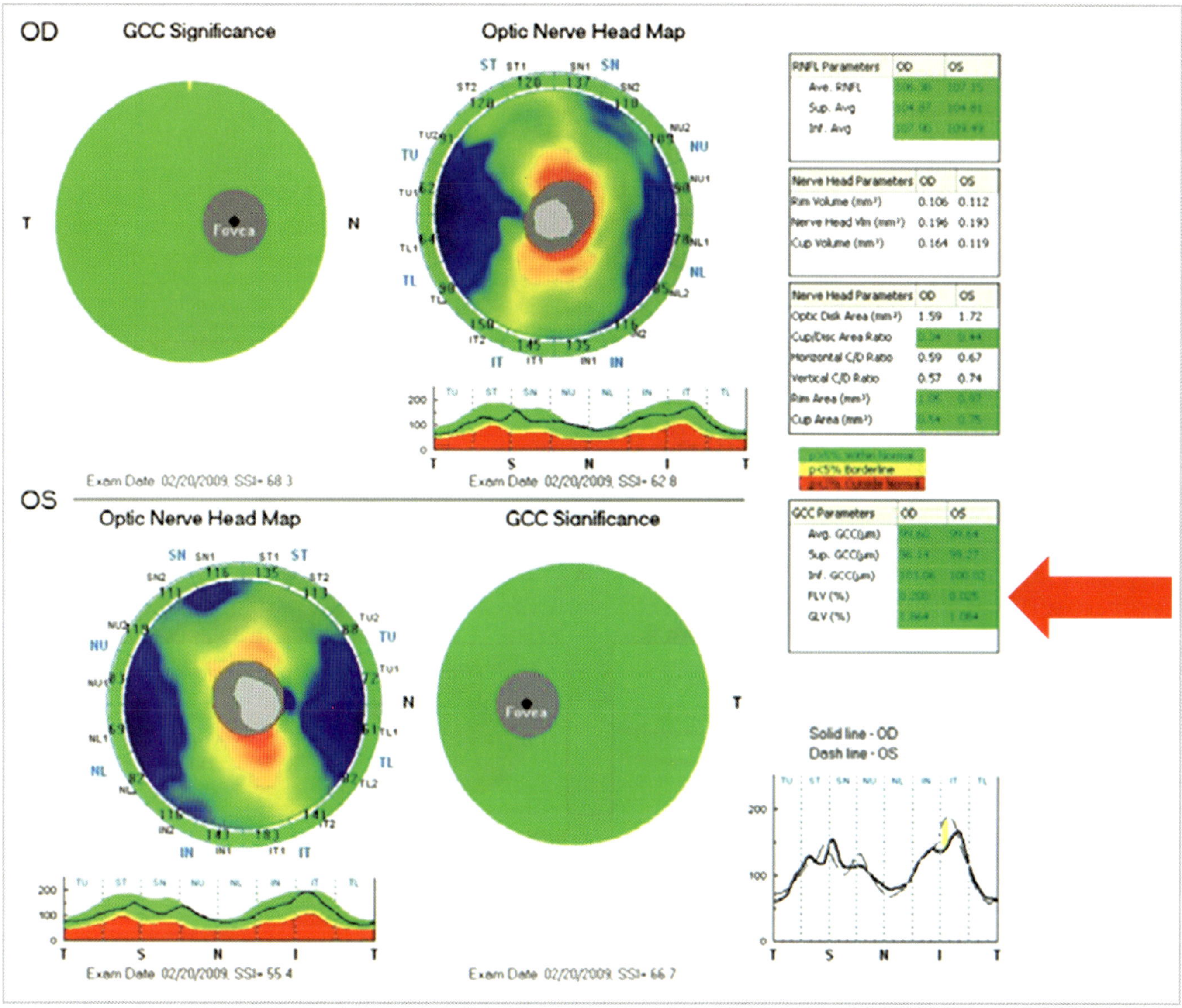

Figure 15.11 RTVue spectral domain optical coherence tomography (SD-OCT) printout. RTVue SD-OCT is designed to measure the inner retinal thickness. The red arrow shows ganglion cell complex parameters.

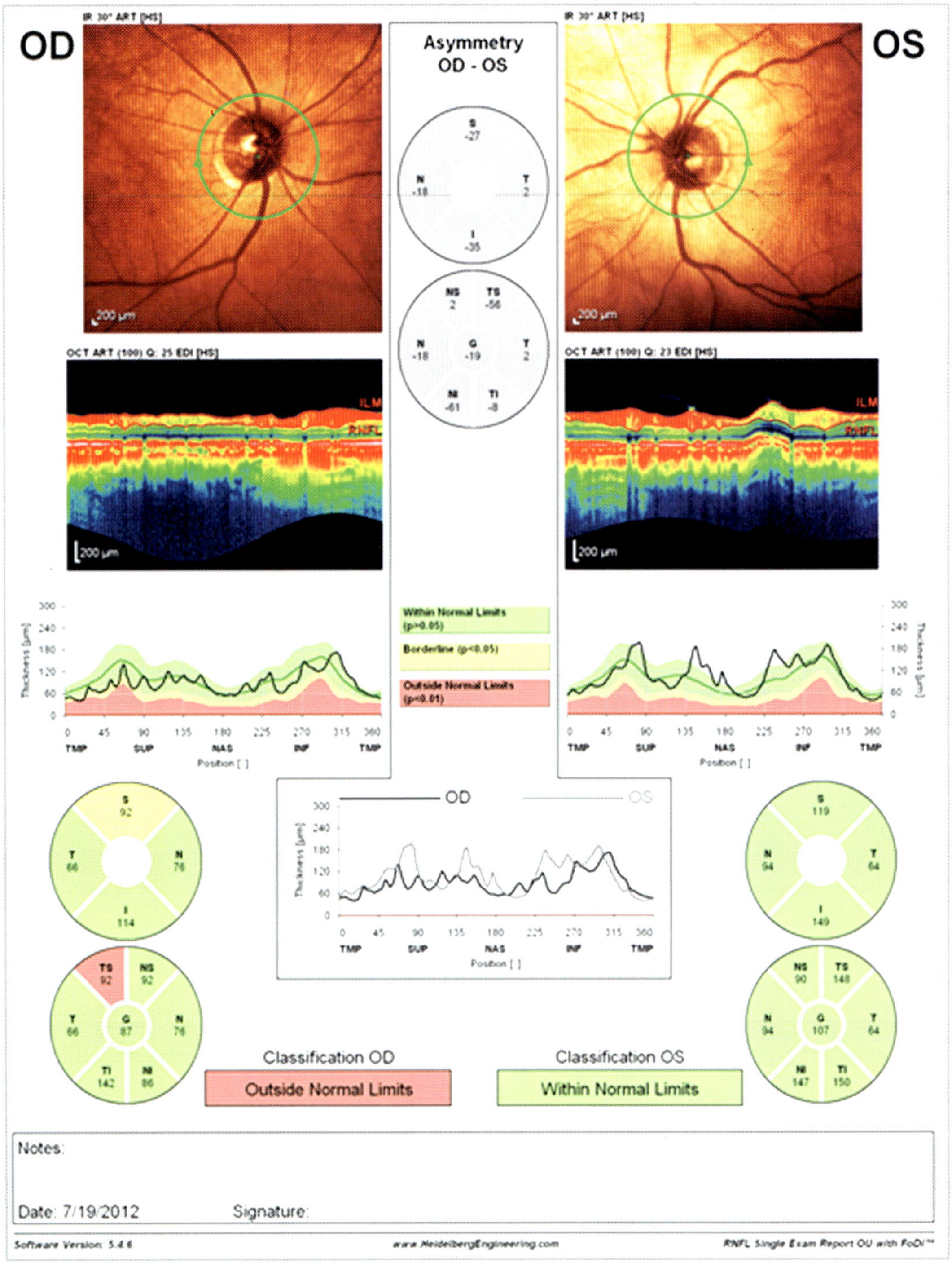

Figure 15.12 Spectralis spectral domain optical coherence tomography printout. The retinal nerve fiber layer thickness around the optic disc is measured in six sectors corresponding to the sectors generated by the Heidelberg Retina Tomograph.

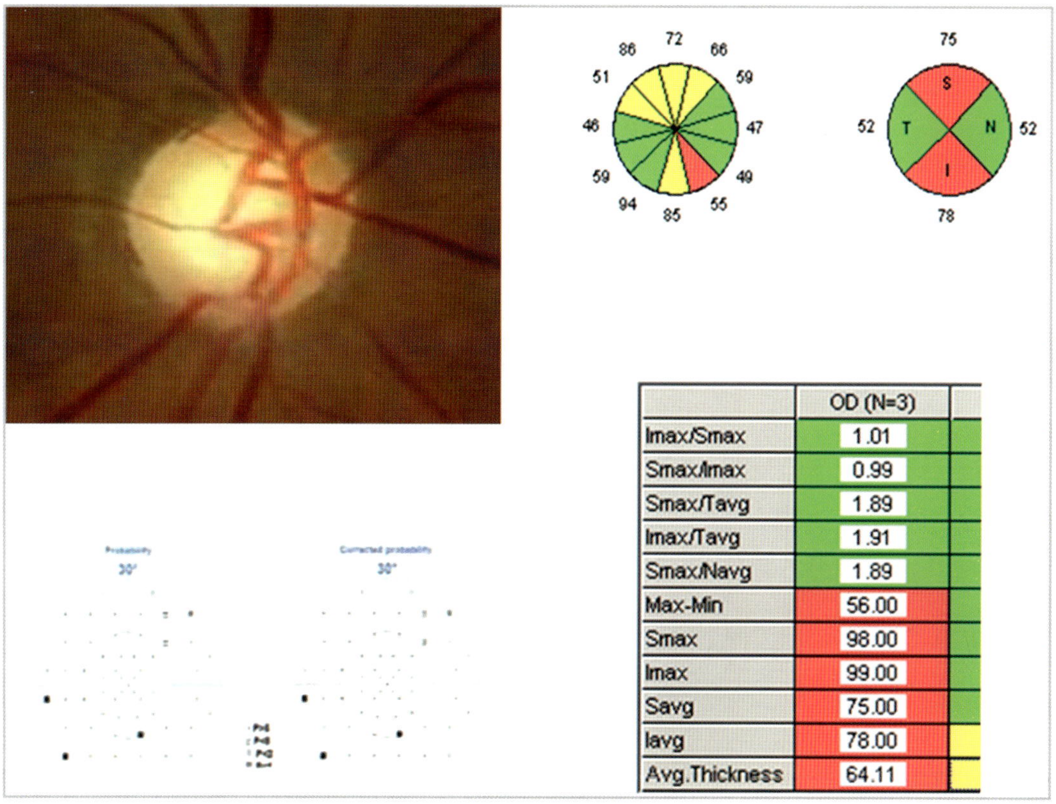

	OD (N=3)
Imax/Smax	1.01
Smax/Imax	0.99
Smax/Tavg	1.89
Imax/Tavg	1.91
Smax/Navg	1.89
Max-Min	56.00
Smax	98.00
Imax	99.00
Savg	75.00
Iavg	78.00
Avg.Thickness	64.11

Figure 15.13 Pre-perimetric glaucoma. Spectral domain optical coherence tomography (SD-OCT) shows good glaucoma diagnostic capability with no statistically significant differences between time domain OCT and the newer SD-OCT.

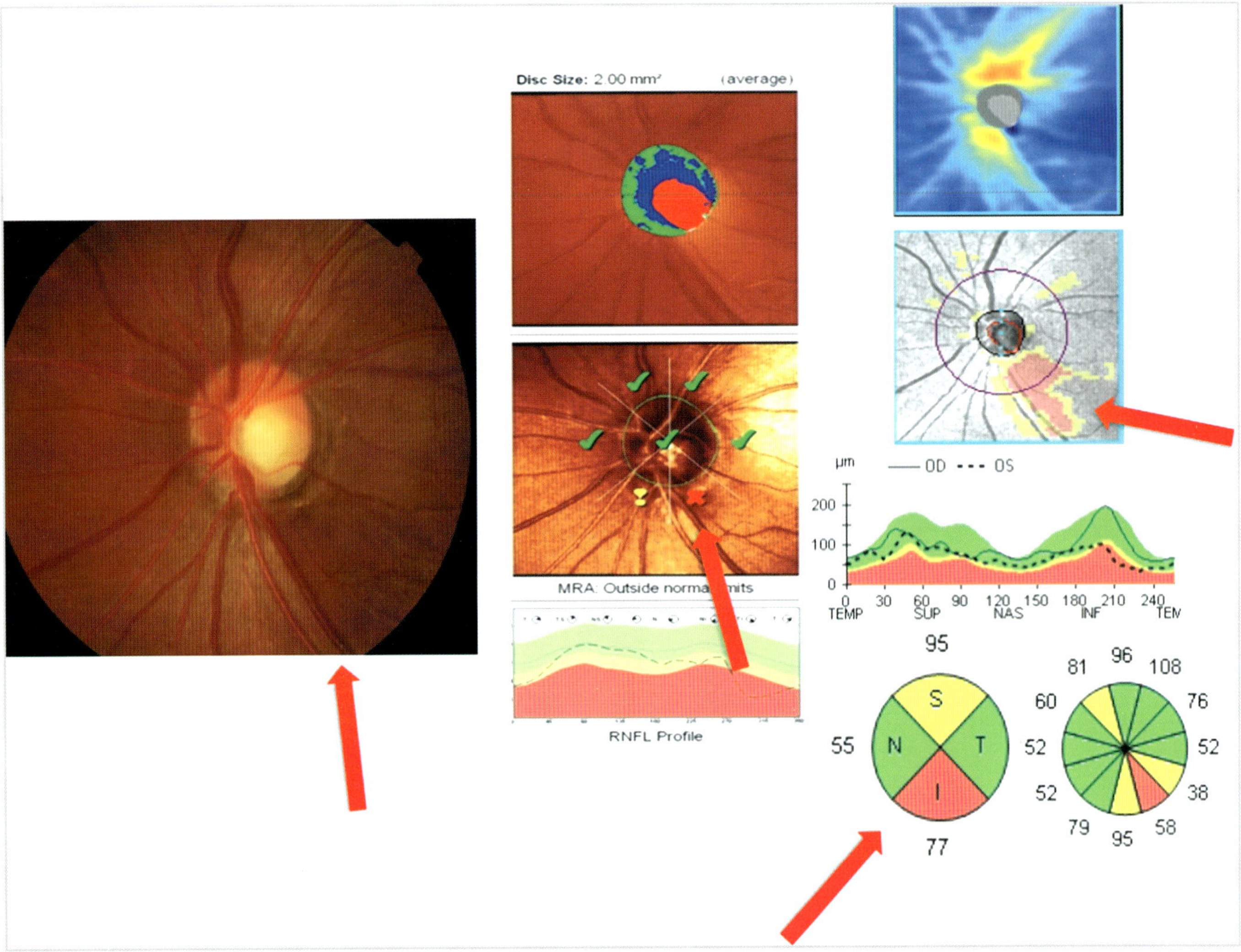

Figure 15.14 A spectral domain optical coherence tomography emphasizes structural correlation of an inferior retinal nerve fiber layer (RNFL) defect with an inferior rim notch/RNFL defect on the disc photograph.

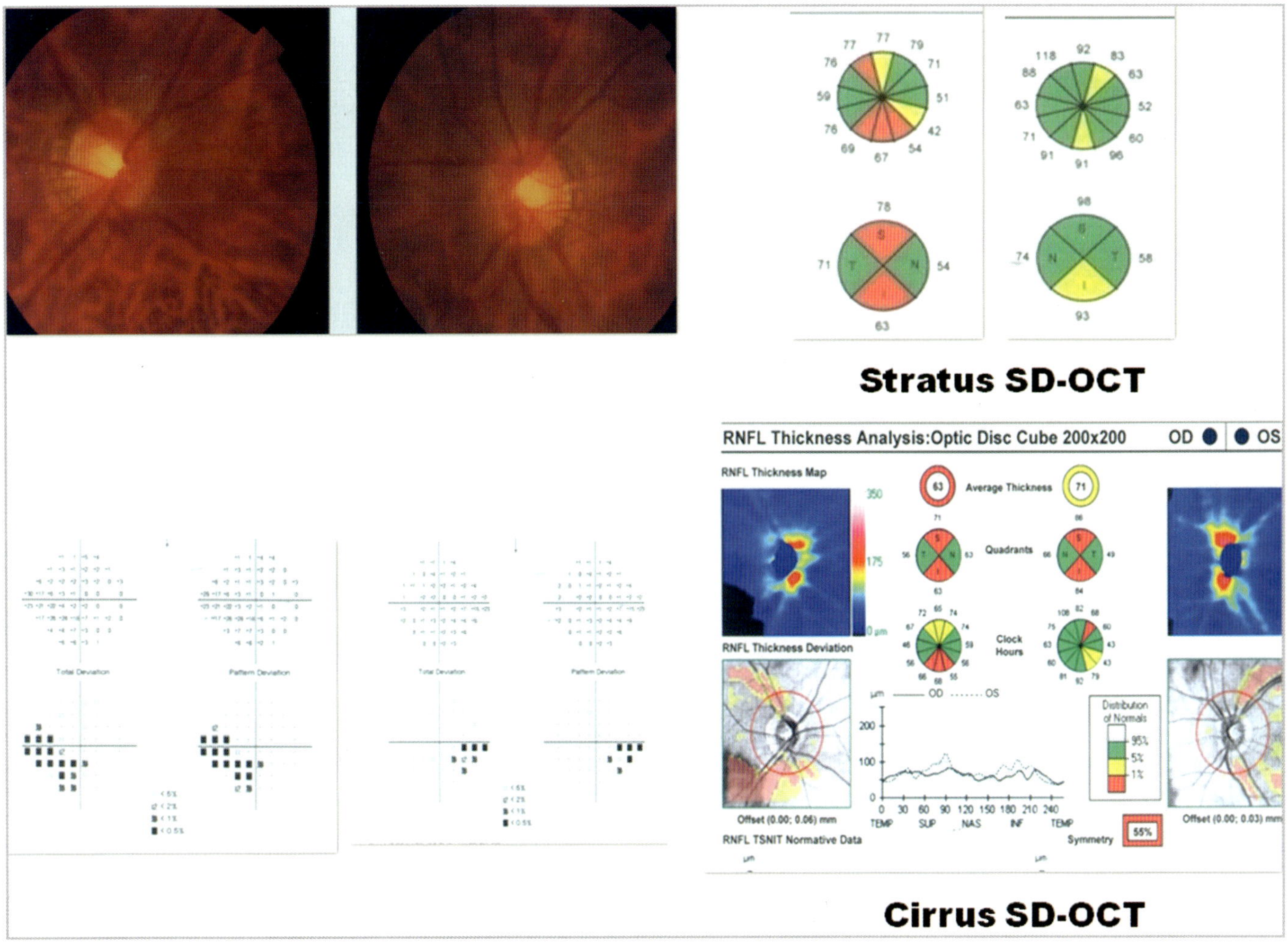

Figure 15.15 A spectral domain optical coherence tomography detects structural losses better than a time domain optical coherence tomography in a small glaucomatous optic disc.

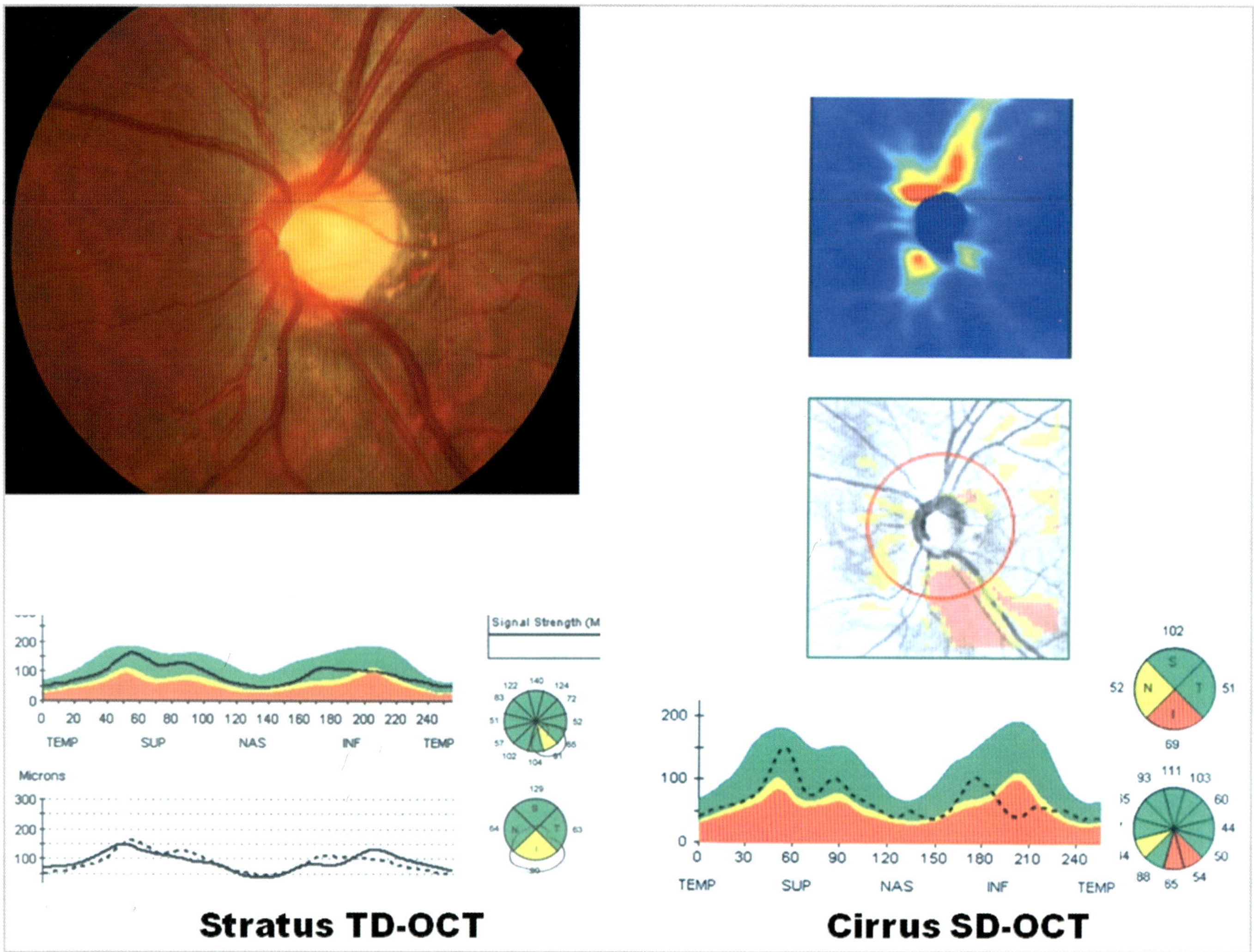

Figure 15.16 Both time domain optical coherence tomography and spectral domain optical coherence tomography (SD-OCT) detect a structural defect that otherwise could be missed clinically. The defect is more clearly seen with the SD-OCT.

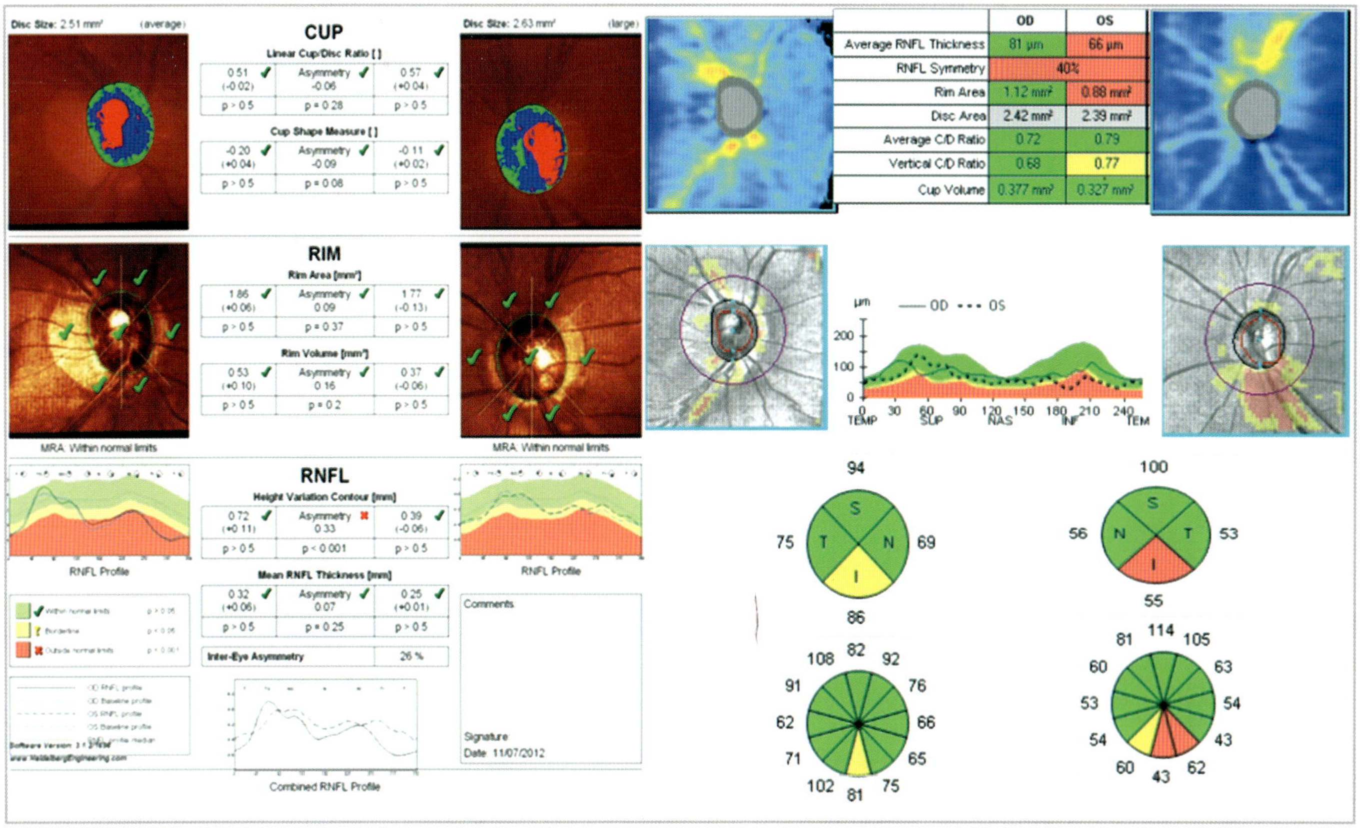

Figure 15.17 Different technologies cannot be compared with each other and some parameters may be flagged as normal in one device but abnormal in another.

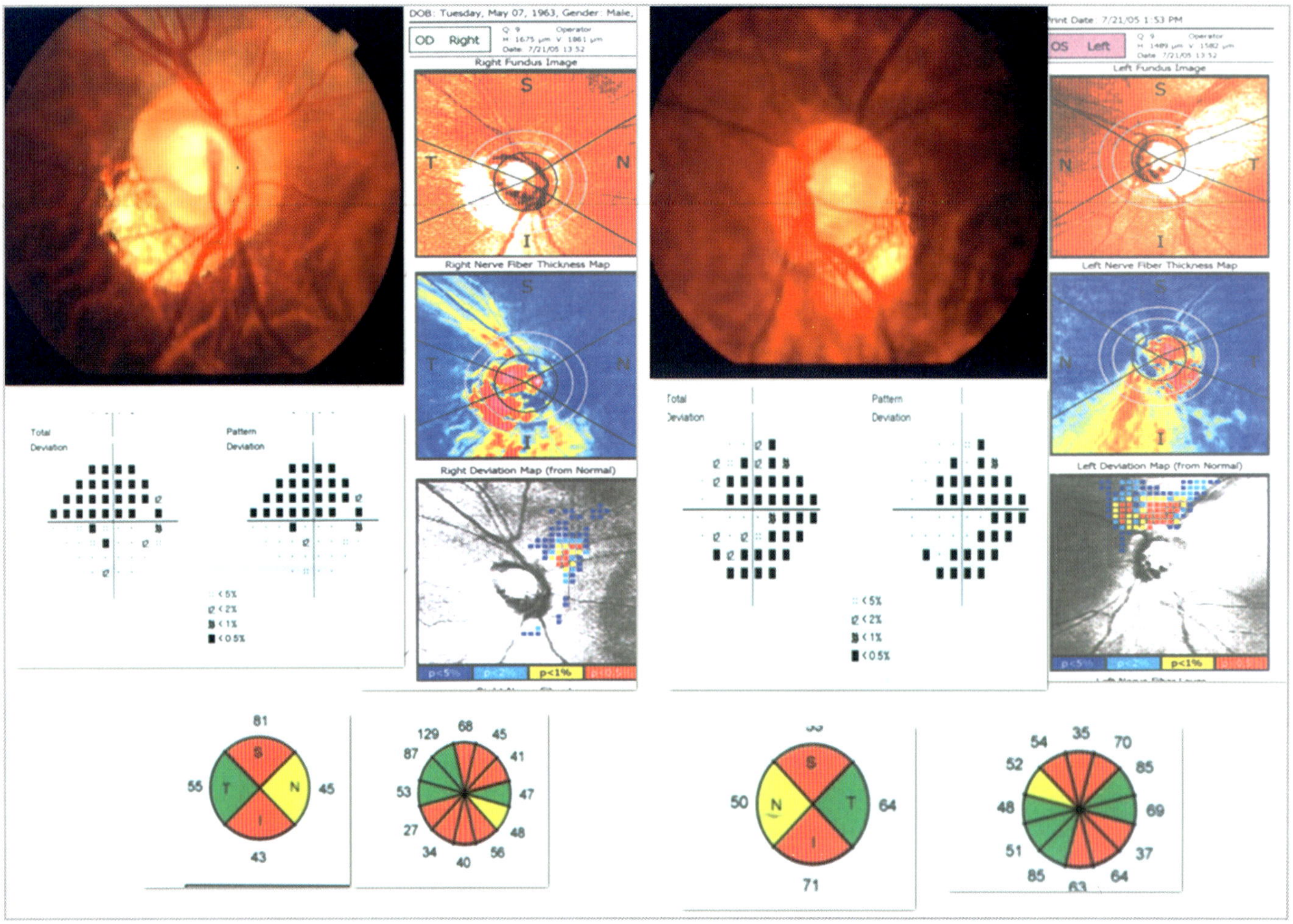

Figure 15.18 Nonglaucomatous myopic and tilted discs are poorly classified by optic nerve head/retinal nerve fiber layer devices.

REFERENCES

Budenz DL, Anderson DR, Varma R, et al. Determinants of normal retinal nerve fibre layer thickness measured by Stratus OCT. *Ophthalmology* 2007; **114**:1046–1052.

Bowd C, Tavares IM, Medeiros FA, et al. Retinal nerve fibre layer thickness and visual sensitivity using scanning laser polarimetry with variable and enhanced corneal compensation. *Ophthalmology* 2007; **114**:1259–1265.

Chang R, Budenz DL. New developments in optical coherence tomography for glaucoma. *Curr Opin Ophthalmol* 2008; **19**(2):127–135.

Coops A, Henson DB, Kwartz AJ, Artes PH. Automated analysis of Heidelberg Retina Tomograph optic disc images by Glaucoma Probability Score. *Invest Ophthalmol Vis Sci* 2006; **47**:5348–5355.

De Leon-Ortega JE, Sakata LM, Monheit BE, et al. Comparison of diagnostic accuracy of Heidelberg Retina Tomograph II and Heidelberg Retina Tomograph 3 to discriminate glaucomatous and nonglaucomatous eyes. *Am J Ophthalmol* 2007; **144**:525–532.

Ferreras A, Pablo LE, Pajarín AB, et al. Diagnostic ability of the Heidelberg Retina Tomograph-3 for glaucoma. *Am J Ophthalmol* 2008; **145**:354–359.

Foo L, Perera SA, Cheung CY, et al. Comparison of scanning laser ophthalmoscopy and high-definition optical coherence tomography measurements of optic disc parameters. *Br J Ophthalmol* 2012; **96**:576–580.

Lemij HG, Reus NJ. New developments in scanning laser polarimetry for glaucoma. *Curr Opin Ophthalmol* 2008; **19**:136–140.

Lin, SC, Singh, K, Jampel, HD, et al Ophthalmic technology assessment: optic nerve head and retinal nerve fibre analysis. A report by the American Academy of Ophthalmology. *Ophthalmology* 2007; **114**:1937–1949.

Mai TA, Reus NJ, Lemij HG. Structure-function relationship is stronger with enhanced corneal compensation than with variable corneal compensation in scanning laser polarimetry. *Invest Ophthalmol Vis Sci* 2007; **48**:1651–1658.

Medeiros FA, Zangwill LM, Bowd C, et al. Evaluation of retinal nerve fibre layer, optic nerve head, and macular thickness measurements for glaucoma detection using optical coherence tomography. *Am J Ophthalmol* 2005; **139**:44–55.

Miglior S, Guareschi M, Albe E, et al. Detection of glaucomatous visual field changes using the Moorfields regression analysis of the Heidelberg retina tomograph. *Am J Ophthalmol* 2003; **136**:26–33.

Schuman JS, Pedut-Kloizman T, Hertzmark E, et al. Reproducibility of nerve fibre layer using optical coherence tomography. *Ophthalmology* 1996; **103**:1889–1898.

Strouthidis NG, White ET, Owen VM, et al. Factors affecting the test–retest variability of Heidelberg retina tomograph and Heidelberg retina tomograph II measurements. *Br J Ophthalmol* 2005; **89**:1427–1432.

Tan O, Chopra V, Lu ATH, et al. Detection of macular ganglion cell loss in glaucoma by Fourier-domain optical coherence tomography. *Ophthalmology* 2009; **116**:2305–2314.

Wollstein G, Garway-Heath DF, Hitchings RA. Identification of early glaucoma cases with the scanning laser ophthalmoscope. *Ophthalmology* 1998; **105**:1557–1563.

Wollstein G, Garway-Heath DF, Fontana L, Hitchings RA. Identifying early glaucomatous changes. Comparison between expert clinical assessment of optic disc photographs and confocal scanning ophthalmoscopy. *Ophthalmology* 2000; **107**:2272–2277.

Wollstein G, Ishikawa H, Wang J, et al. Comparison of three OCT scanning areas for detection of glaucomatous damage. *Am J Ophthalmol* 2005; **139**:39–43.

Zangwill LM, Jain S, Racette L, et al. The effect of disc size and severity of disease on the diagnostic accuracy of the Heidelberg Retina Tomograph (HRT) Glaucoma Probability Score and Moorfields Regression Analysis. *Invest Ophthalmol Vis Sci* 2007; **48**:2653–2660.

Index

Note: Page numbers in **bold** or *italic* refer to tables or figures respectively.